Exploring the Role of ICTs in Healthy Aging

David Mendes
Universidade de Évora, Portugal

César Fonseca
Universidade de Évora, Portugal

Manuel José Lopes
Universidade de Évora, Portugal

José García-Alonso
Universidad de Extremadura, Spain

Juan Manuel Murillo
Universidad de Extremadura, Spain

A volume in the Advances in Medical Technologies and Clinical Practice (AMTCP) Book Series

IGI Global
PUBLISHER of TIMELY KNOWLEDGE

Published in the United States of America by
IGI Global
Medical Information Science Reference (an imprint of IGI Global)
701 E. Chocolate Avenue
Hershey PA, USA 17033
Tel: 717-533-8845
Fax: 717-533-8661
E-mail: cust@igi-global.com
Web site: http://www.igi-global.com

Library of Congress Cataloging-in-Publication Data

Library of Congress Cataloging-in-Publication Data

Names: Mendes, David, 1966- editor. | Fonseca, César, 1973- editor. | Lopes, Manuel José, editor. | García-Alonso, José, 1984- editor. | Murillo, Juan Manuel, 1967- editor.
Title: Exploring the role of ICTs in healthy aging / David Mendes, César Fonseca, Manuel José Lopes, José García-Alonso, Juan Manuel Murillo, editors.
Other titles: Exploring the role of information and communication technologies in healthy aging
Description: Hershey, PA : Medical Information Science Reference, [2020] | Includes bibliographical references and index. | Summary: "This book explores models and processes of domiciled care for the elderly and the development of applied technological edge computing solutions"-- Provided by publisher.
Identifiers: LCCN 2019035884 (print) | LCCN 2019035885 (ebook) | ISBN 9781799819370 (h/c) | ISBN 9781799819387 (ebook)
Subjects: MESH: Information Technology | Aged | Medical Informatics Applications | Quality of Life | Independent Living
Classification: LCC R855.3 (print) | LCC R855.3 (ebook) | NLM WT 26.5 | DDC 610.285--dc23
LC record available at https://lccn.loc.gov/2019035884
LC ebook record available at https://lccn.loc.gov/2019035885

This book is published in the IGI Global book series Advances in Medical Technologies and Clinical Practice (AMTCP) (ISSN: 2327-9354; eISSN: 2327-9370)

British Cataloguing in Publication Data
A Cataloguing in Publication record for this book is available from the British Library.

All work contributed to this book is new, previously-unpublished material.
The views expressed in this book are those of the authors, but not necessarily of the publisher.
For electronic access to this publication, please contact: eresources@igi-global.com.

Advances in Medical Technologies and Clinical Practice (AMTCP) Book Series

ISSN:2327-9354
EISSN:2327-9370

MISSION

Medical technological innovation continues to provide avenues of research for faster and safer diagnosis and treatments for patients. Practitioners must stay up to date with these latest advancements to provide the best care for nursing and clinical practices.

The **Advances in Medical Technologies and Clinical Practice (AMTCP) Book Series** brings together the most recent research on the latest technology used in areas of nursing informatics, clinical technology, biomedicine, diagnostic technologies, and more. Researchers, students, and practitioners in this field will benefit from this fundamental coverage on the use of technology in clinical practices.

COVERAGE

- Diagnostic Technologies
- Clinical Studies
- Clinical Data Mining
- E-Health
- Neural Engineering
- Biomechanics
- Nursing Informatics
- Telemedicine
- Biometrics
- Clinical Nutrition

The Advances in Medical Technologies and Clinical Practice (AMTCP) Book Series (ISSN 2327-9354) is published by IGI Global, 701 E. Chocolate Avenue, Hershey, PA 17033-1240, USA, www.igi-global.com. This series is composed of titles available for purchase individually; each title is edited to be contextually exclusive from any other title within the series. For pricing and ordering information please visit http://www.igi-global.com/book-series/advances-medical-technologies-clinical-practice/73682. Postmaster: Send all address changes to above address.

Titles in this Series

For a list of additional titles in this series, please visit:
http://www.igi-global.com/book-series/advances-medical-technologies-clinical-practice/73682

Mobile Devices and Smart Gadgets in Medical Sciences
Sajid Umair (The University of Agriculture, Peshawar, Pakistan)
Medical Information Science Reference • © 2020 • 363pp • H/C (ISBN: 9781799825210) • US $245.00

Applications of Deep Learning and Big IoT on Personalized Healthcare Services
Ritika Wason (Bharati Vidyapeeth's Institute of Computer Applications and Management (BVICAM), India) Dinesh Goyal (Poornima Institute of Engineering and Technology, India) Vishal Jain (Bharati Vidyapeeth's Institute of Computer Applications and Management (BVICAM), India) S. Balamurugan (QUANTS IS and Consultancy Services, India) and Anupam Baliyan (Bharati Vidyapeeth's Institute of Computer Applications and Management (BVICAM), India)
Medical Information Science Reference • © 2020 • 248pp • H/C (ISBN: 9781799821014) • US $275.00

Communicating Rare Diseases and Disorders in the Digital Age
Liliana Vale Costa (University of Aveiro, Portugal) and Sónia Oliveira (University of Aveiro, Portugal)
Medical Information Science Reference • © 2020 • 412pp • H/C (ISBN: 9781799820888) • US $295.00

Artificial Intelligence Paradigms in Smart Health Informatics Systems
Abdel-Badeeh M. Salem (Ain Shams University, Egypt) and Senthil Kumar A V (Hindusthan College of Arts and Science, India)
Medical Information Science Reference • © 2020 • 300pp • H/C (ISBN: 9781799811015) • US $265.00

Incorporating the Internet of Things in Healthcare Applications and Wearable Devices
P. B. Pankajavalli (Bharathiar University, India) and G. S. Karthick (Bharathiar University, India)
Medical Information Science Reference • © 2020 • 288pp • H/C (ISBN: 9781799810902) • US $285.00

For an entire list of titles in this series, please visit:
http://www.igi-global.com/book-series/advances-medical-technologies-clinical-practice/73682

IGI Global
PUBLISHER of TIMELY KNOWLEDGE

701 East Chocolate Avenue, Hershey, PA 17033, USA
Tel: 717-533-8845 x100 • Fax: 717-533-8661
E-Mail: cust@igi-global.com • www.igi-global.com

Table of Contents

Section 3
Systemic Approaches of Current ICT Trends and Technology Supporting the Model

Detailed Table of Contents

Class 3 maintained hierarchical and semantic proximity to Class 2, which deals with technologies to ensure the safety of elderly patients in the use of medicines. For nurses, technologies help in the safety of elderly patients, but do not guarantee the extinction of adverse events. The chapter considered the need for patient safety to become an organizational culture favoring the quality of clinical nursing care in the handling of medicines.

Luísa Teixeira-Santos, The Health Sciences Research Unit: Nursing, Nursing School of Coimbra, Portugal
Elzbieta Bobrowicz-Campos, Faculty of Psychology and Educational Sciences, Centre of 20th Century Interdisciplinary Studies, University of Coimbra, Coimbra, Portugal
Filipa Ventura, The Health Sciences Research Unit: Nursing, Nursing School of Coimbra, Portugal
Vitor Parola, The Health Sciences Research Unit: Nursing, Nursing School of Coimbra, Portugal & Faculty of Health Sciences, University Fernando Pessoa, Porto, Portugal
Adriana Coelho, The Health Sciences Research Unit: Nursing, Nursing School of Coimbra, Portugal
Maria de Lurdes Ferreira Almeida, The Health Sciences Research Unit: Nursing, Nursing School of Coimbra, Portugal
Isabel Gil, The Health Sciences Research Unit: Nursing, Nursing School of Coimbra, Portugal
Maria Teresa Moreno-Casbas, Nursing and Healthcare Research Unit, Instituto de Salud Carlos III, Spain
João Apóstolo, The Health Sciences Research Unit: Nursing, Nursing School of Coimbra, Portugal

This chapter focuses on the use of technology on older adult health promotion. During the ageing process, they experience changes in physical, cognitive, psychological, and social domains. Frailty is the most problematic expression of ageing and entails a high risk of adverse outcomes. In order to prevent it, healthcare professionals must intervene on health promotion. However, it's impossible to continuously monitor the health status of thousands of people. Technologies can bridge the gap between older people's home and the hospital. Especially those with sensors, allow healthcare professionals to continuously monitor the older people's health status and evaluate the health parameters to prioritize care and alert to necessary behavioral changes. The seniors become more aware and responsible for their health, increasing their literacy, autonomy, and well-being. They become more engaged in activities that promote successful ageing. In this chapter, the authors address one of many research projects that monitor the health parameters of older people in a community setting through wearable sensors.

Information and communication technologies (ICTs) are important for improving healthcare services worldwide. Using tools related to ICTs such as smartphones (cell phones), video conferencing, computers enhances the delivery of health services as well as electronic health (e-health). Therefore, this study's main objective is to investigate the e-health readiness for higher education institution students in an emerging country (Botswana). The study achieved this by identifying the readiness factors that affect the adoption of e-health using the conceptual framework (technology readiness and acceptance model for e-health). The study established that students' optimism, innovativeness, discomfort, and insecurity influence e-health perceived ease of use. However, only optimism and discomfort influence e-health perceived usefulness whereas innovativeness and insecurity did not influence e-health perceived usefulness. Additionally, the study found out that e-health perceived usefulness and e-health perceived ease of use have an influence on e-health adoption.

In this last section we develop and explore the subtleties and intricacies of deploying a system as complex as this one to a wider public. Different angles of impacts both in the targeted population (co-morbid conditions elderly), in their closest environment (family and neighbors, the informal caregivers) and in the professional healthcare professionals that are responsible for the lifelong process of health and care. The most recent, although stable, technological trends are considered and weighed trying to come as close as possible to a proposal that is simultaneously the most economically viable and appealing to the professionals, trying to relief their heavy

status. The experiments carried out show us that it correctly evaluates these patients and reduces the effort required by health professionals.

Sheila Bonilla, Universidad de Extremadura, Spain
Enrique Moguel, Universidad de Extremadura, Spain
José Garcia-Alonso, Universidad de Extremadura, Spain
Javier Berrocal, Universidad de Extremadura, Spain
Juan M. Murillo, Universidad de Extremadura, Spain

The increase in the elderly population today is a fact. This group of people needs day-to-day care due to their age, and, in addition, they often have health problems. Technology can be used to mitigate these problems. However, it must be borne in mind that most of this population is currently unable to get the most out of electronic devices. To help elders benefit from these devices, systems adapted to their needs, and preferences are needed. In particular, systems that use the elders' contextual information to integrate several aspects of eldercare and adapt them to each elder would provide significant benefits. In this case, the emotions will be used to recognize to what extent an elderly person needs care at certain times of the day and to adapt surrounding IoT systems to their needs and moods. For this purpose, this chapter proposes to use smartphones as the devices that centralize contextual information of the elders, focusing on emotion recognition.

Mara Pereira Guerreiro, UI&DE, Escola Superior de Enfermagem de Lisboa, CiiEM, Instituto Universitário Egas Moniz, Portugal
Isa Brito Félix, UI&DE, Escola Superior de Enfermagem de Lisboa, Portugal
João Balsa, Faculdade de Ciências, Universidade de Lisboa, Portugal
Maria Beatriz Carmo, BioISI, Faculdade de Ciências, Universidade de Lisboa, Portugal
Maria Adriana Henriques, UI&DE, Escola Superior de Enfermagem de Lisboa, ISAMB, Faculdade de Medicina da Universidade de Lisboa, Portugal
Afonso Cavaco, iMed.ULisboa, Faculdade de Farmácia, Universidade de Lisboa, Portugal
Ana Paula Cláudio, BioISI, Faculdade de Ciências, Universidade de Lisboa, Portugal

Preface

Demographic aging is a global reality, albeit with particular expression in the so-called developed countries. In good truth these two facts (i.e., aging and development) are related, i.e. population ageing is clearly a sign of a society development.

Despite this, population ageing poses challenges to societies never equated. In fact, as a result of the lifepath of the current elderly, they are aging with high loads of disease in the form of multimorbidity and dependence. The available data indicate us that the process of population ageing is not only maintained but is expected (United Nations DESA, 2019). But it is also true that the number of years lived with dependence has been increasing (Jagger & Reyes-Frausto, 2003; Jagger et al., 2016; Kingston et al., 2017, 2018).

Such circumstances induce a high consumption of care, a huge pressure on the health and social safety system and, at the same time, an urgent need to change the organizational models of provision and care due to the adjustment to the previous circumstances.

From here two lessons can be withdrawn: 1) we need to develop a strategy that prevents future people from having such a high burden of disease and levels of dependence; 2) we need to make efforts to adapt our ability to respond to the current needs of the elderly.

This book is a contribution to this second illation.

The necessary efforts to adapt the ability to provide care need to be addressed based on two fundamental principles:

1. The dignity of the elderly must prevail under any circumstances and for this it is essential to preserve their autonomy;
2. The most important factor for successful aging depends on preserving proximity relationships.

Having these principles by reference, we structured the book so that the first part was constituted by an innovative proposal that provides centrality to an instrument that allows care planning that integrates all caregivers and ensures continuity of care wherever they are provided: the Individual Care Plan. In the concept of caregivers, we begin by considering the elderly himself, this being a way of highlighting the importance of self-care and its preservation. We also consider informal caregivers and obviously professionals.

This instrument creates conditions to transform care planning into a negotiation process between caregivers and the person cared for, thus giving expression to the integration and co-production of care.

Thus, an innovative instrument is presented, which is intended to complement the electronic health registry and is very useful for all caregivers.

Somehow the other parts of the book are related to the first.

Thus, the second part begins by enunciating the challenges and opportunities for healthy aging in the context of a digital society, and then we are conducted for issues related to social representations of safety in health professionals (physicians and nurses). Later, we are introduced to technology as a way to involve the elderly in the activities promoting a successful aging.

The third part of this book is completely dedicated to a systematic coverage of current ICT trends and technologies that support the model presented in the first part. Several studies demonstrating how ICT are being developed in such a way as to be an aid in the care process in multiple and different health conditions.

From all the chapters presented, there is a very interesting perspective on the contribution of ICT to the adequacy of our ability to respond to the needs of the elderly. It is also evident the long way that we still need to go not only towards this technological development to be done in an integrated way and by reference to principles and a model of care, but also for them to be developed with the objective of their contribution to increasing access to care and, by the way, to make them more effective.

Finally, it is intended with this book that it also constitutes a challenge to knowledge sharing, thus increasing new developments.

Manuel José Lopes
Universidade de Évora, Portugal

REFERENCES

Jagger, C., Jagger, C., & Reyes-Frausto, S. (2003). *Monitoring Health by Healthy Active Life Expectancy–A User's Guide*. Retrieved from https://www.researchgate.net/publication/263943580

Jagger, C., Matthews, F. E., Wohland, P., Fouweather, T., Stephan, M., Robinson, L., ... Brayne, C. (2016). A comparison of health expectancies over two decades in England: Results of the Cognitive Function and Ageing Study I and II. *Lancet*, *387*(10020), 779–786. doi:10.1016/S0140-6736(15)00947-2 PMID:26680218

Kingston, A., Robinson, L., Booth, H., Knapp, M., & Jagger, C. (2018). Projections of multi-morbidity in the older population in England to 2035: Estimates from the Population Ageing and Care Simulation (PACSim) model. *Age and Ageing*, *47*(3), 374–380. doi:10.1093/ageing/afx201 PMID:29370339

Kingston, A., Wohland, P., Wittenberg, R., Robinson, L., Brayne, C., Matthews, F. E., & Jagger, C. (2017). Is late-life dependency increasing or not? A comparison of the Cognitive Function and Ageing Studies (CFAS). *Lancet, 390*, 1676–1684. doi:10.1016/S0140-6736(17)31575-1

United Nations DESA. (2019). *World Population Ageing 2019: Highlights*. Retrieved from https://www.un.org/en/development/desa/population/publications/pdf/ageing/WorldPopulationAgeing2019-Highlights.pdf

Section 1

Foundation of a New Care Model and Its Supporting Infrastructure

To properly handle healthcare challenges with population ageing severely in the latest decades, a new model that encompasses health and care process throughout life must be developed. The high impact of co-morbidity amongst the elderly, inducing heavy loads in the health and social security systems, that were developed for centuries responding to highly specialized needs and responding to acute episodes, need a reformed response that takes good account of the occurrence of systemic chronic conditions. In this first section we lay the foundation of a full developed care model that promotes the usage of the proximity relations while preserving the self as owner of the care process. The suggested model targets the domiciled care keeping the patient at the center of the dialogue hub that promotes the activation of the less differentiated caregiver. This strategy induces the biggest saving capabilities and promotes the proper handling of co-occurrence of different chronic conditions. We state that a computable framework to support this model must rely upon very recent developments in Artificial Intelligence techniques and capabilities and put forward a highly fail resistant framework to implement the automatic reasoning model.

Chapter 1
The Individual Care Plan as Electronic Health Record:
A Tool for Management, Integration of Care, and Better Health Results

Manuel José Lopes
http://orcid.org/0000-0002-7554-8041
Universidade de Évora, Portugal

César Fonseca
https://orcid.org/0000-0001-6975-612X
Universidade de Évora, Portugal

Patrícia Barbosa
Escola Nacional de Saúde Pública, Universidade Nova de Lisboa, Portugal

ABSTRACT

The idea of the need for healthcare planning, whether in the individual or collective dimensions, is consensual among all health professionals. Despite this consensus, as well as a discourse that values teamwork, planning focused on health professionals has prevailed. Due to the current circumstances, particularly those resulting from changes in the epidemiological profile of the population, a new way of planning individual healthcare is required that must meet the following criteria: be of an individual nature, integrate the active participation of the citizen/family caregiver, be focused on care in the course of life, safeguard interdisciplinarity, assist in decision making about care, and be able to record decisions about care.

DOI: 10.4018/978-1-7998-1937-0.ch001

DEFINITION OF ICP

ICP is defined as

1. A person-centered tool that
2. Constitutes a space for dialogue among all caregivers[1] that
3. Supports and facilitates the management of pathways and
4. The integration of care.

These four dimensions are assumed fundamental. The fact that ICP is defined as person-centered means that it will not be the plan of any profession or sector, but rather the plan of that person, who is primarily responsible for their life and health self-care and autonomous regarding the care process. These may be delegated to other caregivers when the person so wishes or when the requirement of care exceeds their abilities. Because of this centrality in the person, the ICP will always be a space for dialogue between caregivers with the sole objective of building a personalized intervention instrument.

This dialogue will have to be a permanent exercise to be congruent with the evolutionary nature of the health-disease process and the inherent care process. The person appointed by him/her must carry out the management of courses or the care coordinator or case manager, depending on the case; should understand the integration of care as the integration between multiple levels, sectors and / or care providers.

ICP as a care-planning tool is useful whether we equate care to the sick person, with or without dependence, or to the healthy person, with a promotion or prevention perspective.

In this context, the person, sick or healthy, will be the main protagonist and will bring to this space of dialogue and negotiation his narrative, which is based on his experiences and concerns. The centrality conferred on the person stems from the principle of self-determination as a basic dimension of human dignity (Baez & Reckziegel, 2013; Takayuki, 1999). It will also bring your expectations, or if you will, your goals (see Figure 1, right side). These will play a key role in that it will be based on them that care will be planned, e.g. through an approach that uses people's life and health goals to guide health professionals in creating personalized care plans that attends to priorities, needs, preferences and shared values (Nagykaldi, Tange, & De Maeseneer, 2018).

In their narratives, people will use a common language, in contrast to professionals who will use classified languages. However, the former needs to be approximated to some sort of classified language; otherwise, it will not be possible to be treated systematically by information systems. For this purpose there are multiple possibilities, one of the most investigated being the Omaha System (Gao & Kerr, 2016; Topaz,

Figure 1. Construction model of the individual care plan

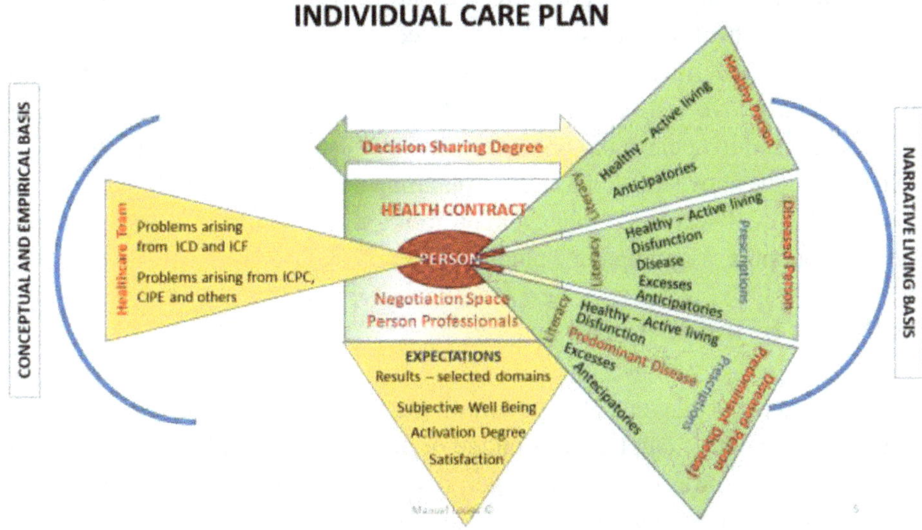

Golfenshtein, & Bowles, 2014). This terminology has the advantage of being cross professional, having a conceptual and empirical basis and being interoperable with other classified languages.

In turn, the various professionals will bring a conceptual and empirical narrative based on the scientific basis of their respective areas of knowledge, but also on the knowledge about that particular person and his problems (see Figure 1, left side). The languages to be used by professionals will be chosen by them, however, through semantic interoperability processes, they need to be doubly translated into the language of the WHO International Classification Family Reference Classifications (Madden, Richard; Sykes, Catherine; Ustun, Bedirhan, nd), and for the language of the Omaha System (Gao & Kerr, 2016; Topaz et al., 2014). The first ensures that WHO's requirements for language uniqueness are met; the second ensures an adequate level of communication among all caregivers, so as to ensure the necessary dialogue space.

This space for dialogue and negotiation has multiple dimensions to consider. First, it is essential in the process of activating the person through the empowerment that results from the dialogue itself. Second, it is essential in the process of managing expectations, an increasingly important dimension in the care process, especially in complex situations of multimorbidity. Third, it is one of the ways of embodying the concept of coproduction of care, that is, the involvement and responsibility of all actors in the care process.

This tool is particularly useful for people with multiple health problems, enabling them to better manage the health care they need. It also allows them to record, according to the health professionals who accompany them, the current situation and the objectives defined for a certain period, thus sharing work and responsibility among all those involved in this process. The ICP allows monitoring actions and behaviors agreed to achieve the objectives and evaluate the results achieved.

In view of the above, the ICP is a care-planning instrument that will integrate the contributions, will serve as a management tool for all providers, and may include treatment, support or anticipatory plans.

Attributes of the ICP

As mentioned above, anyone at any point in the life cycle and at any stage of their health-disease process can take advantage of an ICP. This can be initiative of the own or any health professional. However, it will always be the result of a person-centered process of negotiation between the actors.

The ICP may be of a generic nature or be focused on a specific health condition or condition.

In the first case, we will be thinking about healthy people, but concerned about maintaining their health, with long-term goals and actions of an anticipatory nature. This ICP should highlight the steps needed to maintain health, list the expectations of the person and each caregiver with whom it interacts and include tools such as decision support and a library of standard care plans. These plans should include the recommended care at each stage of the life cycle in which the person meets and incorporate the anticipatory recommendations of the regulatory bodies (e.g. Portuguese General Directorate for Health).

In the second case, the ICP will focus on specific health problems. In this case, we can and should have an ICP library, which will contain the recommended care for the various health problems. In this way, we would align the ICPs contained in the library with the highest quality standards for each situation. All ICPs included in said library will be editable to enable health professionals to tailor them to the concrete situation of each person.

Thus, by way of example, we can previously define an ICP for the most common hip prosthesis surgery, defining the goals to be achieved and the actions to be taken by all caregivers during the hospitalization period, according to the most demanding recommendations. This would save professionals a lot of time since they would only have to edit what different situations each patient may require.

According to what has been stated all ICPs should be based on evidence of better care and health practices. On the other hand, the effectiveness of a plan either must be measurable, in terms of completed plan stages or in terms of desired outcomes actually achieved.

According to this logic, all ICPs are based on an approach in which all resource decisions and allocations are made in order to create value. Health value is defined as the quotient of health outcomes on costs to achieve them (may include costs that are beyond health). Health outcomes can be categorized as follows:

1. Disease prevention;
2. Early detection;
3. Correct diagnosis;
4. Early and timely treatment;
5. Correct treatment for the right patients;
6. Early treatment in the causal chain of the disease;
7. Fast and less delayed care delivery process;
8. Reduced invasive treatment methods;
9. Less and less complications;
10. Fewer errors and repetitions in treatment;
11. Faster recovery;
12. More complete recovery;
13. Reduced disability;
14. Fewer relapses or acute episodes;
15. Progression of the slower disease;
16. Reduced need for long-term care;
17. Reduced disease-induced care.

We are aware that the adoption of an ICP with these characteristics has a strong likelihood of attracting citizens and health professionals as they participate in its preparation. On the other hand, if, in this way, each citizen as a self-caregiver is provided with the information that allows him to make the best decisions, we are contributing to his / her capacity and consequently to preserve his / her health, reducing the use of services.

In spite of this, we also know that not all care will be subject to a predefined plan. Multiple health situations will continue to require trained professionals to make the best decisions possible at the time.

The Relationship Between the Electronic Health Record and the ICP

The Electronic Health Record (EHR) aims to gather essential information from each citizen to improve the delivery of health care; EHR is constructed by clinical data collected electronically for each citizen and produced by health care providers.

EHR allows the registration and sharing of clinical information between the user, health professionals and health service providers, in accordance with the requirements of the Portuguese National Commission on Data Protection (Authorization No. 940/2013).

EHRs have been used for decades by health professionals, who have believed from the outset that they would achieve greater effectiveness of their intervention, the quality of records, ease of access and transmission of information, and support for clinic decision. Despite this initial optimism, there is now some dismay, if not resistance, to the extent that many of these goals were never met (Martin & Sinsky, 2016, Nagykaldi et al., 2018).

However, the issue is more complex than this. According to the above definition, EHR is no more than the clinical data set of a citizen. Although we are aware that these data will need to continue to exist, as they will be essential for taking many of the decisions, they may not be understandable by many non-professional caregivers (e.g., the patient himself or his caregiver). However, for professional caregivers, there may be difficulties in turning data into useful information for decision-making. In other words, it may not be sufficient to have all the data collected in an electronic record if it does not function as a decision support system.

In this context, we believe that all data should continue to be systematized in the form of a personalized and integrated health record. However, we need to broaden the concept of health data with the aim of integrating the patient narrative, as mentioned above, on the one hand, and integrating all the data collected by the multiple devices used by citizens in their daily life -day, in particular those related to heart rate, weight, blood pressure, physical activity (measured by number of steps). All this information will now need to be subjected to automatic analysis processes, ideally using Artificial Intelligence, in the sense that it can be used to support the decision of the professionals, thus creating a decision support system. It can be defined as any tool that provides caregivers, both professional and non-professional, with information filtered or directed to a specific person or situation. Thus, if we equate a decision support tool inserted in the health information system, it should provide:

- Correct information (evidence-based guidance, response to clinical need);
- For the right people (entire care team - including the patient);
- Through the correct channels (e.g. EHR, mobile device, patient portal);

- In the correct intervention formats (for example, order sets, flow sheets, control panels, patient lists);
- At the right points in the workflow (for decision making or action) (Bresnick, 2017).

In this way, it is possible to envisage a decision support system based on the clinical information of each person as the appropriate instrument to help in the construction of its ICP in what it has of more specific. Thus, we would be making life easier for health professionals because they would have standardized ICP libraries on the other, they would benefit from an instrument that, acting as decision support, would suggest the specific elements of each person.

In this framework, but also taking into account the goal of integration and continuity of care, we propose a redefinition of EHR functioning as the back office of all the clinical information of a particular person and the ICP as the front office shared by all caregivers mode. In this way, any additional information in the EHR, added by any sector, level of care or caregiver, will be passed on to the ICP if it is relevant in terms of care to be provided. The ICP so constructed will ensure that all caregivers are aware of and are able to contribute to the plan under way, embodying the integration of care and the concept of person-centered care; will still be an inducer of effectiveness insofar as it will prevent repetition or gaps in the intervention process, and minimize clinical risk.

In this framework, the ICP assumes a nuclear importance insofar as it constitutes an essential tool in the concentration, integration and continuity of care, and at the same time, it transforms clinical information into the raw material of care planning for each person. To this end, and in addition to what has already been said, a dynamic of innovation is generated at various levels, among which we highlight:

1. The need to develop a library of generic plans, anticipatory or related to certain health problems. This library will include anticipatory plans that consider the care to be taken to maintain health and which can range from caring for food and physical activity to the type of health examinations that are recommended at a given age (e.g., breast cancer screenings in the women or colon and prostate cancer in man). It will also include specific plans for specific health situations. As an example, and knowing that the most frequent multimorbidity cluster is cardio metabolic, which includes hypertension, diabetes and obesity (Prazeres & Santiago, 2015), it would be appropriate to develop an ICP for this health condition.
2. The need to develop intelligent algorithms that allow a dynamic combination of, on the one hand, the clinical information of the person, on the other hand, their expectations and the objectives that the same has defined, in order to

contribute to the respective ICP in what the even have to be specific. The algorithm will have to conjugate the way in which each one of the elements of this cluster (e.g., hypertension, diabetes and obesity) manifests itself in that person, assigning them meaning in function of the relative weight that they have in each moment in the health condition, with the expectations and the objectives of the same.

3. The above algorithms will also be the basis of a health decision support system, which will have to be thought to be useful to all care providers. It is recalled that most people with some health problem are in their homes and take almost all of their care. Thus, it is they who make the most decisions and who need the most support in this decision-making.
4. Due to the foregoing, there is a need to develop interoperability, not only data, but also semantics, which allows the full effectiveness of the algorithm referred to above, but also an adequate response to the needs of the person, regardless of the level of care or the (geographical) location in which he/she is located.
5. The development of coproduction dynamics of care to the extent that, integrating all caregivers in the process of building the ICP we, in practice are embodying this concept. The coproduction of care has a direct impact on the qualification of the person and their caregiver, but also on adherence to the prescribed therapeutic measures, once these have been jointly defined.
6. From the previous one, a new dynamic of integration of care at the micro level and, consequently, a redefinition of the relationships within the health team is developed. The latter will essentially stem from the fact that the ICP clearly defines not only the various stages of the care process, but also the role of each in the process.
7. Development of summary screens appropriate to the profile of each caregiver. These screens will present the status of the current plan, the next steps, and the most relevant data regarding both the care you have and the latest outcome indicators.
8. Development of analytical capacity to evaluate each plan individually, but also to evaluate several dimensions of groups of people with health situations similar or integrated into a region. This analytical capacity should make it possible to analyze not only the outcome indicators but also the effectiveness of care, that is, to combine the results achieved with the respective costs.

Pathway Management and Care Integration

The ICP was once defined as a person-centered instrument, which constitutes a space for dialogue among all caregivers and supports and facilitates the management of pathways and the integration of care. It is therefore appropriate to consider the aforementioned route management and care integration.

In order to understand the explanation about care pathways, it is important to fit them into the theorizing of the course of life. For this purpose, we use the "conceptual framework of the age stratification life course" which includes historical and biographical time, incorporating personal change (ie, human development and / or aging), life cycle stages and life, transitions and trajectories throughout life (Alwin, 2012).

In this context, care pathways can be understood here in a double and complementary perspective. On the one hand, the sequence of health events and their care that takes place throughout life; on the other hand, the organized response of the health services and others to the events and transitions of health or with repercussions on health that occur throughout the life cycle, considering their different stages. Combining both, we can affirm that care pathways are defined as a complex intervention for mutual decision-making and organization of care processes for a well-defined person or group of patients over a well-defined period (Vanhaecht, 2007). They are task-oriented care plans that detail essential steps in the care of patients with a specific clinical problem and describe the expected clinical course of a patient (Li, Liu, Yang, & Yu, 2014).

The defining characteristics of care pathways include:

- An explicit statement of the objectives and key elements of evidence-based care, best practices and expectations of patients and their characteristics;
- Facilitating communication between team members and patients and family members;
- Coordinating the care process, coordinating the roles and sequencing the activities of the multi-professional team, patients and their families;
- Documentation, monitoring and evaluation of variations and results, and identification of appropriate resources
- Theoretical advantages and disadvantages of care pathways for patients, professionals and others

It can thus be said that the main objective of a care pathway is to improve the quality of care throughout the continuum, improving the outcomes of risk-adjusted patients, promoting safety, increasing satisfaction and optimizing resource use (Vanhaecht, 2007).

Combining what was said above about the ICP with this route management perspective, it can be affirmed that there is a bi-univocal and systematic relationship between the two. That is, if a particular course of care is defined in advance (e.g. for people with dementia), then the ICPs to be developed for these people should materialize the respective course. If the course of care is not defined, it can be sketched from the ICPs developed for a given population with certain type of characteristics. This may be particularly useful if we consider multimorbidity situations such as the cardio metabolic cluster already mentioned several times, for which it is more difficult to define a path of care.

With regard to responsibility in the management of the course of care and in accordance with the principle of autonomy, the first and most important person is the person. Obviously, this does not mean that we are not aware, on the one hand, of the low levels of literacy of people, on the other, the high requirement that certain health situations pose with regard to their management. Consequently, in the management of the course of care each citizen can mobilize resources that he considers appropriate to his health situation. For this, it will have the supplementary aid of the NHS, which can be equated as follows:

Level 0: Corresponds to people with a high level of literacy and, predominantly, with low complexity health situations. In this case, each person searches for the "providers" needed to help him or her complete their care plan;

Level 1: Complementary from the previous level, but in this case the information needed for the identification of the "providers" necessary to carry out the care plan is made available by the NHS;

Level 2: By combining the complexity of the health situation and people's literacy, at this level, the NHS (i) provides the necessary information to identify the "providers" needed to carry out the care plan and also (ii) on how best to use the resources of the NHS for this purpose;

Level 3: In the extreme situation of high complexity and / or low literacy, the NHS (i) pre-defined and contractualized routes are made available by the NHS in order to carry out the health plan (ii) and, in addition, the necessary information for the identification of private providers in case they do not exist in the NHS.

REFERENCES

Alwin, D. F. (2012). Integrating varieties of life course concepts. *The Journals of Gerontology. Series B, Psychological Sciences and Social Sciences*, *67*(2), 206–220. doi:10.1093/geronb/gbr146 PMID:22399576

Baez, N. L. X., & Reckziegel, J. (2013). O direito humano fundamental de autodeterminação e os seus limites éticos frente ao princípio da proteção da dignidade humana. *Prisma Juridico*, *12*(1), 225–252. doi:10.5585/prismaj.v12n1.3427

Bresnick, J. (2017). *Understanding the Basics of Clinical Decision Support Systems*. Retrieved January 6, 2019, from https://healthitanalytics.com/features/understanding-the-basics-of-clinical-decision-support-systems

Deshpande, P. R., Rajan, S., Sudeepthi, B. L., & Nazir, A. (2011). Patient-reported outcomes: A new era in clinical research. *Perspectives in Clinical Research*, *2*(4), 137–144. doi:10.4103/2229-3485.86879 PMID:22145124

Gao, G., & Kerr, M. (2016). Documentation of Patient Problems and Strengths in Electronic Health Records. *Internal Medicine: Open Access*, *6*(3). doi:10.4172/2165-8048.1000221

Li, W., Liu, K., Yang, H., & Yu, C. (2014). Integrated clinical pathway management for medical quality improvement - Based on a semiotically inspired systems architecture. *European Journal of Information Systems*, *23*(4), 400–417. doi:10.1057/ejis.2013.9

Madden, R., Sykes, C., & Ustun, B. T. (n.d.). *World Health Organization Family of International Classifications: definition, scope and purpose*. Retrieved from https://www.who.int/classifications/en/FamilyDocument2007.pdf?ua=1

Martin, S. A., & Sinsky, C. A. (2016). The map is not the territory: Medical records and 21st century practice. *Lancet*, *388*(10055), 2053–2056. doi:10.1016/S0140-6736(16)00338-X PMID:27125861

Nagykaldi, Z. J., Tange, H., & De Maeseneer, J. (2018). Moving from problem-oriented to goal-directed health records. *Annals of Family Medicine*, *16*(2), 155–159. doi:10.1370/afm.2180 PMID:29531108

Prazeres, F., & Santiago, L. (2015). Prevalence of multimorbidity in the adult population attending primary care in Portugal: A cross-sectional study. *BMJ Open*, *5*(9), e009287. doi:10.1136/bmjopen-2015-009287 PMID:26408832

Takayuki, M. (1999). Human Rights, the Right of Self-Determination and the Right to Freedom - Munakata Takayuki; The International Journal for Peace Studies. *International Journal of Peace Studies*, *4*(1). Retrieved from http://www.gmu.edu/programs/icar/ijps/vol4_1/takayuki.htm

Topaz, M., Golfenshtein, N., & Bowles, K. H. (2014). The Omaha System: A systematic review of the recent literature. *Journal of the American Medical Informatics Association*, *21*(1), 163–170. doi:10.1136/amiajnl-2012-001491 PMID:23744786

Vanhaecht, K. (2007). *The impact of Clinical Pathways on the organisation of care processes*. Katholieke Universiteit Leuven.

ENDNOTE

1 In this sense the first and most important caregiver is the user patient as responsible for self-care. All others provide care by delegation of this and only when the same cannot or does not know. In this context, the dialogue between caregivers should reflect this logic.

Chapter 2
Resilient Software Architecture Platform for the Individual Care Plan

David José Murteira Mendes
https://orcid.org/0000-0002-7664-8597
Universidade de Évora, Portugal

Manuel José Lopes
https://orcid.org/0000-0002-7554-8041
Comprhensive Health Research Centre, Universidade de Évora, Portugal

José Manuel García-Alonso
https://orcid.org/0000-0002-6819-0299
Universidad de Extremadura, Spain

Jorge Santos
https://orcid.org/0000-0003-1000-8252
Universidade de Évora, Portugal

Luís Manuel Mota Sousa
https://orcid.org/0000-0002-9708-5690
Comprehensive Health Research Center, Universidade de Évora, Portugal

ABSTRACT

The individual care plan (ICP) is a metamorphic being. The only steady reality that it maintains is its final objective, stated and explained in the previous chapter where the ICP is thoroughly introduced and debated. It is a fantastic beast, better described as a system of systems that is severely polymorphic due to its coverage both in level

DOI: 10.4018/978-1-7998-1937-0.ch002

of care as well as sources of data to handle. Patient monitoring generates large volumes of data. There is the evident need of an advanced approach that can deal with these huge amounts of healthcare data extracted from various sources such as the wearable sensors, medical, and nursing records that are currently called big data. The purpose of this chapter is to introduce and discuss the software platform that is adequate to develop and deploy the system paying attention to the needs of high-availability, sensitive information security; service-level agreements for multiple healthcare interoperability; law and ruling conformance; as well as other technical and ethical aspects.

INTRODUCTION

In the previous chapter we introduced our concept of an innovative model of care that maintains a double time series of the care needs history and provided actions as well as the clinical antecedents in a care contract that enables the communication among all the levels involved. The ICT framework architecture able support the ICP (integrated Care Plan), defined in the previous chapter, is described in this one at its different levels. We try an approach using subsequent refinements from more general to more detailed explanations and diagrams to fully cover the proposal. When appropriate, we present several types of diagrams to better illustrate the ideas. Our proposal, at the end, is based in specific POSS[1] technologies that are proven both effective globally in technology as well as the less costly to maintain.

Methodology

Resilient Software Platform Reference Architecture

In a complex system of systems like this one, the responsibility of leading and coordinating the technical activities and artifacts development rests is a software architect's shoulders.

Although the different artifacts shown in the Figure 1 are all heavily dependent of each other, we stress the focus in this article to present and discuss the software architecture, it will be used as the foundation for the platform's software architecture document. All of the features discussed arise from the user requisites for the system that will function as a helping tool for all the healthcare ecosystem that involves the actors presented in the section 1.3.1. The requisites conform the system that has to

Figure 1. Software architect responsibilities

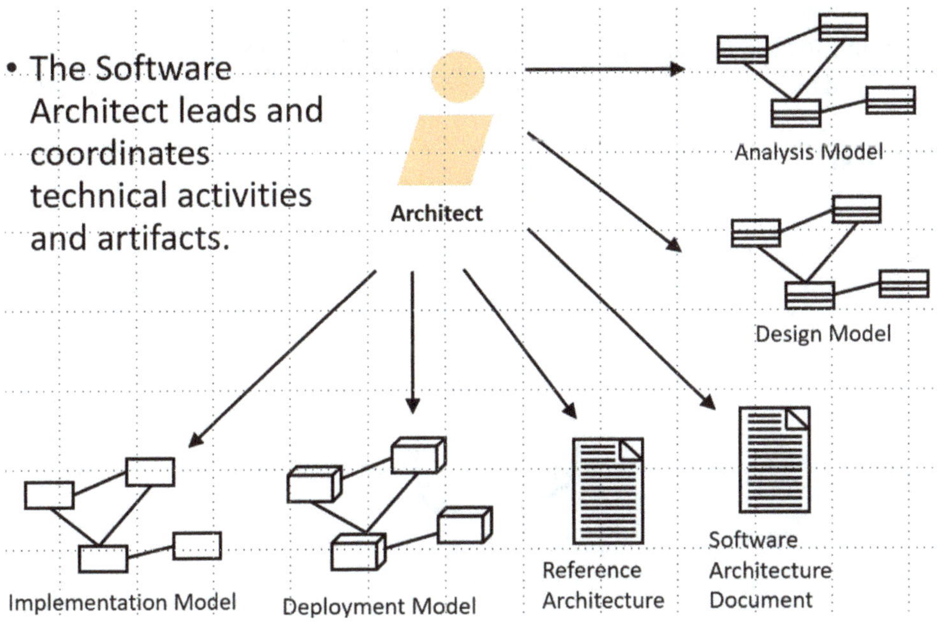

be deployed in a advanced architecture that has to be already proven in the field. There is no space for relying upon futuristic novel concepts because the system of systems has no room for failure. These possible advances are presented in section 5 - Future Developments.

The proposed architecture relies in a highly resilient structure with no single point of failure and several failover redundancies all using POSS projects.

The C4 Model for Visualizing Software Architecture

Software architecture diagrams are a fantastic way to communicate how a complex software system is built. The C4 software architecture model was invented by Simon Brown (Brown, 2018) and we strongly support and use it for the sake of communicating the architectural concepts and implementation options about the ICP. The C4 model consists of a hierarchical set of software architecture diagrams for context, containers, components, and code. The hierarchy of the C4 diagrams provides different levels of abstraction, each of which is relevant to a different audience. Hence, we get a multi audience approach when trying to disseminate the ICP concept.

The Individual Care Plan Architecture Proposal

According to the refinement proposal induced by the C4 system the overall concept is introduced by contextualizing the interaction between the care provider and the ICP

Context

Figure 2. ICP Context

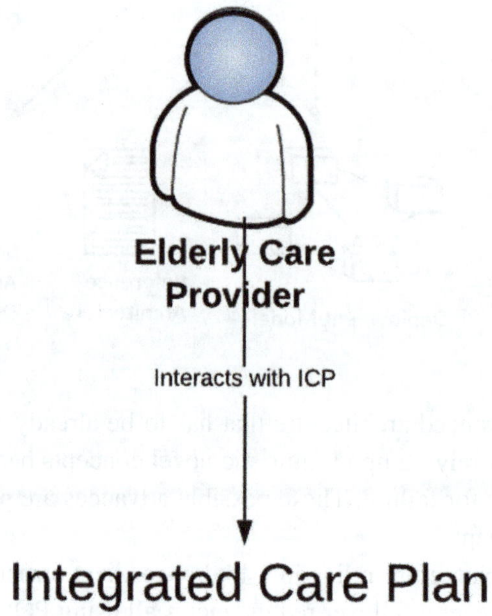

Actors in their Context

Introduced in the previous ICP article, the elderly care provider actors are heterogenous regarding their health and care literacy and responsibilities. A matrix can be formed to position the different stakeholders against each other and relating to the cost of activation.

Containers

In our proposed architecture we suggest containerizing the different components trying to isolate the functionalities and maximize the deploying capabilities. The glue that gathers every container functionality is the REST API for communications.

Table 1.

Care provider	Care level	Care-literacy	Activation cost
Doctor	Tertiary/secondary	High	High
Nurse	Tertiary/secondary/primary	High	High
Formal carer	Primary/continued/nursing home	High/Medium	Medium
Informal carer	Home	Medium/Low	Low
Self-care	Home	Unknown	Low/none

Figure 3. ICP container

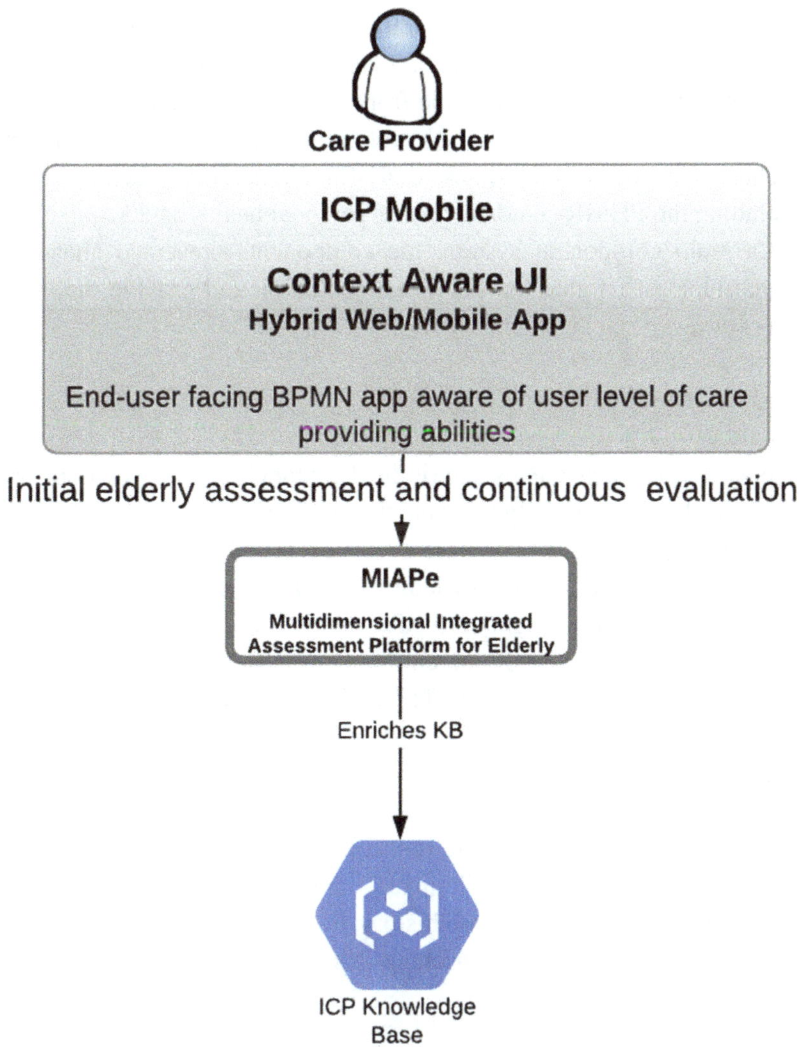

Instead of building solely on top of kubernetes we opted to deploy an open source virtualization infrastructure, Charmed OpenStack from CANONICAL, that provides the tooling needed for complete infrastructure and communications management. The OpenStack charms deliver fast and repeatable OpenStack deployments with loose coupling between OpenStack services (CANONICAL, 2020) and everything deployed over a virtual data center (Graupner et al., 2002).

Components

The ICP is a multi-component piece of software. The interactions amongst the components are based mainly in RESTful (Fielding, 2000) messaging. This is the option assumed in order to make the overall system as much evolutive as possible. The goal is to be possible for the ICP to be adaptable to different environments from the broad range of healthcare landscape from primary, home, tertiary, continuous or whatever level of care providing. Notably regarding the new model approach proposed here is the focus on the standard FHIR interoperability technology (Dodd, 2016) including the PHMR standard for IoT personal health data acquisition.

Being a multi component system, the components presented ahead are the fundamental blocks that glue the ICP data foundation and provide the intelligent operation over it.

ICP Model Creator

Running only once for each ICP instance is the ICP Model Creator. This bootstrapping component has the responsibility to create the ontological terminological relations, the TBox[3], forming the knowledge base over the (Hyperledger) Business Network to which all the future enriched knowledge, the ABox[4], must conform. The TBox models a virtual elder with a highly effective representation of the Aging Ontology (Hsieh, 2015) suitable for fast online enrichment, reasoning and accommodating recent AI[5] techniques like DL[6], RL[7] and TL[8] in a life course healthcare process model.

ICP Healthcare Janitor

For handling each person's healthcare process the responsibility is handled by the Janitor. The Healthcare Janitor is built up of 2 components. One that is invoked only once for the initial creation of the care history, the initial ICP of a given person and the other that keeps updating and enriching this infrastructure.

Figure 4. ICP model creator

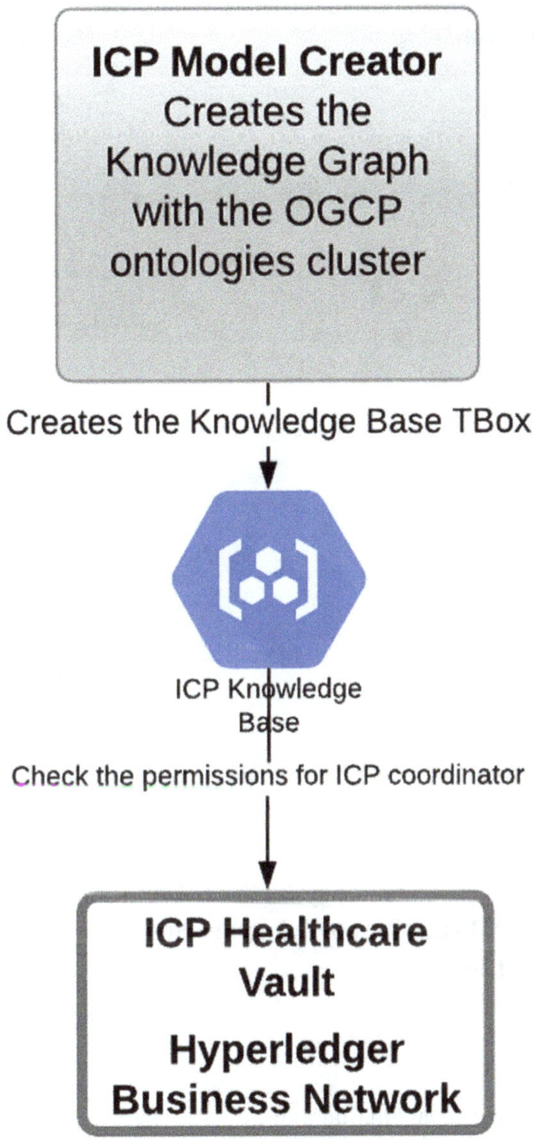

Initiator

When initially invoked for some new patient the Janitor creates the ICP knowledge base by gathering the care history by interrogation of all the involved partners (stakeholders) in the blockchain. It's the first time we encounter the ICP Coordinator who is the care professional assigned to this profile. In fact, the creation, if we think

Figure 5. ICP healthcare janitor initiator and housekeeper

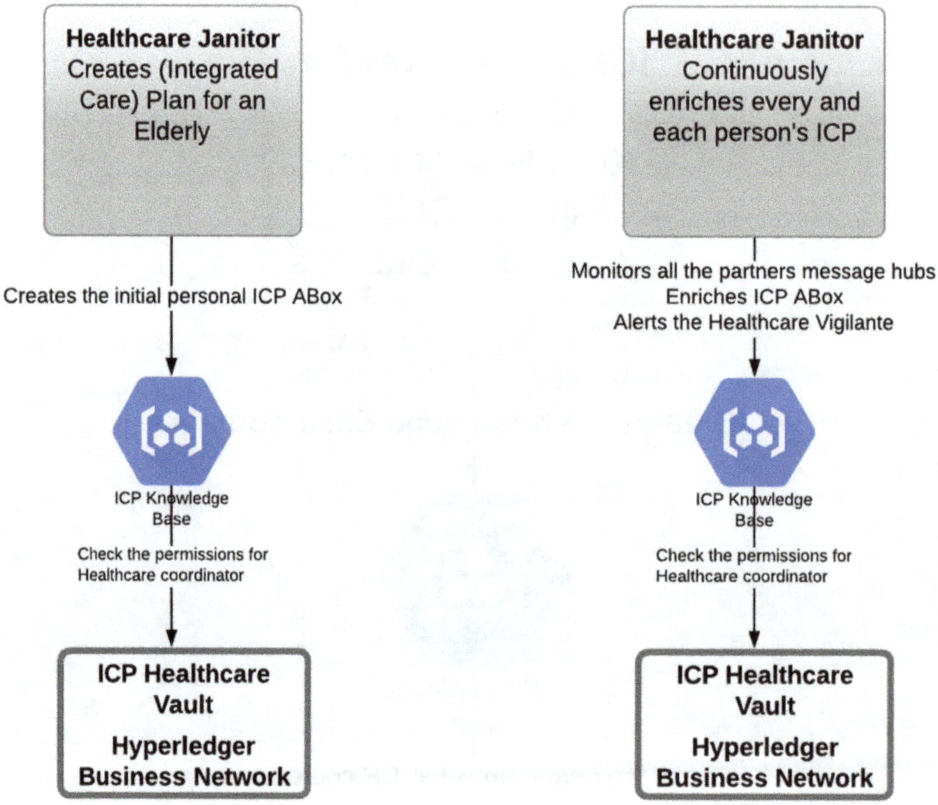

of the knowledge base as an ontology, of the ICP at this moment corresponds to the generation of an ABox for that pseudonymized person that encompasses his or her care and clinical history.

Housekeeper

A continuously functioning agent that monitors the stream of events occurring in the controlled living environments the ALIEs (Assisted Living Intelligent Environments). The streaming flow of events have to be dealt with an information fusion (Nweke et al., 2019; Open Access King et al., 2017) handler that pseudonymizes, purifies, cleanses and homogenizes data from sensors. The stream feeds the permissioned blockchain (Ichikawa et al., 2017; D. Mendes et al., 2018) that is based in Hyperledger currently offered by the Linux Foundation. We refer to this highly secure environment as the ICP healthcare vault. After creating a new axiom, a clinically relevant fact, the Housekeeper alerts the healthcare vigilante that possibly triggers some alerts if needed.

ICP Healthcare Vigilante

The vigilante understands the clinical relations stated in the ICP that provides restrictions to any clinically relevant event. Perhaps better understood with an example, a given event in face of some person's care and clinical history is not problematic or even relevant at all, while for some other person it may be very important and

Figure 6. ICP Healthcare vigilante

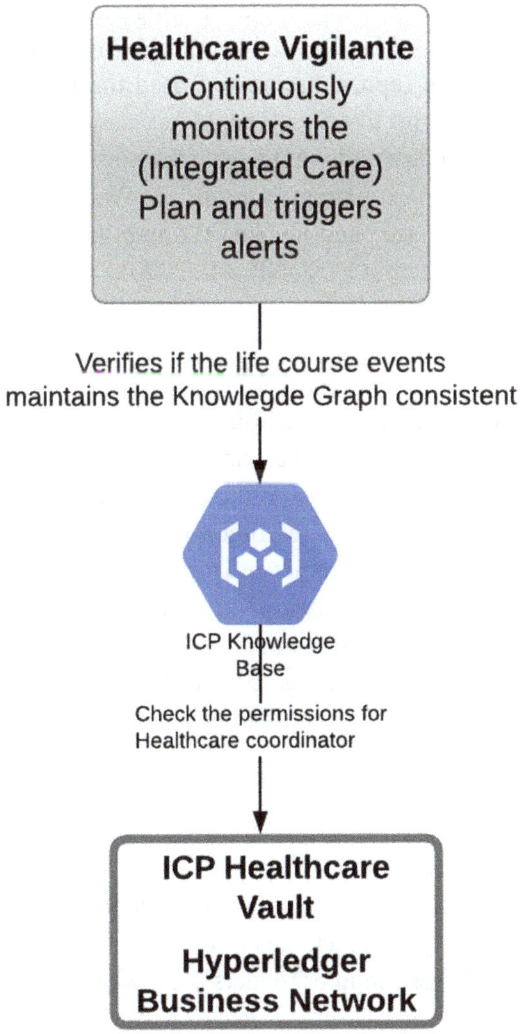

urgent to generate an alert and take the necessary actions for the adequate care to be provided. The Healthcare Vigilante is the continuously monitoring agent that checks any event occurrence against the ICP and triggers the alert based in the consensus automatically verified by the stakeholders in the Hyperledger Business Network.

ICP Mobile Context Aware UI

The app that is the main human interface for caregivers is sensible to each user's clinical literacy and acts accordingly. It is based in a dialogue driven natural interface that has natural language understanding and generation (NLU and NLG) capabilities (Hirschberg & Manning, 2015; Roukos, 2008; Tur et al., 2018)and, being context/ user aware "speaks" a language appropriate for each user to understand. Instead of using domain oriented clinical language understanding and generation like the authors suggested in prior works (D. Mendes, 2014; D. J. M. Mendes et al., n.d.) based in ontology based knowledge representation, we used the more recent capabilities available in assistant platforms like Siri, Google Assistant or Cortana to provide the general conversation structure and we delegate the specific clinical dialogue to a specialized agent developed extending SuperGLUE (Wang et al., 2019) using CCL (Clinical Controlled Language) and invoked through the microservices structure available in OpenStack Charm (CANONICAL, 2020).

ICP Analytics

Diverging the focus to another level of usability in our platform, it is noticeable that the system must provide insights to other kind of users who are not the patients or their caregivers but the managerial and political as well as the research community. That can be viewed as a BI (Business Intelligence) and statistical analysis layer but, however, it has progressed to be a predict and forecasting tool. In fact, the modeling nature of the ICP is an optimum foundation for usage of forecasting and classification ML[9] techniques. Using the underlying authorization and authentication blockchain structure, the suitable usage of aggregated information provides invaluable pre-processed secondary knowledge for these higher-level users.

DISCUSSION

The previously introduced agents provide an intelligent tool to help the healthcare providers to better do their job. In fact, the number of diverse sources of information and the heterogeneity of these sources renders the care provider a formidable clerk

Figure 7. ICP mobile context aware UI

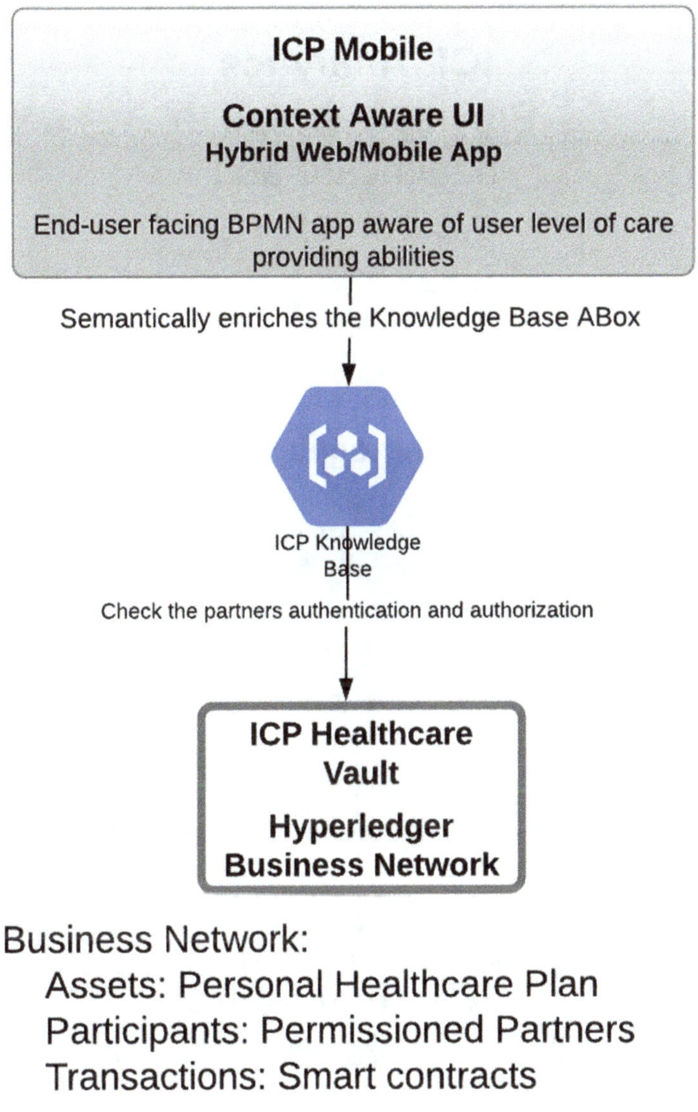

work to be sustained. One of the main objectives of our proposal is to release both the professional and the informal carer of this heavy burden burnout and let him/her focus on the noble chores of the health professionals. By gathering some consensual **clinical guidelines and clinical orientation norms, we** devised some initial "*ICP rules*". These are further refined in face of the healthcare vault enrichment, automatically generated by consensus and validated by scientific evidence. These refined rules generate the key performance indicators (KPI) that are used to evaluate

Figure 8. ICP analytics

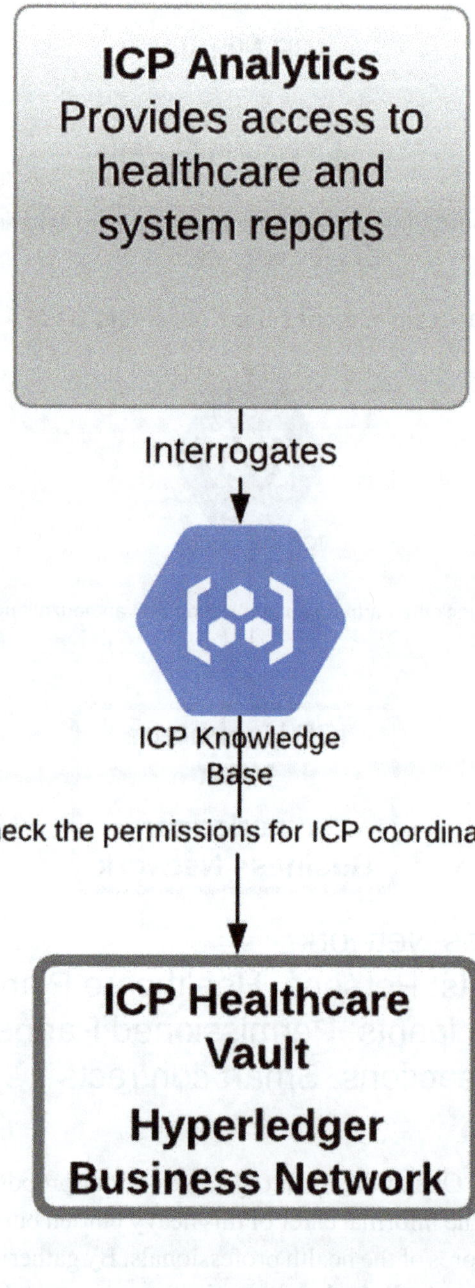

how effective the framework is as a precision and value-based medicine support tool. The platform induces in refining the healthcare pathways in a personalized fashion not possible using the usual, former, manual methods, thus paving the way for a much easier accomplishment of a carer duties.

IMPLEMENTATION

Implementation Overview

This type of critical mission software has to be up and running 24/7 without failure. With such a complex mix of stakeholders there is the additional complexity of surpassing the interoperability issues. The implementation has to follow strict modern software architecture guidelines in order to aspire to be successful. However, all the infrastructure has to be proven in the field and not to recent, thus prone to immaturity issues.

When referring to principles abiding to these constraints, we get a high techie list of architectural options:

1. Distributed containerized platform of platforms.
2. Design by contract lightweight APIs interfacing.
3. Standardized messaging interoperability.
4. Highly secure communication when out of militarized environment.

We can name each option because one of the principles is the usage of proven technology:

1. Kubernetes
2. REST, Blockchain Smart Contracts
3. FHIR, HL7
4. Secured communication (https) with TLS certificates at least 2048 bit.

All these options are thumb rules, several are not applicable when in the real environment. For instance, the encryption in the Edge computing (IoT) layer is not possible since the devices are low power consumption and low computing capability hence the real implementation is based in token passing and acceptance for the vital signs and activities of daily living data communication. Thus, we must take advantage of an edge computing platform infrastructure and we picked up the open-source framework for IoT edge computing EdgeX Foundry. EdgeX Foundry is a vendor-neutral open source project hosted by The Linux Foundation building a common open framework for IoT edge computing. It's packaging scheme, a snap, contains all of the EdgeX core, security, and support reference services, as well as Consul, Kong, MongoDB, Vault, a JRE for the remaining Java services, and a set of basic device services.

For the virtualization approach, we are aware that organizations have started virtualizing their IT workloads and migrating from legacy monolithic infrastructure to cloud environments. Many choose VMware as a provider for their virtualized infrastructure. However, due to the costs associated with VMware licensing, support and professional services, many are not able to significantly reduce the TCO.

In search of alternative solutions, we opted by (Charmed) OpenStack. The OpenStack platform, originally from Ubuntu, as evolved to be fully scripted with charm scripts and became fully DevOps friendly.

Figure 9. ICP overall architecture

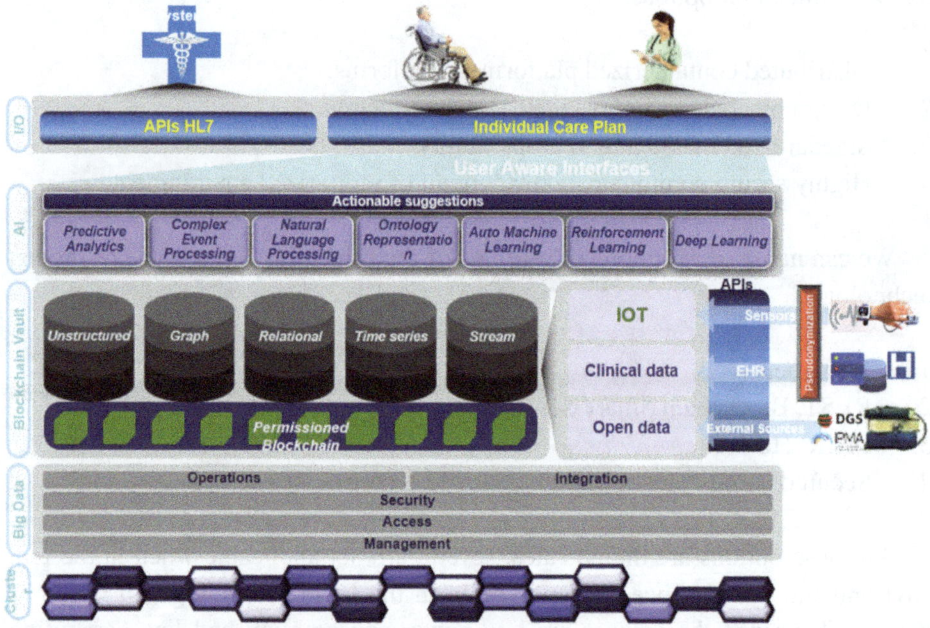

Figure 10. Cluster virtualization structure

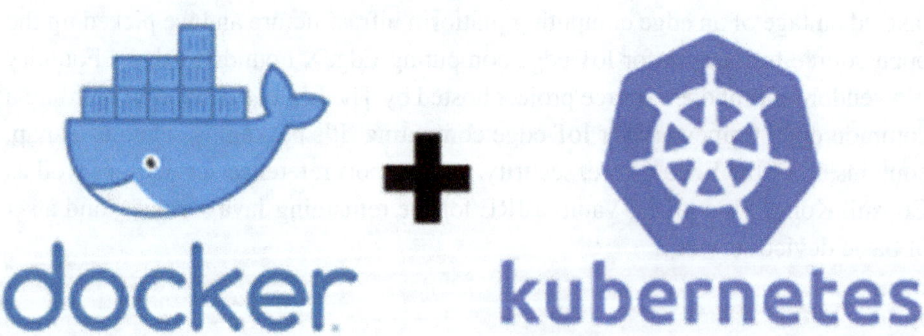

The overall 4IE PIC infrastructure may be depicted like in the following figure:

This multi-layer architecture has several platforms in each of its levels. Going in the bottom-up direction we have in the bottom cluster layer a microK8s structure based in **Kubernetes** managing docker images:

The Big Data layer hosts a complete Apache Hadoop Ecosystem that encompasses all the subsystems shown in the image gently provided by Packt:

This ecosystem handles part of the communications for data extraction, namely with the EHR and other knowledge sources shown in the upper layer. The file system of the different stakeholders appears as a consolidated HDFS, virtualizing the underlying specific systems. We get hence the possibility of application of the frameworks in the ecosystem like the MapReduce (YARN) or SQL Query

Figure 11. Apache hadoop ecosystem

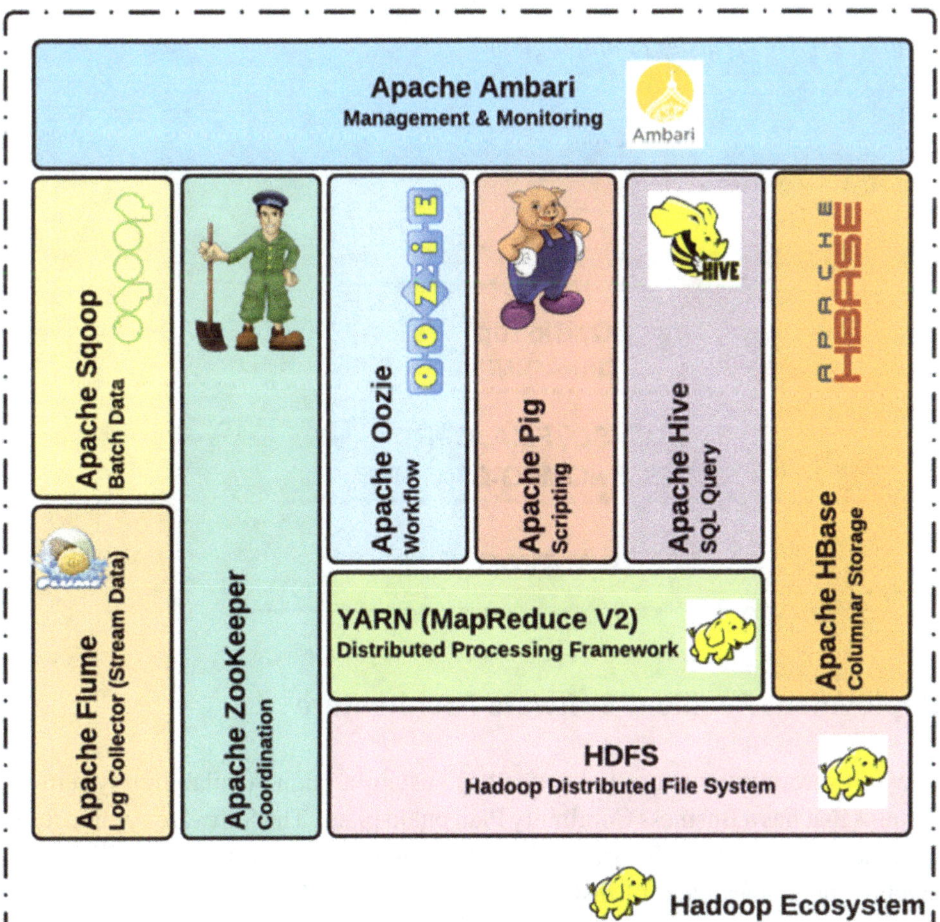

(HIVE), notably the Stream Data collector (Flume) that infuses and "purifies" the heterogeneous data coming from IoT sensors. All the coordinating activities spanning the various stakeholders' systems are kept by the proven Zookeeper in a centralized managed, distributed way. If intended, one can filter, sequence and consume data by Sqoop and, finally, the management and monitoring is performed by the Ambari overhaul addon.

The permissioned blockchain is based in the Linux Software Foundation Hyperledger offering whose implementation ranges from Mainframes to Microsystems like those present in the EdgeX Foundry computing IoT layer. We have successfully implemented it in a cluster formed by heterogeneous Raspberry PI boards (3 model B, B+ and others).

The reasoning (AI) layer holds the knowledge representation based in the Ontology of General Clinical Practice (OGCP) (D. Mendes & Rodrigues, 2013) that is formed by a well architected cluster of plug-in ontologies shown is the following figure:

Figure 12. OGCP cluster of ontologies

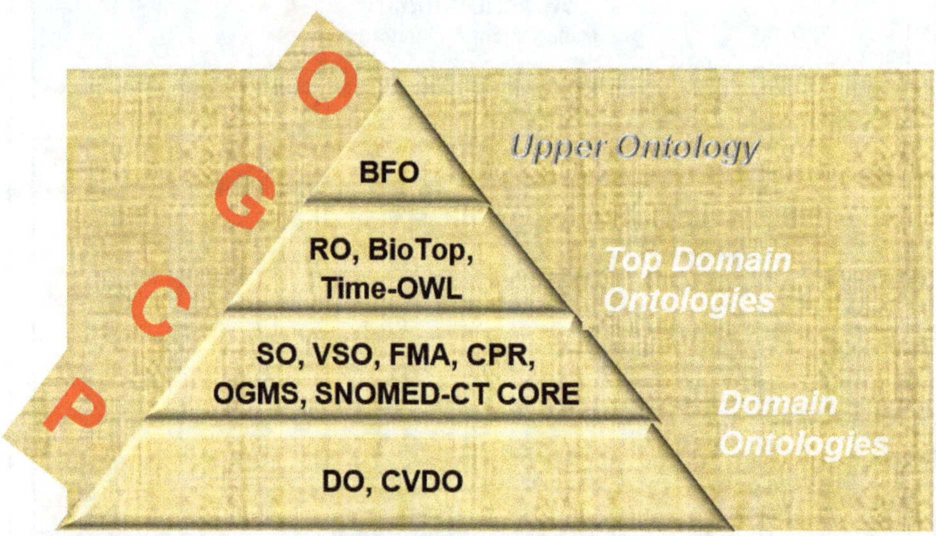

Deployment Resilient Software Architecture

The software infrastructure is intended to sustain a High Availability system of systems that has a Business Continuity Plan put in place. The Software Architecture document generates a Software as a Service architecture proposal. The architecture handles the management of distributed components. There is no distinction in a distributed component architecture between clients and servers. Each distributable entity is an object that provides services to other components and receives services from other components. Component communication is through a middleware system. 4IE+ partnership institutions and platforms users form a highly distributed system.

Resiliency induces special concerns about data privacy (Clinical personal data) and Business Continuity. In the deployment of the system, a series of management guarantees must be assured:

- The Distributed component architecture with BCP (Business Continuity Planning) is guaranteed by SLA (Service Level Agreement).
- Support of full ALM (Application Lifecycle Management) including agnostic development and CI/CD (Continuous Integration/Continuous Development) functionality.
- Agnostic regarding components like programming languages, application servers, databases, Blockchain DLA (Distributed Ledger Architecture), etc.

The above-mentioned contractual guarantees are an absolute need to support the High Quality of Service with Minimal Downtime, Stability, Redundancy and thus the intended Resilience in deployment.

CONCLUSION

In the present chapter we showcase our already implemented proposal for the ICP infrastructure. It is, however, a moving target because each implementation must be able to conform to big tradeoffs having to use the already installed systems in the healthcare, social partners and any other different organizations involved in a person's healthcare process throughout life. We tried to standardize the install infrastructures by defining some controlled ALIEs, trying to use CoC (Convention over Configuration) (Chen, 2006) rules but the real implementations have to be configured with a high level of detail.

The care model implemented, as well as the suggested computing infrastructure is our best effort to develop what can be considered the ignitor of the self-ownership and control by a person of his/hers care process throughout lifetime in line with (Halfon & Hochstein, 2002).

FUTURE DEVELOPMENTS

In the immediate future the research group intends to consolidate some larger proof of concept implementations. The presented infrastructure is working in a VDC (Virtual Data Center) (Graupner et al., 2002) in the DECSIS Datacenter located in Évora. The regional hospital in Évora is developing its implementation of the ICP along with the local primary care health centers and some local retirement homes with the support of Universidade de Évora and DECSIS. The ICP implementation is being developed in the hospital premises. A very important recognition has been awarded to DECSIS as the leader in the regional ALICE project by the EIP on AHA European partnership by awarding the project as a 2 stars reference site in February 2020. This large scale pilot implementation is to be developed involving all the Alentejo Central (Évora district) involving several counties, the regional health administration, the central hospital (Hospital do Espírito Santo de Évora), the local healthcare centers, the integrated care teams and selected ALIEs to be implemented throughout the district in the 3 major multimorbidity clusters chosen (OCPD, Diabetes and Chronic Coronary Disease).

ACKNOWLEDGMENT

We want to express our deepest gratitude to DECSIS, SA[10] in the person of its CEO Eng. Manuel Silva and the DTD[11] Director Eng. Rui Barroso for the continuous support of the authors work that rendered this article and its scientific and technological innovations possible.

REFERENCES

Brown, S. (2018). *The {C4} Model for Software Architecture*. InfoQ.

CANONICAL. (2020). *OpenStack Docs: Welcome to the OpenStack Charm Guide*. https://docs.openstack.org/charm-guide/latest/

Chen, N. (2006). *Convention over Configuration*. Academic Press.

Dodd, J. C. (2016). *Healthcare IT Transformation : Bridging Innovation, Integration, Interoperability, and Analytics*. CRC Press. doi:10.1201/9781315366876

Fielding, R. T. (2000). *Architectural Styles and the Design of Network-based Software Architectures*. Academic Press.

Graupner, S., Kotov, V., & Trinks, H. (2002). *Resource-Sharing and Service Deployment in Virtual Data Centers*. Academic Press.

Halfon, N., & Hochstein, M. (2002). Life Course Heath Development: An Integrated Framework for Developing Health, Policy, and Research. *The Milbank Quarterly*, *80*(3), 433–479. doi:10.1111/1468-0009.00019 PMID:12233246

Hirschberg, J., & Manning, C. D. (2015). Advances in natural language processing. *Science*, *349*(6245), 261–266. doi:10.1126cience.aaa8685 PMID:26185244

Hsieh, N. (2015). *Ontology Based Integration of Residential Care of the Elderly System in Long-Term Care Institutions*. doi:10.12720/jait.6.3.96-102

Ichikawa, D., Kashiyama, M., & Ueno, T. (2017). Tamper-Resistant Mobile Health Using Blockchain Technology. *JMIR mHealth and uHealth*, *5*(7), e111. doi:10.2196/mhealth.7938 PMID:28747296

Mendes, D. (2014). *Clinical Practice Knowledge Acquisition and Interrogation using Natural Language*. Universidade de Évora. https://www.rdpc.uevora.pt/bitstream/10174/12553/1/dissertation_Dm_PhDi.pdf

Mendes, D., Rodrigues, I., Fonseca, C., Lopes, M. J., García-alonso, J. M., & Berrocal, J. (2018). *Anonymized distributed PHR using Blockchain for openness and non- repudiation guarantee*. Academic Press.

Mendes, D., & Rodrigues, I. P. (2013). OGCP - A new ontology for clinical practice knowledge representation and a proposal for automated population. *Proceedings of JIUE 2013 - Jornadas Do Departamento de Informática Da Universidade de Évora - Évora, Portugal.*

Mendes, D. J. M., Rodrigues, I. P., & Fonseca, C. (n.d.). *Clinical Decision Support Systems Question and Answering*. doi:10.4018/978-1-5225-4944-4.ch009

Nweke, H. F., Teh, Y. W., Mujtaba, G., & Al-garadi, M. A. (2019). Data fusion and multiple classifier systems for human activity detection and health monitoring: Review and open research directions. *Information Fusion*, *46*, 147–170. doi:10.1016/j.inffus.2018.06.002

Open Access King, R. C., Villeneuve, E., White, R. J., Sherratt, R. S., Holderbaum, W., & Harwin, W. S. (2017). Application of data fusion techniques and technologies for wearable health monitoring. *Medical Engineering & Physics*, *42*, 1–12. doi:10.1016/j.medengphy.2016.12.011 PMID:28237714

Roukos, S. (2008). Natural Language Understanding. Springer Handbooks. doi:10.1007/978-3-540-49127-9_31

Tur, G., Celikyilmaz, A., He, X., Hakkani-Tür, D., & Deng, L. (2018). Deep Learning in Conversational Language Understanding. In *Deep Learning in Natural Language Processing* (pp. 23–48). Springer Singapore. doi:10.1007/978-981-10-5209-5_2

Wang, A., Pruksachatkun, Y., Nangia, N., Singh, A., Michael, J., Hill, F., . . . Bowman, S. R. (2019). *SuperGLUE: A Stickier Benchmark for General-Purpose Language Understanding Systems*. https://arxiv.org/abs/1905.00537

ENDNOTES

1 Professional Open Source Software.

2 Professional Open Source Software.

3 Terminology Box.

4 Axiom Box.

5 Artificial Intelligence.

6 Deep Learning.

7 Reinforcement Learning.

8 Transfer Learning.

9 Machine Learning.

10 www.decsis.eu

11 Digital Transformation Department.

Section 2
Scientific Evidence Foundations for the Lifetime Evolution of Healthcare

The scientific evidence that guides us to the proposal stated in the first section was thoroughly scrutinized and is presented in this section in all and every aspect that must be considered. The challenges that the current state of the art ICT landscape poses to the elderly as well as the fabulous new possibilities arising from the simultaneous dawn of big data, IoT, Machine Learning, open source software and others have to be carefully considered and brought into the table in order to target a system in the edge of all the current computing possibilities. However, many professional, social and ethical considerations have paramount importance for a system that is intended to be a real functional tool instead of an IT toy. All the considerations presented in the present section will mold the system as an effective aid encompassing the full caregiver spectrum from the self to the highly specialized tertiary provision of care.

Chapter 3
Ageing and Health in the Digital Society:
Challenges and Opportunities

Elzbieta Bobrowicz-Campos
https://orcid.org/0000-0001-5889-5642
Faculty of Psychology and Educational Sciences, Centre of 20th Century Interdisciplinary Studies, University of Coimbra, Coimbra, Portugal

Armanda P. M. Matos
https://orcid.org/0000-0003-0802-5870
Faculty of Psychology and Educational Sciences, Centre of 20th Century Interdisciplinary Studies, University of Coimbra, Coimbra, Portugal

ABSTRACT

This chapter describes the innovative solutions generated by the digital society in the field of health and reflects on the effectiveness of the mechanisms implemented in the last decade to increase the adoption of these solutions by the aged population. This reflection begins with the analysis of the digital divide-related issues, relying on the assumption that the lack of a joint multi-stakeholder effort to reduce existing differences in access to digital resources may result in deepening inequality in health. The opportunities and risks for ageing and health in the digital era are presented considering different healthcare purposes, contexts, and end-users' perspectives. Finally, the recommendations to maximize the impact of strategic actions to increase digital literacy and to reinforce digital engagement are presented.

DOI: 10.4018/978-1-7998-1937-0.ch003

INTRODUCTION

Today's society faces digital transformation in almost all its sectors and levels of action. The use of digital resources to create digital solutions is profoundly embedded in the context of personal and professional life, being transversal to different individual, community and social challenges (Dufva & Dufva, 2019; Martin, 2008). Over the last decade, the policy decision-makers have undertaken a substantial effort to increase the availability and accessibility of the digital resources, creating opportunities for their wide and impactful adoption by different community members (Rantala & Suoranta, 2008). Simultaneously, strategic actions have been proposed to increase digital literacy and to reinforce digital engagement in the creation of new products and services in both the public and private sectors. Healthcare and well-being, education, labor market and economy, governance and civic engagement, or public safety are examples of areas targeted by innovation trends. The joint multi-stakeholder effort towards digital inclusion aimed to reduce inequalities existing in the effective participation of citizens in the life of society, attempting to scale up the benefits resulting from the educational, economic, and social opportunities offered by digital innovation. Nevertheless, the gaps in empowerment in the informed use of the digital resources have not yet been overcome, which prevents many citizens from conscious contributing to the formation of the society of the future (Organisation for Economic Cooperation and Development; OECD, 2019).

The concerns on equal adherence to benefits resulting from the products and services offered by the digital society are not recent. For example, the discussion around the digital divide (a phenomenon opposed to digital inclusion) and its consequences for democracy, economic equality and growth, social inclusion, educational attainment, life-course outcomes or personal and public security was at its peak at the beginning of the 21st century (Bucy, 2000; DiMaggio, Hargittai, Celeste, & Shafer, 2004; van Dijk, 2005). At that time, the focus of interest of social science researchers was predominantly on the material, intellectual, motivational and social access to ICT (Yu, Ndumu, Liu, & Fan, 2016), with the most significant barriers to the adoption of new technologies being identified in relation to the reduced possession of technological devices or the permission for their use (material access), and the reduced possession of competences and knowledge supporting ICT acceptance (intellectual access). Other issues found crucial to narrowing/widening the digital divide have considered the level of willingness to adopt ICT in daily life (motivational access), and the level of readiness to create social identities, relations, and conditions that allow for the satisfaction of needs at the personal and/or professional levels (social access). In a broader perspective, the propagation of the digital divide was examined under the restricted availability vs tangibility of material, mental, social, temporal, and cultural resources (van Dijk, 2005). The unequal distribution of those resources was pointed out as one of the indirect causes of unequal participation in society, and therefore as one of the factors responsible for perpetuating the existence of unequal opportunities and rewards for different personal and positional categories within society (van Dijk, 2012). Finally, from the macro perspective, the higher order mechanisms, such as socio-economic, political or cultural forces, leading to direct or indirect changes in ICT acceptance and usage were acknowledged (Yu et al., 2016). This broader approach allowed to define a framework for developing a shared community understanding of digital inclusion and for creating action plans to reinforce digital transformation.

Nowadays, the analysis of issues related to digital inclusion and exclusion, carried out by international entities that aim at the sustainable growth of society, is mainly focused on the opportunities and risks that digital innovation brings to the well-being of individuals and communities (OECD, 2019). In this new panorama, digital disengagement and digital exclusion are considered to be relevant risks to the citizens' well-being and quality of life, as they often lead to different forms of deprivation, especially with respect to employment and income, living conditions, education, and health, as well as access to products and services that guarantee the satisfaction of the individual and social needs (OECD, 2019). The vulnerability for digital disengagement seems to be particularly linked with advanced age, low qualifications, reduced mobility and economic inactivity (Helsper, 2008). It is common for people with these characteristics to suffer from some form of social exclusion. Thereby, it can be said that digital exclusion and social exclusion mutually support each other, exacerbating the consequences of the marginalization in the use of benefits of digital innovation.

Inequalities in access to products and services offered by society have been particularly impactful in the population of older adults. On the one hand, this population is more affected in terms of material, intellectual, motivational and social access to ICT. On the other hand, it presents a very high demand for health services. It is a fact that the application of digital tools to support healthcare (such as electronic health records, telehealth, and mobile health solutions, or wearable devices and sensors to collect health-related data and monitor health status) have multiple vantages for the aged population (European Commission, 2017; McAuley, 2014; OECD, 2019). First, it allows for a person-centered and individually tailored approach by facilitating communication of data to health professionals and by enabling an integrated view of the older person's health status. Second, it contributes to the enhancement of the medical treatment effectiveness by providing accurate and comprehensible data, monitoring the impact of the prescribed intervention program and notifying the adjustments needed to be introduced into that program. Third, it creates opportunities for implementation of early prevention programs by allowing the collection of data on vital signals in the course of daily activities and at home place, and helping older person to engage more with his/her own health. The use of digital tools to support healthcare services was also shown to be cost-effective (European Commission, 2017; McAuley, 2014), which is crucial to increasing the sustainability of health systems threatened in the last decade by demographic ageing. Despite all these vantages in removing physical barriers to access and utilization of health services by older adults, digital innovation in the health sector is not risk-free, leading to differences in up-take of digital solutions and exacerbating health inequalities. Those risks are precisely related to the fact that in a case of a significant number of older citizens, the ownership of technological devices is quite reduced, and/or the knowledge, motivation and/or readiness to use them for improving health-related outcomes is not sufficient (McAuley, 2014).

This chapter will provide a space for reflection on the effectiveness of the mechanisms integrating the aged population in the strategic plans of action proposed by digital society in the field of health. It will also critically analyze whether those strategic plans accomplish with the assumptions of the European Community's smart, sustainable and inclusive growth, informed by the historical and contemporary diversity of different cultures, and based on the creative and productive potential of all generations, allowing older citizens to participate actively in the today's society. This reflection will highlight the challenges and opportunities offered by digital transformation in the sector of health, being supported in the model of digital inequality.

BACKGROUND

In the last years, the European policy-makers have recognized the creation of mechanisms for the wide diffusion of ICTs-based tools and services used to improve the health of European citizens as one of the priority issues on the political agenda. Digital solutions have been identified as essential for expanding access to health and social services and enhancing the quality of care (European Commission, 2018), with their positive impact being expected either in the prevention, or diagnosis, treatment, and monitoring of different clinical conditions. To streamline the process of digital transformation, three pillars of actions have been proposed.

The first of the three pillars focuses on secure access and exchange of health data between citizens and health providers across Europe. The promotion of policies towards cross-border interoperability and portability of personal health data was justified with the possibility of extending access to data-sets and increasing the secondary use of health data, which is particularly relevant for defining new health prevention strategies and personalized medicine. Progress in the fields of data-driven healthcare research has also been pointed out as a targeted issue. The second pillar highlights the need for polling health data for advanced research, disease prevention, and personalized medicine. The rationale for linking data-sets from a wide range of sources, including human, animal, environmental and societal, is related to the possibility of improving early warning and detection of health threats from infectious diseases, strengthening the tracking and control of infectious diseases outbreaks, and enabling timely and personalized treatment of infected patients. In addition, the actions proposed within the second pillar addressed the diagnosis and personalized treatment of rare diseases. Regarding the third pillar, its conceptualization included supplying and up-taking of digital tools and data for citizen empowerment and person-centered healthcare. In this case, the action plan addressed the epidemic and chronic conditions, reinforcing the need for placing the person at the heart of innovative models for health and social care (European Commission, 2018).

One of the greatest challenges addressed by this three-pillar strategic action plan is the rapid increase in the number of older citizens (European Commission, 2017). Digital transformation is intended to facilitate the satisfaction of the increasing health and well-being needs of the aged population, fostering a shift to the connected patient and home-care delivery, and thus alleviating the pressure on the current model of healthcare. It is also intended to enhance the opportunities for active participation in society and independent living through the development and implementation of measures that enable the maximization of a healthy and autonomous life (Council of the European Union, 2012). The spreading and scaling up of digital transformation with the purpose of guaranteeing the successful ageing of the European population is highly supported by the European Innovation Partnership on Active and Healthy Ageing (EIP on AHA). In the EIP on AHA approach, successful aging is related to the maximum possible functioning in the physical, psychological and social dimensions of the individual's life, regardless of the existing health comorbidities, and to the ability to manage and take advantage of the resources that are available in the community to maintain or improve health-related outcomes (Wong, 2018). The EIP on AHA also pursues a goal of supporting the long-term sustainability and efficiency of the health and social care system, and a goal of enhancing the competitiveness of EU industry through the expansion of the silver market and of the digital single market (https://ec.europa.eu/eip/ageing/home_en).

Due to limited material, intellectual, motivational and social access to digital resources, older adults are identified as one of the most vulnerable groups in terms of benefiting from the digital products and services offered by society, including those related to healthcare (Helsper, 2008). According to Survey of Adults Skills (PIAAC) administrated by OECD (2015a) in 28 OECD countries, more than 50% of the adult population can only perform the simplest set of computer tasks or have no ICT skills at all, and in the group of persons aged 55-65 years, only one in ten is able to complete tasks that require the use of specific technology application or that involve multiple steps. With regard to the ICT use to connect with different public services, data provided by Eurostat (2019) show that in 2018 only 38% of European Community population aged 55-74 years interacted with public authorities through the Internet, 31% obtained information from public authorities' web sites, 21% downloaded official forms and 24% submitted completed forms. These numbers depend on the levels of formal education. That is, persons with low formal education, compared to persons with medium and high formal education, connect online with public services less frequently; and the persons with high formal education are those who most often use ICT to interact with public authorities. The numbers mentioned above also vary from country to country, with the highest values being found in Denmark and the lowest in Bulgaria (e.g.: for the age range of 55-74 years, interactions with public authorities were identified in 87% of the Danish population and in 11% of the Bulgarian population).

It is a fact that in the last 10 years the percentage of active Internet users has increased exponentially (in most cases doubling the values registered in 2008, as presented by Eurostat, 2019); however, the presented statistics show that there is still much work to be done. Without the continuous and joint effort of the different stakeholders, inequalities in the access to public services will not be reduced, which in the field of the health may lead to altered (and often more limited) pattern of access to the determinants of health, an intensification of psychosocial stressors, and a subsequent increase in the disease risk factors (McAuley, 2014). The reduction of well-being in this age group with the simultaneous increase in morbidity and mortality rates is one of the possible consequences of these changes.

To avoid this negative scenario, the European Commission has begun to implement the new education strategy, establishing a work plan for the dissemination of flexible and operable solutions that respond to the real needs and challenges of society and that can be provided in the context of lifelong learning (European Commission, 2012). This new education strategy has recognized digital competence as one of the eight core competencies required for personal fulfillment and development, employability and social inclusion (Council of the European Union, 2018). It has also stressed the relevance for active citizenship of non-formal and informal learnings gained through personal experiences in a variety of approaches and learning contexts. The non-formal and informal education were indicated as being particularly fruitful in adulthood since it allows covering the gaps that result from typical twentieth-century educational trends, which mainly encouraged the acquisition of knowledge rather than the development of practical skills and conscious and critical attitudes. Nowadays, there are many different learning opportunities that increase the digital inclusion of older adults, and that are suitable for learning style preferences and information processing of this population, respecting age-related changes in cognitive and physical functioning and the special needs of accommodation. However, to be more impacting on the lives of older persons, these opportunities need to be useful and respond to the personal and social needs of the trainees with advanced age (Martínez-Alcalá et al., 2018). They should also create conditions for the achievement of proactive learning, fostering social inclusion and promoting autonomy.

All the above mentioned health- and education-related strategic actions were undertaken to reduce the social inequalities and to support the development of inclusive, innovative and reflective societies (European Commission, 2016), being their long-term consequences extensively and exhaustively discussed, especially in relation to the advanced age. In the following sections, the chapter authors will look at the opportunities and challenges offered by digital society in the field of healthy and active ageing and in the field of healthcare in advanced age.

DIGITAL MEDIA FOR HEALTHY AND ACTIVE AGEING

The ubiquity of digital resources in different domains of life has significantly modified the patterns of media consumption, reducing barriers to active participation in creating new contents and their subsequent sharing among different members of the community (Jenkins, Purushotma, Weigel, Clinton, & Robison, 2009). The shift from the paradigm of mass communication to the paradigm of multimedia communication, besides creating conditions for decentralized social production and interactive consumption of information, also enabled the establishment of communication networks, supporting the rapid circulation of contents in a globalized world. In other words, the digital media users became consumers and also producers of information. The reposition from passive to active participation in the society was aided by the distinct characteristics of new media, such as interactivity, multimodality of contents and instruments, portability and high connectivity (Livingstone, 2004). As a consequence, the explosion of knowledge was observed.

The amount and availability of published information contributed significantly to the increase of informed choices, including in the field of health. As an example, health websites and expert forums, observatories, mobile applications or digital platforms aiming at promoting healthy lifestyles and preventing chronic diseases or raising awareness about the need to seek medical help in the presence of warning signs can be listed. However, an overabundance of data made the search of required information and the selection of relevant and valid contents quite difficult (Fieldhouse & Nicholas, 2008). To identify information that addresses knowledge gaps and allows the creation of new understandings, the individual must know how to use digital resources, but also be able to compare and critically evaluate information obtained from different sources (Matos, Festas, & Seixas, 2016). He/she also needs to have the capacity to incorporate gathered information into his/her knowledge base and value system (Fieldhouse & Nicholas, 2008; Martens, 2010). It means that media user needs to have the capacity to distinguish between media products that share evidence-based contents and media products that present personal opinions and comments or expose data without caring about its validity (e.g. debates on the benefits and disadvantages associated with the caffeine or red wine consumption). He/she needs to know how to defend against persuasive commercial content presented either in the explicit or implicit form, which promotes unhealthy behaviors (e.g. related to substance use) or incites to purchase the products that promise (often misleadingly) long and healthy life. Another challenge is related with a capacity to not be tied to the form of data presentation (text vs graphics, animations, audio, video or other easy to process elements), and to prefer information based on their content and not on their graphical form (e.g. health websites authored by the legal entities that present exhaustive information on certain health issues vs personal blogs that present partial information, seeking to arouse certain emotions in a reader and get a fast feedback). Finally, media user must be able to make an unbiased choice, avoiding to search for preference- or expectation-supporting information (e.g. conscious response to the trends promoting the increase or reduction of consumption on certain types of foods or to the actions that sensitize to the need for physical exercise).

In the case of older adults, this panorama is much more complicated. Older adults belong to the generation that, by not being born in the digital era, may have some difficulty accepting new technology or even resists it (Prensky, 2001). This generation gap (Fieldhouse & Nicholas, 2008) is not irrelevant for levels of digital fluency. According to Wang, Com, Myers and Sundaram (2013), the main constraints related to the use of digital resources in advanced age are the low accessibility to digital infrastructure and technological support, and the reduced opportunity to participate in digital content creation, but also the low levels of willingness or need to perform this kind of actions. Age as a moderator of digital skills and digital engagement levels was also identified by van Deursen, Helsper, Eynon and van Dijk (2017). These authors have established that older persons have fewer skills and engage less with the Internet for personal, social, cultural and economic purposes. They have also shown that this disengagement have a negative impact on the achievement of tangible outcomes in different domains of life, including health. Based on these findings, the authors confirmed the exacerbating effect of digital exclusion on existing offline inequalities.

Interestingly, in another study addressing digital divide (van Deursen, & van Dijk, 2010), it has been demonstrated that the relationship between age and different levels of Internet skills (operational, formal, information and strategic) is not so simple. Namely, with regard to basic skills in using internet technology, as well as formal skills of navigation and orientation, the performance of older adults, when compared to the performance of the younger generations, was shown to be poorer.

However, for the internet skills that support actions of fulfilling the information needs and drive decision-making and reaching relevant goals, age was not shown to be a predictor. The level of all internet skills was revealed to be associated with the level of education. Moreover, while longer internet experience seem to contribute to the improvement of the operational internet skills (van Deursen, & van Dijk, 2010), the capacity of communicating through the Internet may compensate for the lack of information skills (van Deursen, Courtois, & van Dijk, 2014). Tirado-Morueta, Aguaded-Gómez and Hernando-Gómez (2018) have also demonstrated that age is not a factor that within itself predicts the Internet access and use. According to these authors, the physical access to the Internet and its use in the simple tasks of everyday life are associated to the socio-demographic status of the older person and his/her access to socio-economic resources. However, both these variables are influenced by age. Thus, it can be said that the influence of age on internet usage is not direct.

The above-mentioned findings prove that the evolution towards a knowledge-based society must necessarily be accompanied by the increase in media literacy levels. However, to avoid the propagation of digital inequalities, media education have to encompass all citizens, including older adults, even if they do not look for formal opportunities for new learnings. When the older adults decide to use digital resources for health purposes, they need to know why they are making this. And after finding required contents, they need to think about who is communicating the health-related information and with whom, how this information is produced and what does it mean, who is supposed to receive it and with what purpose, and, finally, how does the information presents its subject (Sheibe & Rogow, 2012). This is the path to active participation in the digitally transformed society.

DIGITAL MEDIA FOR HEALTHCARE IN ADVANCED AGE

Many of the strategic objectives proposed by the World Health Organization (2017) to support actions on health in advanced age require the use of digital resources for their successful achievement. The digital technology is seen as a valuable means to support the development of age-friendly environments (home places, cities and communities), alignment of health systems to the needs of older populations, development of sustainable and equitable systems for long-term care and improvement of measurement and monitoring of health-related variables. The great potential of the digital technologies stems from their abilities to eliminate or at least reduce physical and social barriers to healthcare and to create pathways for community engagement to strengthen person-centered geriatric care (Bobrowicz-Campos, Couto, Teixeira-Santos, & Apóstolo, 2019). The wide and regular use of these technologies is also relevant because of their capacity to improve the accessibility of older adults to comprehensive and reliable health-related information and to increase the number of quality communication channels with the health professionals and other stakeholders (World Health Organization – Regional Office for Europe, 2017). These technologies, when implemented in different health services in the synergistic and integrated manner, are also expected to allow the collection of data that are highly accurate, reproducible and useful for clinical diagnosis and for defining clinical treatment, that enable monitoring of overall health status and that contribute to the prediction of health-related outcomes. In other words, the deployment of digital innovation is expected to enhance the operational efficiency of health systems and to improve patient experiences (OECD, 2019). The integrated and personalized approach to health in advanced age, which prioritize the encouragement and empowerment of older people and their family members to take responsibility for their own independence and well-being, and which tailor the patients individual needs and preferences, is crucial for increasing the sustainable and successful response by health systems (Cano et al., 2018; Gwyther et al., 2018).

In practical terms, digital solutions may be implemented at the level of primary and long-term care services in order to strengthen the connectivity of the aged person with health professionals. For example, telehealth, eHealth or mHealth services, and other similar, are nowadays recognized as an important factor of patient involvement on health-related actions and of health professional commitment to ensure affordable access to quality care (World Health Organization – Regional Office for Europe, 2017). The digital technology can be used in the home environment to gather information on vital signs of older adults with chronic diseases (blood pressure cuffs, heart rate monitors, respiratory and breath analysis flow meters and blood glucose-level analyzer), allowing continuous remote monitoring and activation of alarms and triggering of appropriate responses when values of monitored variables transgress the pre-established thresholds. This achievement is particularly relevant for the establishment and improvement of a sustainable and equitable long-term care system. However, its impact may be also observed in the reduction of the use of primary health services, and this because of the moderating influence of the immediate feedback to the users' anxiety levels (World Health Organization – Regional Office for Europe, 2017). Moreover, the technology-based measurements may significantly improve patient-centered screening and assessment by providing quality information, which will be reflected in both clinical decision-making and medical assistance.

The use of digital resources for self-management also seems to be very promising. Presently, there are many interactive device applications that enable an assessment of symptoms and behaviors (gait, sleep, movement), providing additional knowledge regarding their management, motivational messages, and/or educational, learning and training material. The great innovation of these applications is related to their ability to obtain data from the user's natural environment and individual and social contexts and enrich the feedback provided based on this complementary information (World Health Organization – Regional Office for Europe, 2017). For integrated and efficient care that tailors individual needs and preferences, this holistic view of individual functioning seems to be indispensable. The implementation of the last mentioned solutions is additionally expected to contribute to the maximization of older persons' autonomy and enable their engagement in activities that promote their own well-being, as well as the well-being of their families and communities (World Health Organization, 2017).

Besides reinforcing person-centered care and improving healthcare performance and quality, digital resources may also contribute positively to patient safety (OECD, 2019). It is true that the implementation of these resources does not substitute the clear definition of safety standards, education, and training of professionals or patient engagement in the prevention of risky behaviors. However, it may assist in the monitoring of possible adverse events, delivering alert messages whenever necessary. This achievement is particularly important in the case of healthcare-associated infections or pressure injuries (Slawomirski, Auraaen, & Klazinga, 2017). Digital resources may also aid health professionals in conducting medical exams or surgeries, enhancing the precision of processed information or applied procedures, and thus diminishing diagnostic or treatment errors. Another benefit is related to the reduction of risk of delayed diagnosis or failure to timely follow-up. Finally, digital technology may be used to reduce significantly adverse drug events either in primary and ambulatory care or hospital care (OECD, 2019; Slawomirsky et al., 2017).

There is also a debate about the use of digital innovation for the creation of health data infrastructure, including big datasets that link information on patient health outcomes, primary and long-term care provision, prescription of medicine, emergency and hospital inpatient records, mortality registers, among others (European Commission, 2017; OECD, 2015b). However, the first implementation of this innovation has shown that is necessary to strengthen mechanisms of confidentiality and protection of personal data. The approval procedures for the use of personal records, public disclosure, and transparency, effective consent and choice mechanisms, as well as training and skills development in privacy and security are other issues that require profound reflection (OECD, 2015b). The protection of data from ransomware and other types of malicious software programs that cause hindering or disrupting the delivery of care is not less relevant (ECRI Institution, 2017).

The vantages of the deployment of digital innovation in healthcare are multiple. The beneficiaries of this innovation are older adults and their families, but also health professionals and health organizations. To enhance this innovation positive impact, it is necessary to create a cultural ecosystem that is user-driven and that address equity, social cohesion, solidarity, social justice and sustainability (Tziraki-Segal et al., 2018). It is also necessary to reinforce the co-development of technological solutions with end-users, providing a response that is suitable for these end-users needs, preferences, and expectations. According to Tziraki-Segal and colleagues (2018), there are significant failures on the transfer of the new technologies from the research field to the clinical practice. The reasons for these failures are immature or not appropriate development of technological solutions, the low level of user-friendliness associated with the lack of sufficient skills to use the new technology or to the long learning curve required for that technology use, and rapid loss of interest in using innovative resources with a subsequent return to the usual behaviors. Other risks are related to technology acceptance, subjective and objective usefulness and costs (World Health Organization – Regional Office for Europe, 2017). As suggested by Tirado-Morueta and colleagues (2018), the belief that innovative solutions can be useful in performing daily routines explains, at least partially, the decision of the older adults to employ them in the tasks and activities. However, when older adults do not have the ability to make easier the use of technology, their acceptance of the technology-based innovation is significantly delayed. Moreover, the quality of access to social and economic resources seems to be a strong predictor of the frequency of technology usage in daily life (Tirado-Morueta et al., 2018). Psychological factors, such as feeling old, having greater technology-related anxiety and having lower levels of venturousness also negatively influence the use of digital resources, especially in terms of producing new contents and their communication to others (Peral-Peral, Arenas-Gaitán, & Villarejo-Ramos, 2015).

DIGITAL MEDIA AND RISKS FOR ACTIVE PARTICIPATION IN HEALTH

Although there is a lot of effort to involve relevant stakeholders in projects and initiatives that enable older adults to join these new health and educational trends (e.g., the EIP on AHA, https://ec.europa.eu/eip/ageing/home_en), today's media tend to marginalize seniors (Rozanova, Northcott, & McDaniel, 2006) and present ageing processes in a tendentious and stereotyped fashion (Milner, van Norman, & Milner, 2012). This discriminative approach, especially towards individuals who do not correspond to the normative concepts of successful ageing (Rozanova et al., 2006), make older adults more vulnerable to social exclusion and loss of control over decision making (World Health Organization, 2017), having a subversive effect on their engagement in the proposed actions. For example, public communication often addresses the topic of the economic burden to society that results from increased health and social care costs in the advanced age (Lumme-Sandt, 2011), identifying a phenomenon of demographic ageing in terms of a threat to the sustainability of the public health system. It also confers upon the aged population, in comparison with economically active adults, less social value, thus promoting negative images about the older persons and encouraging intentional and unintentional ageism (Milner, et al., 2012; Rozanova et al., 2006). The patronizing messages on ageing based on the prejudices regarding the cognitive and physical capacity of older persons (Milner, et al., 2012), as well as the underrepresentation of the opinions, interests, and needs of seniors as media consumers, are other examples of narratives that shape social discourse. The representation of aged population advocated by media may have a very harmful effect on society, leading on the one hand to the unequal treatment of older persons by politicians and decision makers (Officer & de la Fuente-Núñez, 2018), and on the other to the disinvestment in the involvement of seniors in opportunities driven by societal and digital transformations.

According to some authors (Milner, et al., 2012; Officer & de la Fuente-Núñez, 2018; Schreurs, Quan-Haase, & Martin, 2017), the negative images on ageing promoted by media influence self-esteem and self-efficacy of the older adults, impacting their perception of control over health-related outcomes and affecting their will or determination to change attitudes and adopt healthier behaviors. The discourse on ageing prevailing in media may also increase the resistance of older adults in experimenting with new digital tools or services. This resistance can be expressed at the level of motivation for (not) using ICTs to support health- and healthcare-related choices. It can also be manifested through the quality, quantity, and ubiquity of digital tools and services accessed, and through their use, which involves engaging with existing digital content or creating a new one (van Deursen et al., 2017).

As it was previously mentioned, all these components (motivation, access, and use) are closely related to the skills of operational and formal manipulation of the media themselves and to the skills of informational and strategic manipulation of the media-provided contents (van Deursen, & van Dijk, 2010), having a substantial impact on achieving (or failing to achieve) tangible and desired outcomes (Deursen et al., 2017). Therefore, at the time of the widespread implementation of the digital economy model, the resistance to experimenting with new digital tools or services seems to be particularly pernicious as it prevents aged citizens from benefiting from simplified procedures and the provision of low-cost quality health and social care services, reinforcing inequality that exists in society.

In this context, it becomes a priority to change the narratives promoted by the media and to create possibilities to discuss ageing from a broader perspective that reflects the diversity of this phase of life. There is also a need to arrange supportive environments where participative learning and active and conscious involvement of aged citizens in the use of digital solutions is possible. It is crucial these supportive environments respect the heterogeneity of the aged population, offering the training opportunities that consider factors of motivation, access, and use, and that enable the improvement of different kinds of skills (operational, formal, informational and strategic). This multi-faceted approach seems to be the only way to enhance the digital inclusion of older adults and reduce social inequality with regard to the expected health outcomes.

SOLUTIONS AND RECOMMENDATIONS

It is incontestable that, to improve health in advanced age, the digital generational gap needs to be addressed. To maximize the impact of the effort made or planned to be made in the field of health, a collaborative framework should be user-driven (Tziraki-Segal et al., 2018), it means, fit the specific needs, expectation and preferences of the aged population and be linked to the older adults' daily practices, supporting their current activities and goals (Quan-Haase, Williams, Kicevski, Elueze, & Wellman, 2018). This framework should also involve multiple stakeholders, including older adults and their families, health professionals, scientific and academic experts, public authorities, community leaders, industry partners and civil society organizations (Bobrowicz-Campos et al., 2019). The efficient implementation of digital solutions in preventive and diagnostic actions, and in treatment, and monitoring processes, requires the establishment and development of strategies to improve media and digital literacy. These strategies can compensate for the age-related barriers to the technology use and the lack of social and economic resources, fostering the adoption of technological innovation in daily life and reinforcing its usage in simple and complex everyday activities (Tirado-Morueta et al., 2018).

Enhancing the operational, formal, information, communication and strategic competences (van Deursen, & van Dijk, 2010; van Deursen et al., 2014) of older adults, but also of health professionals and formal and informal care providers is essential to prevent health inequality (OECD, 2017). However, without simultaneous action aiming at improving material, motivational and social access to new technologies (van Dijk, 2005), the influence of enhanced knowledge and skills on the adoption of innovative solutions might be not sufficient. Thereby, it is recommended to encourage policy decision-makers to implement practical means that extend the material access of the aged population to innovation-based health solutions. It is also recommended to create opportunities for non-formal and informal learning that are suitable for the different trainees' profiles (older adults, health professionals, and formal and informal care providers) and that address both skills and competencies needed to use the digital technologies and willingness and readiness to adopt these technologies in daily life.

The WHO's Regional Office for Europe (2017) has proposed several initiatives to address the digital gap. These initiatives include, among others, the creation of Internet portals and platforms on activities and support services aiming at improving older adults' health, creation of websites for family caregivers with information on available support and opportunities for peer exchange, dissemination of online expert forums and consultation, or reinforcement of access to age-friendly strategies and action plans. Obviously, the quality of information accessible online cannot always be ensured. Thus, to improve adequacy and safety of the information searched and found, it is recommended that educational opportunities, in addition to considering usage-related issues, focus additionally on critical thinking competences, such as competences of analysis, evaluation, and organization. This approach will empower the older person in the search for reliable sources, in the identification of information that adequately addresses his/her problem, and in the proper decoding and interpretation of the information found (Buckingham, 2007; Matos et al., 2016). It will also enable the effective use of this information to achieve health-related goals, simultaneously avoiding the cognitive and emotional consequences of harmful or misleading messages. Another recommendation is related to the improvement of online communication skills, since active participation in social networks may facilitate access to relevant information (Quan-Haase et al., 2018). Communication online is also seen as a means to strengthen social relationships and increase social capital, being a protective factor for loneliness (Quan-Haase et al., 2018).

The authors of this chapter remind that to reach high levels of effectiveness, the above mentioned educative opportunities should acknowledge the older adult history of media use and consider his/her cultural and social environment (Abad, 2014). They should also be based on principles that guide the learning process in advanced age, such as the usefulness of learning, cooperativeness, and collaboration, fostering social inclusion and promoting autonomy (Martínez-Alcalá, 2018). The reduction of age-related barriers to technology use is another issue that should be addressed by these opportunities. More specifically, in the learning context, instructions and guidelines should be provided to deal with the complexity of the technological innovative tools. There should also be conditions for the use of learning strategies that enhance feelings of technology-related self-confidence and that respect age-related cognitive and sensorial changes and difficulties at the level of fine motricity (Gitlow, 2014; Peral-Peral et al., 2015; Vaportzis, Clausen, & Glow, 2017). Furthermore, the educative opportunities should focus on practical and successful employment of skills related to the use of digital resources, but also on the enjoyment and use of these skills for personal and social benefits (Abad, 2014). This latter aspect is particularly relevant for improving the receptiveness of the technology-related procedures and increasing the motivation to their future implementation in different contexts and for different purposes. Finally, the educative opportunities should assist in the identification of digital tools that are approachable, useful and suitable for older adults' needs, that have recognized functional benefits, and that may be easily integrated into daily life activities (Martínez-Alcalá et al., 2018; Quan-Haase et al., 2018).

CONCLUSION

Over the last decade, a substantial joint multi-stakeholder effort has been made to increase the adoption of innovative technologies in different fields of life, including health. Simultaneously, strategic actions have been developed to increase digital engagement and enable the integration of technology-based solutions in daily life. Older adults constituted one of the target audiences covered by these actions. The rationale for the choice of the aged population for inclusion in actions promoting digital competences is related to the fact that this group, as compared to younger adults, has reduced material, intellectual, motivational and social access to ICT, and enhanced need for health products and services. The existence of these differences is at the origin of health inequality, being necessary to mitigate its adverse consequences.

Digital society brings multiple benefits to older adults' well-being and health. In this chapter, those benefits were described in detail, taking into account different healthcare purposes (screening, diagnosis, treatment and monitoring), different healthcare contexts (home place, primary healthcare services and long-term healthcare services) and different end-users' perspectives (older adults, formal and informal caregivers, health professionals and health organizations). Simultaneously, the risks to the satisfactory and efficient use of innovative technologies in actions that promote successful ageing and support healthcare in advanced age were analyzed. In the final part, the authors provided recommendations to maximize the impact of the effort made or planned to be made in the field of health. These recommendations encourage the creation of educational opportunities that aim to improve the access and use of digital resources by older adults, but also their critical thinking and communication skills. The user-driven framework that involves actors from different community sectors was additionally suggested. The implementation of this framework in educational opportunities will allow for a wider generalization and transfer of learning outcomes in daily life.

ACKNOWLEDGMENT

The development of the COMEDIG project (PTDC/CED-EDG/32560/2017) is supported by FEDER funds through the COMPETE 2020, Portugal 2020 and

European Union Program, and by National Funds (PIDDAC) through the Portuguese Foundation for Science and Technology.

REFERENCES

Abad, L. (2014). Media literacy for older people facing the digital divide: The e-inclusion programmes design. *Media Education Research Journal*, *21*(42), 173–180.

Bobrowicz-Campos, E., Couto, F., Teixeira-Santos, L., & Apóstolo, J. (2019Accepted for publication). Community-led ecosystem - a promising strategy to strengthen person-centered geriatric care in preventing age-related dependency. In C. Fonseca, M. Lopes, D. Mendes, F. Mendes, & J. García-Alonso (Eds.), Handbook of Research on Health Systems and Organizations for an Aging Society. Academic Press.

Buckingham, D. (2007). Digital media literacies: Rethinking media education in the age of the Internet. *Research in Comparative and International Education*, *2*(1), 43–55. doi:10.2304/rcie.2007.2.1.43

Bucy, E. P. (2000). Social access to the internet. *The Harvard International Journal of Press/Politics*, *5*(1), 50–61. doi:10.1177/1081180X00005001005

Cano, A., Dargent, G., Carriazo, A., López-Samaniego, L., Apóstolo, J., Bobrowicz-Campos, E., ... Obbia, P. (2018). T ackling frailty and functional decline: Background of the action group A3 of the European innovation partnership for active and healthy ageing. *Maturitas*, *115*, 69–73. doi:10.1016/j.maturitas.2018.06.009 PMID:30049350

Council of the European Union. (2012). Council Declaration on the European Year for Active Ageing and Solidarity between Generations (2012): The Way Forward. *European Commission*. Retrieved from http://register.consilium.europa.eu/doc/srv?l=EN&f=ST%2017468%202012%20INIT

Council of the European Union. (2018). Recomendação do Conselho de 22 de maio de 2018 sobre as Competências Essenciais para a Aprendizagem ao Longo da Vida (Texto relevante para efeitos do EEE). *Jornal Oficial da União Europeia, C 189*, 1-13.

DiMaggio, P., Hargittai, E., Celeste, C., & Shafer, S. (2004). From unequal access to differentiated use: a literature review and agenda for research on digital inequality. In K. Neckerman (Ed.), *Social inequality* (pp. 355–400). New York: Russell Sage Foundation.

Dufva, T., & Dufva, M. (2019). Grasping the future of the digital society. *Futures*, *107*, 17–28. doi:10.1016/j.futures.2018.11.001

ECRI Institution. (2017). *Executive brief: Top 10 Health Technology Hazards for 2018. A Report from Health Devices.* Retrieved from: https://www.ecri.org/Resources/Whitepapers_and_reports/Haz_18.pdf

European Commission. (2012). *Commission presents new Rethinking Education strategy. Press Release.* Brussels: European Commission. Retrieved from https://europa.eu/rapid/press-release_IP-12-1233_en.htm

European Commission. (2016). *Europe in a changing world – Inclusive, innovative and reflective societies.* Retrieved from https://ec.europa.eu/programmes/horizon2020/en/h2020-section/europe-changing-world-inclusive-innovative-and-reflective-societies

European Commission. (2017). *Digital Transformation Monitor: Uptake of digital solutions in the healthcare industry*. European Commission. Retrieved from https://ec.europa.eu/growth/tools-databases/dem/

European Commission. (2018). *Communication from the Commission to the European parliament, the council, the European economic and social committee and the committee of the regions on enabling the digital transformation of health and care in the digital single market; empowering citizens and building a healthier society*. Brussels: European Commission. Retrieved from https://eur-lex.europa.eu/legal-content/EN/TXT/?uri=CELEX:52018SC0126

Eurostat. (2019). *Individuals using the internet for interacting with public authorities*. Retrieved from http://appsso.eurostat.ec.europa.eu/nui/mainPage.do

Fieldhouse, M., & Nicholas, D. (2008). Digital literacy as information savvy: The road to information literacy. In C. Lankshear & M. Knobel (Eds.), *Digital literacies: Concepts, policies and practices* (pp. 47–72). New York: Peter Lang Publishing.

Gitlow, L. (2014). Technology Use by Older Adults and Barriers to Using Technology. *Physical & Occupational Therapy in Geriatrics*, *32*(3), 271–280. doi:10.3109/02703181.2014.946640

Gwyther, H., Bobrowicz-Campos, E., Apóstolo, J., Marcucci, M., Cano, A., & Holland, C. (2018). A realist review to understand the efficacy and outcomes of interventions designed to minimise, reverse or prevent the progression of frailty. *Health Psychology Review*, *12*(4), 382–404. doi:10.1080/17437199.2018.1488601 PMID:29916302

Helsper, E. (2008). *Digital inclusion: an analysis of social disadvantage and the information society*. London: Department for Communities and Local Government.

Jenkins, H., Purushotma, R., Weigel, M., Clinton, K., & Robison, A. (2009). *Confronting the Challenges of Participatory Culture. Media education for the 21st Century.* Massachusetts Institute of Technology. doi:10.7551/mitpress/8435.001.0001

Livingstone, S. (2004). What is media literacy? *Intermedia, 32*(3), 18–20.

Lumme-Sandt, K. (2011). Images of ageing in a 50+ magazine. *Journal of Aging Studies, 25*(1), 45–51. doi:10.1016/j.jaging.2010.08.013

Martens, H. (2010). Evaluating media literacy education: Concepts, theories and future directions. *The National Association for Media Literacy Education's Journal of Media Literacy Education, 2*(1), 1–22.

Martin, A. (2008). Digital Literacy and the "Digital Society". In C. Lankshear & M. Knobel (Eds.), *Digital literacies: Concepts, policies and practices* (pp. 151–176). New York: Peter Lang Publishing.

Martínez-Alcalá, C., Rosales-Lagarde, A., Alonso-Lavernia, M., Ramírez-Salvador, J., Jiménez-Rodríguez, B., Cepeda-Rebollar, R., ... Agis-Juárez, R. A. (2018). Digital inclusion in older adults: A comparison between face-to-face and blended digital literacy workshops. *Frontiers in ICT, 5*, 21. doi:10.3389/fict.2018.00021

Matos, A. P., Festas, M. I., & Seixas, A. M. (2016). Digital media and the challenges for media education. *Applied Technologies and Innovations, 12*(2), 43–53. doi:10.15208/ati.2016.04

McAuley, A. (2014). Digital health interventions: Widening access or widening inequalities? *Public Health, 128*(12), 1118–1120. doi:10.1016/j.puhe.2014.10.008 PMID:25458115

Milner, C., van Norman, K., & Milner, J. (2012). The Media's Portrayal of Ageing. In J. Beard, S. Biggs, D. Bloom, L. Fried, P. Hogan, A. Kalache, & J. Olshansky (Eds.), *Global Population Ageing: Peril or Promise?* (pp. 28-31). World Economic Forum.

Officer, A., & de la Fuente-Núñez, V. (2018). A global campaign to combat ageism. *Bulletin of the World Health Organization, 96*(4), 295–296. doi:10.2471/BLT.17.202424 PMID:29695887

Organisation for Economic Co-operation and Development. (2015a). *Adults, Computers and Problem Solving: What's the Problem?* Paris: OECD Publishing. doi:10.1787/9789264236844-

Organisation for Economic Co-operation and Development. (2015b). *Health data governance: Privacy, monitoring and research.* Paris: OECD Publishing. doi:10.1787/9789264244566-

Organisation for Economic Co-operation and Development. (2017). *Preventing Ageing Unequally*. Paris: OECD Publishing. doi:10.1787/9789264279087-

Organisation for Economic Co-operation and Development. (2019). *How's life in the Digital Age?: Opportunities and risks of the digital transformation for people's well-being*. Paris: OECD Publishing. doi:10.1787/9789264311800

Peral-Peral, B., Arenas-Gaitán, J., & Villarejo-Ramos, A.-F. (2015). From digital divide to psycho-digital divide: Elders and online social networks. *Media Education Research Journal*, *23*(45), 57–64.

Prensky, M. (2001). Digital natives, digital immigrants. *On the Horizon*, *9*(5), 1–6. doi:10.1108/10748120110424816

Quan-Haase, A., Williams, C., Kicevski, M., Elueze, I., & Wellman, B. (2018). Dividing the grey divide: Deconstructing myths about older adults' online activities, skills and attitudes. *The American Behavioral Scientist*, *62*(9), 1207–1228. doi:10.1177/0002764218777572

Rantala, L., & Suoranta, J. (2008). Digital Literacy Policies in the EU - Inclusive Partnership as the Final Stage of Governmentality? In C. Lankshear & M. Knobel (Eds.), *Digital literacies: Concepts, policies and practices* (pp. 91–117). New York: Peter Lang Publishing.

Rozanova, J., Northcott, H., & McDaniel, S. (2006). Seniors and Portrayals of Intra-generational and Inter-generational Inequality in the Globe and Mail. *Canadian Journal of Aging*, *25*(4), 373-386.

Scheibe, C., & Rogow, F. (2012). *The teacher's guide to media literacy: Critical thinking in a multimedia world*. Thousand Oaks, CA: Corwin. doi:10.4135/9781483387581

Schreurs, K., Quan-Haase, A., & Martin, K. (2017). Problematizing the Digital Literacy Paradox in the Context of Older Adults' ICT Use: Aging, Media Discourse, and Self-Determination. *Canadian Journal of Communication*, *42*(2), 359–377. doi:10.22230/cjc.2017v42n2a3130

Slawomirski, L., Auraaen, A., & Klazinga, N. (2017). The economics of patient safety: Strengthening a value-based approach to reducing patient harm at national level. *OECD Health Working Paper, 96*. Retrieved from: https://www.oecd-ilibrary.org/docserver/5a9858cd-en.pdf?expires=1562940862&id=id&accname=guest&checksum=1E1B38EC433983A757038ADADA17CA82

Tirado-Morueta, R., Aguaded-Gómez, J. I., & Hernando-Gómez, A. H. (2018). The socio-demographic divide in Internet usage moderated by digital literacy support. *Technology in Society*, *55*, 47–55. doi:10.1016/j.techsoc.2018.06.001

Tziraki-Segal, Ch., de Luca, V., Santana, S., Romano, R., Tramontano, G., Scattola, P., ... Illario, M. (2019). Creating a Culture of Health in Planning and Implementing Innovative Strategies Addressing Non-communicable Chronic Diseases. *Frontiers in Sociology*, *4*, 9. doi:10.3389/fsoc.2019.00009

van Deursen, A., Courtois, C., & van Dijk, J. (2014). Internet skills, sources of support and benefiting from internet use. *International Journal of Human-Computer Interaction*, *30*(4), 278–290. doi:10.1080/10447318.2013.858458

van Deursen, A., Helsper, E., Eynon, R., & van Dijk, J. (2017). The compoundness and sequentiality of digital inequality. *International Journal of Communication*, *11*, 452–473.

van Deursen, A., & van Dijk, J. (2010). Internet skills and the digital divide. *New Media & Society*, *13*(6), 893–911. doi:10.1177/1461444810386774

van Dijk, J. A. (2005). *The deepening divide: Inequality in the information society*. SAGE Publications.

van Dijk, J. A. (2012). The evolution of digital divide. The digital divide turns to inequality of skills and usage. In J. Bus, M. Crompton, M. Hildebrandt, & G. Metakides (Eds.), Digital Enlightenment – Yearbook 2012 (pp. 57-74). Amsterdam: IOSS Press.

Vaportzis, E., Clausen, M. G., & Glow, A. (2017). Older Adults Perceptions of Technology and Barriers to Interacting with Tablet Computers: A Focus Group Study. *Frontiers in Psychology*, *8*, 1687. doi:10.3389/fpsyg.2017.01687 PMID:29071004

Wang, Q., Com, B., Myers, M., & Sundaram, D. (2013). Digital natives and digital immigrants: Towards a model of digital fluency. *Business & Information Systems Engineering*, *6*(6), 409–419. doi:10.100712599-013-0296-y

Wong, R. (2018). A new strategic approach to successful ageing and healthy ageing. *Geriatrics*, *3*(4), 86. doi:10.3390/geriatrics3040086 PMID:31011121

World Health Organization. (2017). *Global strategy and action plan on ageing and health*. Geneva: World Health Organization.

World Health Organization – Regional Office for Europe. (2017). *Age-friendly environments in Europe. A handbook of domains for policy action*. Copenhagen: World Health Organization.

Yu, B., Ndumu, A., Liu, J., & Fan, Z. (2016). E-inclusion or digital divide: An integrated model of digital inequality. *Proceedings of the Association for Information Science and Technology*, *53*(1), 1–5. doi:10.1002/pra2.2016.14505301099

KEY TERMS AND DEFINITIONS

Digital Divide: Differences on the user's access to the digital infrastructure and its use to achieve personal and professional outcomes, caused by socio-demographic, socio-economic or geographical factors.

Digital Inclusion: Phenomenon describing issues of opportunity to access, adopt and applicate digital innovation in daily life.

Digital Society: Refers to society in which digital technologies are widely used to respond to different individual, community and social challenges.

Digital Transformation: Phenomenon describing the innovative and creative expansion of digital usages ate the society level related to the substantial increase in digital knowledge, skills, and attitudes.

Health Inequalities: Systematic differences in access to health services and products caused by the unequal position of healthcare users in society.

Media Literacy: Effect of media education focused on the development of skills needed to access, analyze, evaluate and create media contents.

Successful Ageing: Refers to ageing that, despite the existence of age-related diseases and disabilities, is lived with satisfaction and meaning of life, being filled by valued activities.

Well-Being: Experience of health, life satisfaction and a sense of meaning.

Chapter 4
Social Representations of Nurses on Medical Safety Culture in Clinical Care for Elderly People

Maria do Céu Mendes Pinto Marques
Comprehensive Health Research Center (CHRC), Universidade de Évora, Portugal

Francisca Tereza Galiza
Universidade Federal do Piauí, Brazil

Maria Célia Freitas
Universidade Estadual do Ceará, Brazil

Maria Vilani Cavalcante Guedes
Universidade Estadual do Ceará, Brazil

ABSTRACT

Evaluating the culture of drug safety, of certain services, and specific subjects, especially for the elderly population, makes it possible to identify gaps in clinical nursing care. The study aimed to analyze the social representations of nurses regarding the culture of drug safety in clinical care for the elderly people. This is a descriptive and exploratory research of qualitative nature, having the theoretical support of social representations. The chapter samples 38 nurses via interview and a non-participant observation. Analysis is done using Alceste software. This

DOI: 10.4018/978-1-7998-1937-0.ch004

resulted in seven stable classes, and Class 3 had the largest representation, 23% of the corpus. Class 3 maintained hierarchical and semantic proximity to Class 2, which deals with technologies to ensure the safety of elderly patients in the use of medicines. For nurses, technologies help in the safety of elderly patients, but do not guarantee the extinction of adverse events. The chapter considered the need for patient safety to become an organizational culture favoring the quality of clinical nursing care in the handling of medicines.

INTRODUCTION

The adoption of a safety culture by both health services and the individuals involved in this process requires the sharing of values, commitment to care practice and the development of skills and abilities, highlighting elements such as communication, culture and the know-how process.

Safety culture is important because it is a structural indicator that favors the implementation of good clinical practice, and includes the use of effective strategies. This proposal stimulates people to potential risks or real failures without fear of reprimanding the manager, as it is an internal policy of the institution (Wachter, 2013; Who, 2004).

In this patient safety scenario, implementing actions that sensitize professionals to the culture of correct practice or that minimize errors in medication handling requires cognitive and psychomotor mastery. Therefore, it is a care modality that involves inherent aspects of the patient, such as age and chronic illnesses, as well as subjective factors of the attending professional, even basic care actions with drug preparation and administration.

Studies related to the frequency of errors indicate that 39% of errors occurred in the medication prescription process, 12% in the transcription process, 11% in the dispensing process and 38% in the medication preparation and administration process (Leape, et al, 1995).

Miaso et al (2006) conducted a research involving the observation of nursing actions in drug management, and identified that in the preparation of drugs the errors observed were related to the manipulation technique, time and place. And in the administration of medications the failures in the administration technique, in the records and in the relationship with the patient were considered.

For nursing, the entire process that involves drug practice, as well as the culture to promote patient safety in this regard, must have its specific care for the various age groups, especially the elderly patients, from drug preparation to administration, in order to ensure an effective result and safe assistance.

The aging process leads to a reduction of 10 to 15% in body water and lean mass. In contrast, there is an increase in adipose tissue reaching 48% in women, which causes an increase in the volume of distribution for lipophilic drugs (Bernardi, 2010).

When it comes to metabolism and excretion of the elderly people, there is a reduction in enzyme secretion, directly interfering with drug metabolism, along with detoxification and drug conjugation, allowing the drug to remain in the bloodstream longer. This occurs due to lower efficiency of organs such as the kidneys that have a reduction in glomerular filtration rate and tubular reabsorption. The liver, the main organ of metabolization through its microsomal enzymatic system, has the activities of this group of reduced enzymes (Eliopoulos, 2011, Bernardi, 2010).

Changes such as these ones directly affect the drug effect and are a predisposing factor for drug interactions and adverse events. It is recommended, however, to learn from the nursing staff about the medications used in the elderly care, allowing knowing the impact of these drugs in this population follow-up and avoiding problems arising from the misuse of medications.

So evaluating the drug safety culture, certain services and specific subjects, especially the elderly people, helps to identify gaps in clinical nursing care; verifying the effectiveness of interventions and setting goals to promote the quality of care, starting from a cohesive professional environment and commitment to the multidisciplinary team. Thus, this study aimed to analyze the social representations of nurses regarding the culture of drug safety in clinical care for the elderly patients.

METHODOLOGY

This is a descriptive and exploratory research of qualitative nature, having the theoretical support of Social Representations. For Jodelet (2001), social representations are the result of the appropriation of the world outside of thought and the psychological and social resignification of this world.

Data were collected at Intensive Care Units of a hospital in Évora-Portugal, from November 2015 to January 2016. 38 nurses participated, who met the following selection criteria: components of the adult/cardiac ICU nursing team who were present during the collection period and provide medication care to the elderly patients hospitalized in the determined sector.

Data were collected through a questionnaire to characterize the social group studied considering sociodemographic and professional questions and structured interview, with the following guiding questions: "What does patient safety in nursing care represent for you?; What do you think about the safety of care in the preparation and administration of medication for the elderly patients?; How do you promote safety in the preparation and administration of a medication for the elderly people?", in addition to non-participant observation.

For researches that use the theoretical framework of social representations, the use of various instruments makes it possible to highlight different aspects, both qualitative and quantitative, in relation to the research problem. Since each instrument may have its analysis modality for the data obtained, thus enabling a deeper and more comprehensive interpretation of the object represented (Nóbrega; Coutinho, 2011).

The interviews were recorded on an electronic and portable tape recorder, transcribed in full, thus ensuring the reliability of the discourses for analysis using the Alceste software (Analyze Lexicale for the Context of a Texte Segments Ensemble), version 2012, of a program that allows to perform textual data analysis or statistical analysis, verifying the main information present in the text, besides allowing the identification of relationships between lexical universes (Camargo, 2005).

Therefore, a database was created that aggregates all the content of the collected material, followed by the coding of the attribute variables determined by the command line researcher, meeting the objectives to be investigated (Saraiva; Coutinho; Miranda, 2011). All interviews, by place of collection, were inserted in a single text file, typed in the Word program, with single space, Courier font, size 10.

In this study, 38 command lines were formed. Each Initial Context Unit (ICU) was separated by a command line, identifying each respondent and seven relevant variables were selected for this research: age, gender, maximum title, time of training, time in ICU, living with the elderly people, and patient safety training.

The research was approved by the Research Ethics Committee of the State University of Ceará, under opinion No. 679,888, in addition to the approval by the Portuguese hospital to host the study.

RESULTS AND DISCUSSIONS

The profile of the investigated nurses was 68% between 20 and 39 years old; feminization remains at 84%, highlighting 58% of respondents with academic education for a maximum of 10 years; even quantitative of nurses with the maximum degree. Regarding length of service in the unit, 71% are allocated between three months and 10 years in the ICUs, 94% said they live with the elderly people daily and 58% indicated participation in training for patient safety.

Regarding the processing of the corpus using Alceste, which generated 72% utilization, consisting of 38 UCIs and 285 Elementary Context Units (UCEs), obtaining 2278 distinct words, with a number of occurrences of 16157. 7 classes were formed from the classification of the words analyzed.

Figure 1. Graphical representation of text processing results by the alceste program - number of ECUs and number of parsable words per class. Évora-PT, 2016.
Source: It was created by the author from the Alceste report

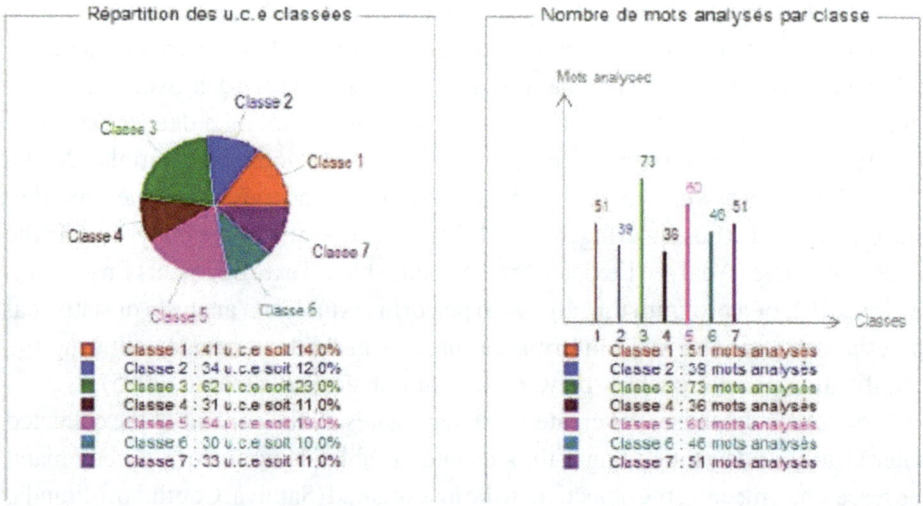

Class 3 was more represented, totaling 62 UCEs, which corresponds to 23% of the corpus, being also the class with the largest number of analyzable words, 73, as shown in figure 01. The main approach of this class has to have possible causes that contribute to the risk or the patient's safety when providing nursing care with medicines in the ICU.

After processing the corpus by Alceste, according to Descending Hierarchical Classification (CHD), the main words generated, considering the occurrence cutoff by the Phi variable greater than or equal to 0.19, as shown in Table 1.

Looking at Figure 2, as for the distribution of radicals according to the proximity of the semantic construction by the Ascending Hierarchical Classification (AHC), two propositions are well defined. The first one concerns the condition of time and stress that lead to failures and, consequently, to adverse events on the part of nurses when providing clinical care to the elderly in drug handling. The second conveys that a secure service depends on the number of professionals.

It can be inferred that feelings of dissatisfaction and improvement in working conditions prevail in the social representation of the nursing community, regardless of culture and social environment.

We follow the same rules here I ask colleagues to check the medicine label. In larger services it must be chaos, as it requires more skill, and the routine is exhausting, more confusing, and more likely to make mistakes (uce # 271 Phi: 0.07 uci # 29: * ind_29 * id_1c * sex_2a * form_3d * max_4a * hosp_5d * oxide_6b * sec_7b).

Table 1. Representative words of class 3 Evora-PT, 2016

WORD	Phi
Nurse	0,29
Stay	0,27
Stress	0,25
Failures	0,24
Error	0,23
Politics	0,22
Compromise	0,22
Cause	0,21
Information	0,22
Hospitals	0,21
Professionals	0,22
Number	0,21
Large	0,20
Routine	0,19
Tools	0,19
Quantity	0,19

Source: Alceste Report

At the hospital in Lisbon, the number of patients and the level of error is different. The more things we have to do, the more mistakes happen and probably more serious. It's complicated with many patients, it has to do with the number of nurses for so many patients (uce # 373 Phi: 0.07 uci # 34: * ind_34 * id_1b * sex_2a * form_3b * max_4b * hosp_5b * ido_6a * seg_7b).

We follow rules, regardless of the service everyone works similarly with a right professional conduct in the care of the medicine. I believe that in larger services the security may be compromised, it depends on the characteristics of each service (uce n°234 Phi: 0.06 uci n°26: * ind_26 * id_1b * sex_2b * form_3b * max_4b * hosp_5b * ido_6a * seg_7a).

The nurse's discourse shows the risk condition in hospital care to the number of professionals below the desired level. In the reality of the Portuguese ICU there is a variation of two to three patients per nurse, considering there are no technicians or nursing assistants in the team. Therefore, nurses' dissatisfaction was inferred as a detrimental factor for safe care.

ECUs are directly related to the problematic issue of the mute zone, revealing the negative and unfavorable feeling that working conditions are imposed on the

Figure 2. Ascending hierarchical classification for class 3 according to the Alceste program, Évora-PT, 2016
Source: Alceste Report

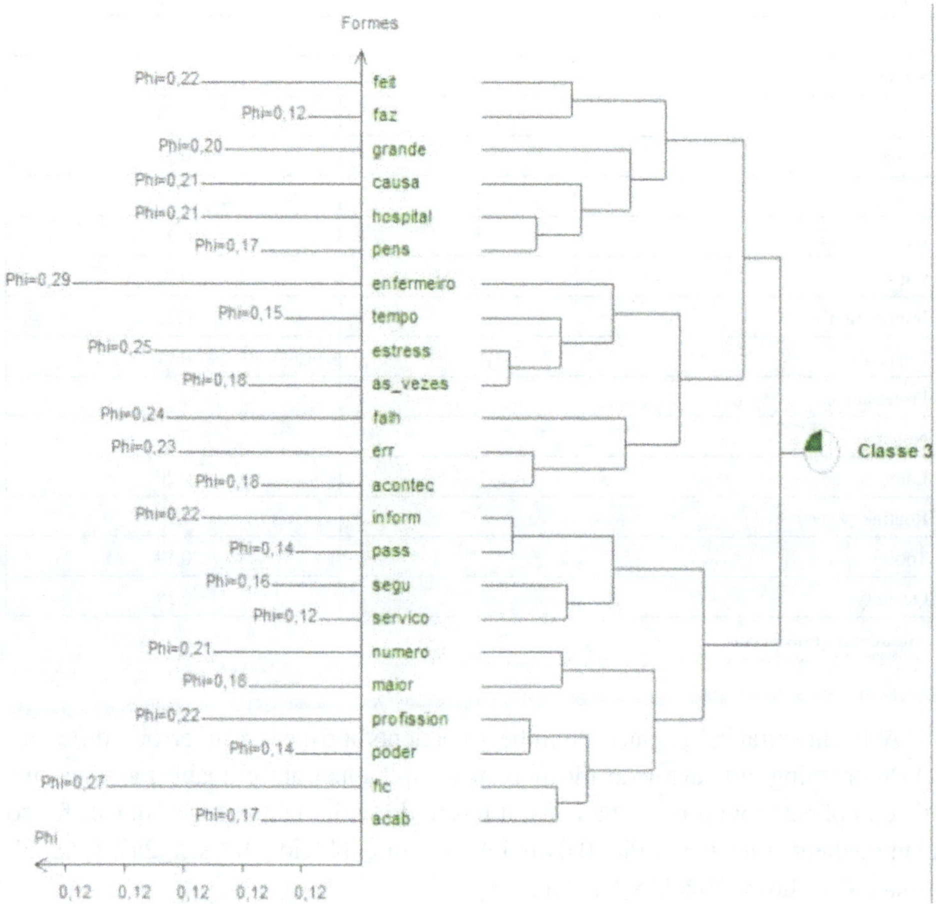

ICU in question. However, the transference of means to express the true meaning of its representative construction, places the individual in a comfortable condition to clearly expose his way of thinking about the object of study.

The main problem around the dimensioning of nursing workers concerns the adverse conditions experienced by the lack of human and material resources. Even with the advent of hard technologies and robotics in the more rigorous monitoring of clinical conditions and therapeutic interventions, the provision of health services has not been able to replace human resources, thus requiring a larger contingent of workers and continuous qualification of these professionals. (Magalhães; Riboldi; Dall'agnol, 2009).

Florence Nightingale was the forerunner of the first method of human resource planning in nursing in the nineteenth century. It was an intuitive method based on subjectivity and proportional relationship between workers and tasks, considering the severity of the patients (Magalhães; Riboldi; Dall'agnol, 2009). Over time, specialties and health services have increased, requiring a more practical tool to determine the ideal number of professionals to meet patient demand. But these new methods still consider the same principle of clinical condition of the elderly plus their number and their conditions of dependence.

I don't know if patient safety in large hospitals is promoted, because they want to reduce professionals to the maximum and this does not promote anything, if it were to reduce the number of patients per nurse I'm sure there would be more care (uce nº181 Phi: 0.04 uci # 19: * ind_19 * id_1a * sex_2a * form_3a * max_4a * hosp_5a * gone_6b * sec_7a).

There is a management policy to consider human resources as the main responsible for high health costs, not valuing their role in the process of care and recovery of the patient. This has led hospital and nursing managers in capturing workers below the evidenced and necessary, for equating this demand in an empirical and particular way, not respecting the effectiveness of care and the work ability of the professional (Magalhães; Riboldi; Dall'agnol, 2009). Therefore, regardless of the care management model, the resoluteness and quality of health care are related to human resources and their physical, mental, emotional and cultural condition to provide this care.

The service may offer appropriate technologies and materials for care, and the professional has the skills and competencies to perform it correctly, but there are other elements that favor the success of work, which in adverse conditions such as work overload, can damage the entire system of security. For example, there are stress, tiredness, inattention and demotivation, elements that directly affect the patient's condition, as a victim of neglect, mistakes and damage.

Whether chaotic or lacking in time, do everything safely. Routines are sometimes stressful. Here in the unit we are two nurses for six patients, if one patient stops we will provide this care, the other patients are left without support, this can compromise safety, as it has happened (uce nº242 Phi: 0.10 uci nº27: * ind_27 * id_1a * sex_2a * form_3b * max_4b * hosp_5b * gone_6a * sec_7b).

Sometimes daily stress and time to do things is not ideal, and in the preparation of medicine, sometimes we are in a hurry to do things (uce nº243 Phi: 0.06 uci nº27: * ind_27 * id_1a * sex_2a * form_3b * max_4b * hosp_5b * gone_6a * sec_7b).

Sometimes other factors end up influencing, such as tiredness. Here a mistake happened because the colleague was tired, took the wrong syringe, prepared all the medicines and changed the syringes. Here tiredness is the most damaging (uce nº180 Phi: 0.0a uci nº19: * ind_19 * id_1a * sex_2a * form_3a * max_4a * hosp_5a * gone_6b * seg_7a).

Study reveals that the main health changes caused by occupational conditions in the hospital environment were pain with 39.64% of inferences, followed by mental tiredness and stress (14.79%) and, to a lesser extent, other changes, such as pain. such as cardiovascular (11.24%), infectious (7.69%) sleep disorders (5.92%) and other types of complaints, nine (5.33%). The highlight for algias has to do with long working hours in unfavorable ergonomic conditions (Dalri; Robazzi; Silva, 2010).

Stress was a word very evidenced in the reports of health professionals as a risk factor for good and safe professional practice. This understanding can be confirmed in ECUs number 242 and 243, and is almost always due to the amount of work done, the ideal working conditions offered to assist the patient and the patient's clinical status. For Dalri, Robazzi e Silva (2010), the work of nursing provides stress situations and causes suffering and illness. It can give rise to psychological distress when meaningless, without social support, unrecognized or in situations that constitute a source of threat to physical and/or mental integrity.

The physical and emotional state of the health professional is not properly valued as a determining factor in the quality of service and patient safety. To promote effective care, a set of aspects that favor such a demand is needed. Perhaps the great difficulty of implementing patient safety policies within health services, goes beyond the lack of organization and incentive of the management sector, goes through the working condition offered to effect basic care with the patient.

There is not someone in the service to allow the national or European security policy that should follow the proposed rules to improve service, but that does not exist (uce n°300 Phi: 0.06 uci n°32: * ind_32 * id_1b * sex_2b * form_3b * max_4b * hosp_5b * gone_6a * sec_7a).

If I think about patient safety the safety policy comes to my mind, I don't know any safety policy inside this hospital, there is no appreciation of the safety policy (uce # 291 Phi: 0.05 uci # 32: * ind_32 * id_1b * sex_2b * form_3b * max_4b * hosp_5b * gone_6a * sec_7a).

In the European Union (EU), it is estimated that between 8% and 12% of hospital inpatients suffer adverse events during their treatment. The EU determined through its Council Recommendation 2009/C 151/01, proposing a comprehensive EU-level strategy to promote patient safety and minimize healthcare-associated infections. This action highlighted on the political agenda of the Member States the national implementation of preventive policies on patient safety. By 2012, ten Member States reported having a national patient safety research program (EU, 2012).

Approximately 3.2 million is the number of patients who contract a healthcare-associated infection each year in the EU, with 20-30% being considered preventable (EU, 2012). In 2006, a study on hospitalization-related adverse effects was carried out in Spain, 9.3% of the inpatients in 2005 suffered adverse events, of which 42.8% were considered preventable. In France, an observational research identified for seven days, per unit, the occurrence of at least one adverse event in 55% of surgical units and 40% of medical units. It is estimated that 35.4% of adverse events could have been prevented (EU, 2008).

In 2009, three public hospitals in the Lisbon region participated in a study involving 1,669 hospitalized patients, that identified an adverse event incidence rate of 11.1%, approximately 53.2% of adverse events were considered preventable (Sousa et al., 2013).

Although the subject's discourse (UCI=32) presented strong dissatisfaction with the managerial conduct of the service, due to the absence of patient safety policies, he stated that he had participated in training on patient safety at the work institution itself. Actions can be considered to happen, but the method of implementation is not meeting the real needs of those involved. Therefore, the importance of knowing the perception of the servers regarding the norms and changes employed, in order to effect the safety culture.

There are worldwide and local initiatives to make patient safety no longer political but culture for managers, healthcare professionals, patients and the entire community involved. It is important to highlight that the breach of safety due to physical and emotional conditions of professionals has represented more risks of adverse events than the lack of normative policies.

CONCLUSION

The results originated from this research show that the social representations regarding the nursing team culture for the safety in the preparation and administration of medication in the elderly, are influenced by the hospital environment and the process of professional formation, linked to a generalist view of care.

For the Portuguese nursing community the responsibility is universal, everyone should assume their role while caring for and ensuring patient safety, but the presence of stressors can interfere with the quality of care provided, as well as the dimensioning of the service, since for the larger the number of patients, the greater the risk of errors in preparing and administering medication.

In addition, during the period of immersion in the field, training and courses were observed to update safety risk indicators or to introduce a new technology or therapeutic approach, promoting the continuous formation of the cultural process for this modality of care.

The use of SRT, as a theoretical framework, made it possible to grasp not only speech, thoughts, but what moves them to be constructed, giving evidence of which beliefs and affections need to be re-signified to promote a change in behavior and culture in the face of aging phenomena, patient safety, clinical nursing care and medication technique.

Therefore, it is considered the need for patient safety to become an organizational culture for managers, healthcare professionals, patients and the entire community involved, thus minimizing health problems of the population, especially the elderly, favoring the quality of clinical nursing care in medication handling.

REFERENCES

Bernardi, R. B., & Barros, H. M. T. (2010). Uso de fármacos em idosos. In *Medicamentos na prática clínica* (pp. 142–153). Porto Alegre: Artmed.

Camargo, B. V. (2005). Alceste: um programa informático de análise quantitative de dados textuais. In A. S. P. Moreira (Ed.), *Perspectivas teórico-metodológicas em representações sociais* (pp. 511–539). João Pessoa: UFPB/Editora Universitária.

Conselho Regional De Enfermagem Do Estado De São Paulo (COREN-SP). (2011). *Erros de medicação: definições e estratégias de prevenção. Rede Brasileira de Enfermagem e Segurança do Paciente (REBRAENSP – POLO SÃO PAULO).* Disponível em: http://inter.coren-sp.gov.br/sites/default/files/erros_de_medicacao-definicoes_e_estrategias_de_prevencao.pdf

Dalri, Robazzi, & Silva. (2010). Riscos ocupacionais e alterações de saúde entre trabalhadores de enfermagem brasileiros de unidades deurgência e emergência. *Cienc. enferm., Concepción, 16*(2), 69-81. Disponible en http://www.scielo.cl/scielo.php?script=sci_arttext&pid=S0717-95532010000200008&lng=es&nrm=iso

Eliopoulos, C. (2011). *Enfermagem Gerontológica* (7th ed.). Porto Alegre: Artmed.

Jodelet, D. (2001). Representações sociais: um domínio em expansão. In As representações sociais. Rio de Janeiro: EdUERJ.

Leape, L. L., Bates D. W., Cullen, D. J., & Cooper, J. (1995). System analysis of adverse drug events. JAMA, 274(1), 35-43.

Magalhaes, A. M. M., Riboldi, C. O., & Dall'Agnol, C. M. (2009). Planejamento de recursos humanos de enfermagem: desafio para as lideranças. *Rev. bras. enferm., Brasília, 62*(4), 608-612. Available from http://www.scielo.br/scielo.php?script=sci_arttext&pid=S0034-71672009000400020&lng=en&nrm=iso

Miasso, A. I., Silva, A. E. B. C., Cassiani, S. H. B., & Grou, C. R. (2006). O processo de preparo e administração de medicamentos: identificação de problemas para propor melhorias e prevenir erros de medicação. *Rev Latino-Am Enfermagem, Ribeirão Preto, 14*(3), 354-63. Available from http://www.scielo.br/scielo.php?script=sci_arttext&pid=S0104-11692006000300008&lng=en&nrm=iso

Nóbrega, S. M., & Coutinho, M. P. L. (2011). O teste de associação livre de palavras. In M. P. L. Coutinho (Ed.), *Métodos de pesquisa em psicologia social: perspectivas qualitativas e quantitativas* (pp. 95–106). João Pessoa: Editora Universitária.

Saraiva, E. R. A., Coutinho, M. P. L., & Miranda, R. S. (2011). O emprego do software Alceste e o desvendar do mundo lexical em pesquisa documental. In *Métodos de pesquisa em psicologia social: perspectivas qualitativas e quantitativas* (pp. 67–94). João Pessoa: Editora Universitária.

Sousa, A. M. D. (2013). *Valiação da cultura de segurança do doente num centro hospitalar da zona centro* (Dissertação). Faculdade de Economia da Universidade de Coimbra, Coimbra, Portugal.

União Européia. (2012). *Comissão ao Parlamento Europeu. Sobre a segurança dos pacientes, incluindo a prevenção e o controlo de infecções associadas aos cuidados de saúde(2009/C 151/01)*. Disponível em: https://ec.europa.eu/health/patient_safety/docs/council_2009_report_pt.pdf

União Européia. (2008). *Direção-Geral da Saúde e da Segurança dos Alimentos da Comissão Européia*. Disponível em: https://ec.europa.eu/health/patient_safety/policy/index_pt.htm

Wachter, R. M. (2013). *Compreendendo a segurança do paciente* (2nd ed.). Porto Alegre: AMGH.

World Health Organization. (2004). *World Aliance for Patient Safety: Forward Programme*. Geneva: WHO Press.

Chapter 5
Technology as a Pathway for Older People to Engage in Activities Promoting Successful Ageing

Luísa Teixeira-Santos
The Health Sciences Research Unit: Nursing, Nursing School of Coimbra, Portugal

Elzbieta Bobrowicz-Campos
https://orcid.org/0000-0001-5889-5642
Faculty of Psychology and Educational Sciences, Centre of 20th Century Interdisciplinary Studies, University of Coimbra, Coimbra, Portugal

Filipa Ventura
https://orcid.org/0000-0001-5722-5612
The Health Sciences Research Unit: Nursing, Nursing School of Coimbra, Portugal

Vitor Parola
The Health Sciences Research Unit: Nursing, Nursing School of Coimbra, Portugal & Faculty of Health Sciences, University Fernando Pessoa, Porto, Portugal

Adriana Coelho
The Health Sciences Research Unit: Nursing, Nursing School of Coimbra, Portugal

Maria de Lurdes Ferreira Almeida
The Health Sciences Research Unit: Nursing, Nursing School of Coimbra, Portugal

Isabel Gil
The Health Sciences Research Unit: Nursing, Nursing School of Coimbra, Portugal

Maria Teresa Moreno-Casbas
https://orcid.org/0000-0001-9061-4628
Nursing and Healthcare Research Unit, Instituto de Salud Carlos III, Spain

João Apóstolo
The Health Sciences Research Unit: Nursing, Nursing School of Coimbra, Portugal

ABSTRACT

This chapter focuses on the use of technology on older adult health promotion. During the ageing process, they experience changes in physical, cognitive, psychological,

DOI: 10.4018/978-1-7998-1937-0.ch005

and social domains. Frailty is the most problematic expression of ageing and entails a high risk of adverse outcomes. In order to prevent it, healthcare professionals must intervene on health promotion. However, it's impossible to continuously monitor the health status of thousands of people. Technologies can bridge the gap between older people's home and the hospital. Especially those with sensors, allow healthcare professionals to continuously monitor the older people's health status and evaluate the health parameters to prioritize care and alert to necessary behavioral changes. The seniors become more aware and responsible for their health, increasing their literacy, autonomy, and well-being. They become more engaged in activities that promote successful ageing. In this chapter, the authors address one of many research projects that monitor the health parameters of older people in a community setting through wearable sensors.

INTRODUCTION

This chapter focuses on the ageing process and the potential impact of the use of technology on the health promotion of older adults. During the ageing process, older adults experience major changes in physical, cognitive, psychological and social domains. These changes can make older people more vulnerable to the onset of diseases and adverse outcomes. Frailty is the most problematic expression of population ageing and is a state of increased vulnerability that entails a high risk of adverse outcomes such as falls, fractures and loss of functionality and autonomy, with subsequent hospitalization and institutionalization. Frailty may also lead to death. When older people experience frailty, they usually resort to healthcare services creating a window of opportunity for healthcare professionals to intervene. In order to prevent adverse events, healthcare professionals must focus their interventions on health promotion and disease prevention of older people. However, to monitor continuously and face-to-face the health status of thousands of older people is an impossible task in the current healthcare service models. Technology has the potential to overcome this barrier by bridging the gap between older people's home and the hospital. Specifically concerning the field of gerontology, the use of technologies can allow the development and delivery of new interventions. Several approaches exist in this area invoking technology as a more comprehensive and dynamic learning process aimed at the physical, emotional and psychological recovery of older people. Among those approaches are the robots, smart homes and ambient assistive living, Internet of Things and sensors.

Technological solutions, especially those which use sensors, allow healthcare professionals to autonomously, proactively and continuously monitor the older' people health status. In this way, seniors can be continuously monitored in their social context, and the professional who evaluates these health parameters can prioritize care and alert to necessary behavioral changes to improve or maintain successful ageing. The older adults become more aware and responsible for their health, increasing their literacy, autonomy, and well-being. Moreover, they become more engaged in activities that promote well-being and quality of life thereby promoting healthy, active and successful ageing. There are many research projects that focus on the use of technologies in health. In this chapter, we address one of them as an example of good practice in monitoring health parameters of older people in a community setting trough wearable sensors.

AGEING IN 21ST CENTURY: TRENDS AT A GLANCE

Ageing is a trend spreading across the world, transforming populations and societies around the globe. In 2015, the world's population aged 60 years and older summed up to 900 million people. By 2050, an increase to 2.2 billion is expected. In 2018, 125 million people were aged 80 years or older in all world. In 2050, 120 million are expected just in China and 434 million worldwide (WHO, 2018). Europe (EU) is not an exception. Almost all European countries are affected by the phenomenon of demographic ageing associated with a significant increase in the average life expectancy, migratory movements and a decrease in birth rate. Demographic ageing is considered one of the greatest social and economic challenges of the 21st century (PORDATA, 2016). From 2016 to 2070 an increase of 9 million people in Europe (EU) is expected. However, the working-age population (people aged 15-64) will decrease by 41 million. This ageing phenomenon in the EU will have a significant implication in the labor force, financial sectors and healthcare systems (European Commission, 2014; Organization for Economic Cooperation and Development, 2017).

Ageing Nowadays

Ageing is a continuous and gradual process of natural adjustments that begin in adulthood and is associated with changes in biological, physiological, environmental, psychological, behavioral, and social dynamic domains. Although the ageing process is associated with decline in the physiologic reserve, older people lose capacities at the physical, psychological and social levels. Changes at the physical level are related to biological factors such as nutrition, mobility, physical activity, strength, balance, mobility, and sensory functions. The psychological changes are associated with cognitive decline, mood liability and exacerbation of depressive and/or anxiety symptomatology, and use of inappropriate and unsuccessful coping strategies. At the social level, older people relations and support tend to weaken as physical and psychological frailty sets in (Gobbens, Van Assen, Luijkx & Schols, 2012).

Some of the age-related changes include cognitive and physical deterioration that result in a decline in sensorial functioning and in daily life activities, leading to an increased susceptibility to disease, disability or frailty. In fact, frailty is the most problematic expression of population ageing and is a state of increased vulnerability that entails a high risk of adverse outcomes (Clegg, Young, Iliffe, Rikkert & Rockwood, 2013).

Frailty is often described as a transitional phase between successful ageing and disability (Chen, Gan & How, 2018). It can be triggered by many external factors, including socio-demographic variables and psychological characteristics, polypharmacy, comorbidities, and lack of physical activity (Dent, Kowal & Hoogendijk, 2016). Frailty progression might lead to increased risk of falls, disability, immobility, hospitalizations, institutionalization, caregiver burden, decreased quality of life and even death (Chen, Gan & How, 2018). However, frailty can be prevented and might be reversible with appropriate interventions, especially if addressed at early stages (Chen, Gan & How, 2018; Monteserin *et al.*, 2010).

Ageing Lifestyles, Chronodisruption and Frailty

People experience ageing with great heterogeneity in their health pathways, therefore to identify which behaviors are associated with healthy and unhealthy ageing processes is crucial (Lowsky, Olshansky, Bhattacharya & Goldman, 2013). The World Health Organization (2015) defines healthy ageing as the process of developing and maintaining the functional ability that enables well-being in older age. Several studies have shown that healthy lifestyle behaviors are consistently associated with better health outcomes in older people. Among the behaviors promoters of healthy lifestyles are not smoking or non-consumption of alcohol, the practice of daily physical activity and daily consumption of fruits and vegetables. In this context, better outcomes are not equivalent to the absence of comorbidities. Improved outcomes only mean that older people with healthier habits have more probability to have a successful ageing, i.e. spend their life with quality with reduced risk of mortality (Kvaavik, 2010; Stenholm *et al.*, 2016; Daskalopoulou *et al.*, 2018)

Modern societies are characterized by a high incidence of chronodisruption, which is a prolonged deterioration of the physiological, behavioral and biochemical rhythms of the organism (Clegg, Young, Iliffe, Rikkert & Rockwood, 2009). Chronodisruption has been related to the inadequate exposure to environmental synchronizers and unhealthy behaviors. Specifically, unhealthy behaviors often disturb circadian rhythms and have a significant and negative impact on individual health status. Currently, there are three major trends in unhealthy behaviors, which are grouped according to changes in eating habits, sleeping patterns and exposure to light. Concerning the eating habits, to eat snacks between meals and lack of meal routines is increasingly common. Sleeping patterns are also changing for the worse. Specifically, there is a tendency to decrease the hours of sleep and to increase the sleep irregularity. The third trend represents an inadequate light exposure with an increase in light exposure at night and a simultaneous decrease in exposure to bright light during the day (Dent, Kowal & Hoogendijk, 2016). These major modifications in lifestyle frequently found in older people, lead to chronodisruption and chronic diseases (e.g. cardiovascular diseases, affective disorders, and some types of cancer) (Davis, Mirick & Stevens, 2011; Pandi-Perumal *et al.*, 2009; Martinez-Nicolas *et al.,* 2018). Essentially, chronodisruption is related with poor lifestyle behaviors, which increase frailty among older people (Brinkman *et al.*, 2018).

Associated with the unhealthy habits described above, older people spend a lot of time alone and have low levels of engagement in integrated social activities potentially increasing social isolation and loneliness, which are both risk factors for poor ageing outcomes (Malcolm, Frost & Cowie, 2019). In fact, loneliness and social isolations can impact older adults' memory, physical well-being, mental health, and life expectancy. Some studies have even found association between the social isolation/loneliness with lower physical activities (Pels & Kleinert, 2016), unhealthy diets (Schrempft, Jackowska, Hamer & Steptoe, 2019; Kobayashi & Steptoe, 2018), and smoking and alcohol consumption (Canham, Mauro, Kaufmann & Sixsmith, 2015). In other words, lack of social relationships predisposes the older adults to the internal chronodisruption. Social interactions provide mental stimulation through complex communication and interaction with others. Social relationships are likely to be intertwined with other health-related lifestyle factors (i.e. a socially, mentally and physically active lifestyle) that may have a synergistic effect on cognitive decline. Therefore, cognitive decline can reduce the social interaction, as it may as well be the consequence of poor social relationships (Kuiper *et al.*, 2016).

The trends alert for the need to consider new solutions to track circadian rhythms, monitor health and social behaviors and provide relevant feedback to health professionals and informal caregivers. Health monitoring will support the enhancement of quality of life, and allow for interventions at the prevention level or to reverse frailty states (Martinez-Nicolas *et al.,* 2018; Apóstolo *et al.*, 2019)

Ageing in a Person-Centered Approach

Ageing populations are often perceived negatively from a social and economic standpoint. However, caring for the older population is not necessarily a burden, especially if they are actively involved and motivated in staying healthy. Beyond active and healthy, older people need to be engaged in having a successful ageing. Specifically, older adults need to be supported in enhancing their possible functioning across the physical, psychological and social dimensions, regardless of existing health comorbidities (Cosco, Prina, Perales, Stephan, & Brayne, 2014). Moreover, successful ageing entails a person's ability to manage and take advantage of the available resources in the community, whereas their involvement has the potential to lead to a more conscious, effective, safe and active ageing process. Focusing on supporting the quality of the ageing process, a successful ageing then reflects ensured levels of autonomy and independence for as long as possible throughout the life cycle, irrespective of existing comorbidities (Wong, 2018).

Current healthcare models however, present several challenges to the implementation of actions and interventions that promote a successful ageing (Beard, 2019; Moore *et al.*, 2017; Sadana & Michel, 2019). Specifically, healthcare services are still centered on disease management, thereby focusing on the disabilities and fragilities more than on the capabilities and resources that are naturally inherent to the person. This is especially happening at the tertiary level of healthcare provision. Here, the empowered and activated older adult only has room for expression while experience exacerbation of symptoms, which are already the manifestation of a crisis situation. Useful interventions at this state might unfortunately have limited benefit in terms of reversing frailty states. Restructuring the current healthcare models towards a successful ageing, while allowing the identification of earlier states of frailty to intervene accordingly is of high importance (Chen, Gan & How, 2018).

Moving from a disease-centered approach, scholars and clinicians in the interdisciplinary field of ageing research and practice are adopting a person-centered perspective to model care processes (Beard, 2019; Kuh, 2019). Irrespective of the varying person-centered models, general consensus reclines on respecting the needs, preferences and personal goals of the older adult despite potential disabilities (McCormack, 2004; Nolan, Davies, Brown, Keady, & Nolan, 2004; Peek, Higgins, Milson-Hawke, McMillan, & Harper, 2007). In a caring context, a collaborative partnership between the older adult and the clinician should then be established and allow for the expression of the uniqueness of each person and his/her life trajectory (American Geriatrics Society Expert Panel on Person-Centered, 2016). In such a context, to understand the older adult's perception of successful ageing is therefore imperative.

Some authors have shed light on the emerging paradox of the successful ageing meaning when looking from the perspectives of older adults against the ones from clinicians (a.k.a. outsiders). From the outsiders' perspective, ageing is generally associated with an increased risk for disease and decline in several functioning domains. Moreover, maintaining health and functioning is crucial for successful ageing. However, evidence shows that overall well-being increases steadily from middle age to very old age. Such trend is reflected on the perspective of older adults themselves, who focus on coping strategies, psychosocial engagement and cultural differences (Kusumastuti *et al.*, 2016). Overall, these aspects considered important to a successful ageing by the older adults will go unnoticed if the healthcare models fail to be person-centered.

In the process of enhancing person-centered practice, there is a need to attend to the heterogeneity in older adults naturally resulting from intra-individual changes throughout the life trajectory and necessarily unique to each person. Some researchers have explored the concept of differential ageing so to emphasize that adults older than 65 years are not a single social group. Inter-individual differences have to be taken into account towards the development of person-centered practice in gerontology. Beyond the usual cognitive and physical functioning, the translation of person-centredness into practice needs to contemplate personality, social networks, lifestyle, beliefs, interests and satisfaction with life (Smith & Gerstorf, 2006). Yet, person-centred practice is not synonymous with good quality of care for older adults. Towards its accomplishment, existing healthcare models should see beyond the person immediate needs and never neglect the importance of knowing the person, his/her values, biography and relationships (McCormack, 2004).

Health Promotion to a Successful Ageing

Maintenance of autonomy and independence requires joint effort of different stakeholders to define and implement strategies for health promotion and prevention of frailty states (D'Avanzo *et al.*, 2017). Health promotion in ageing is based on two basic constructs: one related to daily behavior, and another concerning the conditions in which each person lives (WHO, 2017).

Healthcare professionals take the lid concerning health promotion actions. Additionally, three major groups should be involved in the health promotion of older adults: (i) healthcare professionals representing the role of government and creating a bridge between public sector services and older citizens; (ii) institutions, associations, companies that foster the active role of seniors in the community, answering to the needs and expectations of seniors and creating the conditions for their meaningful involvement; and, finally, (iii) the older person him(her)self and his(her) informal caregivers, including family members, friends and neighbors. The major actions to promote successful ageing must come principally from the individual himself, requiring his active participation in health and conscious responsibility for it (Golinowska, Groot, Baji & Pavlova, 2016).

Moreover, these actions should be designed to enable maintenance and enhancement of functional capacity and self-care of older citizens, and to stimulate their social network, thereby contributing to the improvement of quality of life (Golinowska, Groot, Baji & Pavlova, 2016). The health promotion actions should include exercising, smoke cessation or limit alcohol consumption. Moreover, more positive approaches are also required to address social needs of seniors and create favorable conditions for their inclusion and participation in cultural events and social work, as well as learning activities (idem).

Alongside health promotion comes the prevention of decline associated with ageing. Prevention can be performed in three phases: primary, secondary and tertiary. Primary prevention is performed in the period of pre-pathogenesis, is associated with health promotion, and concerns prevention of diseases in general or of a certain pathology to which the older person may be more susceptible. Such process takes into account the older adult history and the context in which he/she is inserted. Secondary prevention can also be divided into two levels: the first related to diagnosis and early intervention and the second associated with an intervention that delays the evolution of the decline. Finally, tertiary prevention refers to rehabilitation actions in situations of physical or cognitive disturbance.

Successful ageing implies the active and continuous participation of the older adult both in health promotion and in the search for answers in preventing associated physical and cognitive declines. Ageing and lifelong diseases are inevitably conditioned by individual, biological, genetic and psychological determinants. However, in many situations, the decline of cognitive and physical functions is also related to external, behavioral, environmental and social factors. Older people health reflects partially the lifestyles adopted, exposure to outside environments, and the health care the person receives. The participative attitude in the self-care promotion, the adoption of healthier lifestyles with continuous physical activity and cognitive stimulation are essential to live more and better, and decrease the risk of frailty (Apóstolo et. al., 2018).

The knowledge about factors influencing the health status of seniors, such as activity or sedentary lifestyle, eating habits, sleeping pattern, and poor social interactions allows the establishment of a chronodisruption degree (Bonmati-Carrion *et al.*, 2014). Unhealthy lifestyles include the poor social interaction, which in older ages can promote loneliness, isolation and have a negative impact in mental health (Tanskanen & Anttila, 2016).

Data about lifestyle behaviors enables not only the identification of habits that are more susceptible to correction through behavioral changes, but also the definition of strategies that tailor individual needs while considering individual preferences and concerns. The behavioral changes may affect significantly the individual's health and quality of life. However, without encouraging and empowering older adults and their families to take responsibility for these changes, their impact will be quite reduced.

TECHNOLOGY AS A SOLUTION TO A SUCCESSFUL AGEING

The global market is witnessing the growing development of new technologies and devices that can assist older people in their daily living, thereby preventing or delaying institutionalization. Assistive Technologies (ATs) and Information and Communication Technologies (ICTs) are resources that may improve ageing in place for older adults and decrease the caregivers' burden. ATs concern the integration of technology within residences to maintain functional health, security, safety and quality of life (Cook & Polgar, 2014). Usually, ATs are designed to allow individuals to maintain their independence through the performance of tasks, usually related to daily living activities (ADLs) and monitoring behaviors. ATs can eliminate multiple barriers helping people with visual or motor impairments to access services that are traditionally to people without such disabilities. ATs include a wide range of tools, from a simple, low-tech device such as a magnifying glass, to a complex, high-tech device, such as a computerized communication system (Center on Technology and Disability, 2018). ATs include but are not limited to devices with mobility purposes (wheelchairs, scooters, walkers, canes, crutches, prosthetic or orthotic devices), vision, hearing (speech-based systems) or daily living aids, gadgets or small aids to adaptation theirs lives in their own home (Yusif, Soar & Hafeez-Baig, 2016). This kind of technologies promotes the sense of security and independence, while improving users well-being (Blaschke, Freddolino & Mullen, 2009). Another type of technologies is the ICTs, which include computer-based communication devices and Internet applications. ICTs can improve social support and psychosocial well-being. The use of ICT in healthcare, usually named as e-health, is essential to transform healthcare systems and services and complement person-centered and integrated care, that is not only adequate, relevant and significant to the older adult, but also aligned with the Healthy Ageing agenda (WHO, 2015). ICTs have the potential to improve the quality of life of older people, as well as, facilitate cost-effective care by supporting formal and informal care providers (Heart & Kalderon, 2013).

The proximity of technology to gerontology has been emphasized in recent years as a result of technological improvements, leading to the transition from a more traditional approach to a greater focus on an interpersonal relationship with the technology as a supporting resource. This new approach has the potential to manage older adults' care with high levels of efficiency, and also reduce the individual and societal costs of caring (Barbosa, Castro, & Carrapatoso, 2018; Lesauskaitė *et al.*, 2019). To guarantee the quality of life and well-being of people as they grow older while allowing for an healthy and active ageing is challenging.

Digital technologies to tackle health and ageing challenges are increasing and they offer a golden opportunity to restructure the way by which formal and informal caregivers can support and empower the ageing population towards a successful ageing. New technologies that include Robots, Internet of Things (IoT), Smart Home and Ambient Assisted Living (SHAAL) and Sensors (wearable sensors or incorporated in smart homes) are capable to provide assistance, companionship, health and behavior monitoring, improving mental and physical health, and increasing quality of life. Technologies can be used to promote successful ageing in the major achievement areas of health and societal (TASK FORCE ON RESEARCH AND DEVELOPMENT FOR TECHNOLOGY TO SUPPORT AGEING ADULTS, 2019).

Digital Solutions to Assist in Daily Living Activities: Robots, IoT, SHAAL and Sensors

As a complement to increasing healthcare centers, the development of services (i.e. gerontechnology) that can be used in homes and within society, it is extremely relevant. Services capable to increase the independence of elderly's is the key to allow them to age in place (Lesauskaitė *et al.*, 2019).

Living independently requires the ability to perform daily activities, which have the potential to be assisted by technology. The daily activities related to mobility, nutrition, personal hygiene, and medication management can be facilitated with robots, a.k.a. socially assistive robots (SAR), or through smart home technologies. The major goal of SAR is to create a close and effective interaction with end-users to assist and achieved measurable progress in convalescence, rehabilitation, learning, etc. (Feil-Seifer & Mataric, 2005). Smart home technologies are sensors, appliances or devices that can be remotely controlled, accessed and monitored through IoT, used at the person's home (King, 2003).

IoT can be considered both a dynamic and global network infrastructure. It manages self-configuring objects in a highly intelligent way extending internet connectivity beyond traditional devices, like laptop computers, smartphones and tablets, to a diverse range of devices and everyday things, which use embedded technology to communicate and interact with the external environment (Atlam, Walters, & Wills, 2018). The basic idea of IoT is the connectivity of the things through Internet network, where there are: security systems, cars, electronic appliances, lights in household and commercial environments, speaker systems, sensors, actuators, and mobile phones (Srinidhi, Dilip Kumar & Venugopal, 2019).

The use of IoT in healthcare opened up a world of possibilities to monitor older adults in their environment through Smart Home and Ambient Assisted Living (SHAAL). When connected to the Internet, ordinary devices can collect individual data, give extra insight into symptoms and trends, and give feedback to users and formal and informal caregivers about their real-time health or behavior (Islam, Daehan, Kabir, Hossain & Kyung-Sup, 2015). Smart homes with integrated e-health and assisted living technology, is an example of an IoT application in home care for older people (Majumder *et al.*, 2017). Smart home technology is the integration of technology and services through home networking for a better quality of live (Robles & Tai-hoon, 2010). Smart homes integrate different services within a home environment by using communication systems centered on helping residents to live independently. Smart homes may help to enhance the quality of life, promoting independent life and reduce caregivers' time and health costs in general. The benefits of these technologies are not only for older people, but also for their families, formal and informal caregivers. This is what is known as Ambient Assisted Living (AAL) (Ni, Hernando & Cruz, 2015). AAL refers to a system of some auxiliary sensors that make the independent life of a person more comfortable and easier in the home environment. Sensor data can have different formats, such as numerical, categorical, graphics, video, etc. Based on their formats and sensor types, sensors can be classified as vision-based or sensor-based. The sensor with a vision-based approach uses visual sensors, such as video cameras, to monitor movements, while sensor-based approaches use sensors for health and biomedical monitoring. This feature allows them to be located on furniture, appliances, walls, and doors and even used in a wearable way. They can include fall detection systems, monitoring of daily activities, or monitor health parameters (Mshali, Lemlouma, Moloney & Magoni, 2018). In a smart home, sensors are connected through a Personal Area Network or Wireless Sensor Network. Wearable biomedical sensors as body temperature, heart rate, oxygen saturation or blood glucose sensors can be connected by wireless in order to obtain automated, continuous and real-time measurement physiological parameters. Central computing systems manage data, analyze them and send a feedback to the user, caregivers or activate the emergency services if necessary (Majumder *et al.*, 2017).

The major goal is to link the continuous and real-time monitoring of health parameters, through sensors, to healthcare professionals. This is considered a sustainable solution to constantly monitor older adults or people with chronic diseases, at a long distance, without compromising health services and promoting the ageing in place. Nowadays the use of sensors is common to measure parameters such as heart and respiratory rate, blood pressure, blood oxygen saturation, and muscle activity. Such assessments provide indicators of health status with a tremendous diagnostic value. Until recent days, the continuous monitoring of physiological parameters was possible only in the hospital setting. However nowadays, with developments in the field of wearable technology, is possible to obtain continuous and real-time monitoring of physiological signals outside the medical environment (Dias & Cunha, 2018). The obtained data have high rates of accuracy and reproducibility, which facilitates clinical diagnosis and prediction of health-related outcomes. However, to be efficiently used, these data should be gathered based on an integrated approach to health, as the use of devices and applications for monitoring of single disease results in a fragmented view of health condition (Matias, Paixão, Bouça & Ferreira, 2017).

The expansion of wearable sensors that record and track personal data enables active exchange of information between health professionals and the patient and his(her) family, eliminating the physical barriers to knowledge sharing and management. In addition, the evolving trend in using wearable technology enhances understanding of physiological data, and thus offers the potential for patient engagement in the management of his(her) health status (Chiauzzi, Rodarte & DasMahapatra, 2015). The broad use of the wearable technological solutions may ensure an efficient and sustainable response of health and social care systems to the challenges related to demographic ageing. This might be achieved by scaling up preventive strategies on health, identifying the first signs of unpredictable and sudden events (such as falls) and, simultaneously, cutting equipment and reducing of expenditure with unnecessary health services (Dias & Cunha, 2018; Wang, Yang, & Dong, 2017). It also enables ageing at place, without limiting the opportunities for active involvement in family and community life.

How Can Technology Engage Older People in Activities That Promote Successful Ageing?

Older generations are reluctant to adopt new technology into regular life. However, caregivers, family and friends usually support older people in this transition explaining how technology can help in daily living, offering install and setup assistance, guiding them in the use of new devices and helping them to integrate their devices in ways that complement their lives (Vaportzis, Giatsi Clausen & Gow, 2017). The use of technologies in community settings promote the ageing in place because they can simplify daily routines, expand social opportunities, monitor health and improve well-being, while empowering older adults as they connect with the digital solutions and their advantages (Hill, Betts & Gardner, 2015).

Technology is a promising vehicle for promoting health and quality of life. In fact, digital solutions enhance older people's ability to enjoy quality of life by facilitating healthy lifestyles, social connections and access to services (Pak & Collins-McLaughlin, 2018). The significant increase of the use of technology to provide healthcare improves older people's quality of life. For example, technology may serve as the link between older people living at home and their healthcare team at the primary healthcare center or hospital. It may also constitute the bridge to the community and social services allowing to combat loneliness and isolation situations, thereby supporting independence, and facilitating self-management of their health and social conditions (Fischer, David, Crotty, Dierks & Safran, 2014). Older people, together with their caregivers or health professionals, should choose the technological solution that suits them best. The important thing is that it can be a resource to support them to live longer in their homes independently. With this purpose, a needs assessment is necessary to evaluate which capacities most need support.

All technologies that can support monitoring of health status or environmental conditions, promote communication or assist older adults in their regular personal care, engage them in activities that can promote healthy, active and successful ageing. Technologies can help to monitor and support older people in self-management activities to improve physical activity (Zilidou, Douka, Ziagkas, Romanopoulou & Politopoulos, 2018) eating and hydration habits (Halse *et al.*, 2019), sleep patterns (Ko *et al.*, 2015) and social interaction (Khosravi, Rezvani & Wiewiora, 2016). Even the use of digital games and regular applications incorporating game elements can positively impact the physical, cognitive and emotional well-being of the elderly. Game elements can be incorporated into information systems for the elderly in multiple methods, for example, to augment regular tasks, to provide new user experiences and to foster social interaction (Gerling, 2011). Concerning the regular task, it comprises the idea of encouraging elderlies to participate in physical or cognitive therapy by providing game-like experiences, which look like leisure activities and foster the engagement and long-term motivation. In this context, present achievements and high score lists could encourage elderly persons to compete with peers. Additionally, healthcare professionals can use the data provided to monitor and analyze the elderly performance. In that way, decline or improvements in the elderly abilities may be perceived at an early stage. With respect to re-creating inaccessible real-world experiences, it is possible to recreate real-world experiences, which have become unreachable due to age-related changes. Finally, the performance of playful activities and the incorporation of game elements offer the opportunity to promote social interaction between elderlies (Gerling, 2011).

Challenges in the Use of Technologies in the Community

As sensors become smaller, cheaper, and user-friendlier, they can be used more extensively across a wide variety of contexts. Especially in gerontology, with the projected increase in the number of older adults, wearable devices are considered crucial tools to support preventive medicine and self-monitoring (haghi, thurow, & stoll, 2017). In addition to allow for the provision of personalized care, wearable technology is increasing self-engagement with treatment and disease management (baig, gholamhosseini, moqeem, mirza, & linden, 2017). Such behavior is categorized into prevention and health promotion, as older adults who are actively engaged are more likely to maintain health and well-being for a longer life trajectory (zainab & naz, 2017). More generally, technology applications for the older people entail an opportunity for home rehabilitation, to enhance mobility, quality of life and social well-being, as well as, to support family caregivers (armstrong, najafi, & shahinpoorc, 2017; czaja, 2016).

In addition to the mentioned potential applications, technology and specifically wearable devices, have proven to effectively reduce the costs of prevention and health monitoring (Baig *et al.*, 2017; Haghi *et al.*, 2017). In order to promote a successful implementation, the needs, preferences and resources of the users, as well as, the environment where the technology will unfold must be carefully analyzed as potential barriers or facilitators (Barbosa *et al.*, 2018).

Evidence on barriers has been clustered differently depending on the research focus. Yet, common domains emerge in relation to a) user engagement and interaction, b) connectivity and interoperability and c) the sensors themselves (Armstrong *et al.*, 2017; Baig *et al.*, 2017; Haghi *et al.*, 2017).

Attending to the user engagement and interaction, the user group in this domain is extensive and includes, not only older adults, but also their family caregivers, informal care providers and healthcare professionals. Moreover, as wearable devices were initially thought for data collection only, evidence still shows that they lack user-acceptance and are poorly judge in user-interaction aspects as they move towards being more self-engaging and motivating systems (Baig *et al.*, 2017). Additional barriers refer to knowledge insufficiency, negative attitudes, as well as, lack of instructions and guidance associated with the devices complexity, especially when individuals have reduced experience and feel less confident about innovations in health (Vaportzis, Clausen & Glow, 2017; Gitlow, 2014). Age-related cognitive, sensorial and motricity changes are other important barriers to the use of technologies by older adults (Vaportzis, Clausen & Glow, 2017). Considering the divide in terms of access to technology and technology and health literacy skills, attending to the preferences, needs and abilities early on in the system development is imperative (Czaja, 2016). If the benefits offered by technology are clearly perceived and the devices or applications are considered as easy to use, their acceptance among the end-users is higher ((Czaja, 2016) Wallace, Graham and Saraceno, 2013). Moreover, devices and applications need to be carefully thought in order to be unobtrusive and prevent changes in activities of daily life that might put users at risk of isolation.

Along with the increasingly needed integration of care services at different levels of the healthcare chain (i.e. community, primary healthcare centers and hospitals), issues emerge related to interoperability and interconnectivity across technologies and devices (Baig *et al.*, 2017; Czaja, 2016). The ERCCI Institution (2017), for instance, has identified missed alarms that result from inappropriate configuration of notification systems leading to delay in care delivery. Ransomware and other types of malicious software were also pointed out to hinder or disrupt care delivery, becoming a relevant risk inherent to the use of medical technologies (ERCCI, 2017).

Specifically concerning the prominent wearable sensors, the issue of connectivity is a great hinder to its effectiveness as it causes delay in providing results and low quality of data. Further development and research to overcome this hinder is focusing on technological aspects of remote network, low signal strength, low battery lifetime and low transmission speed (Baig *et al.*, 2017).

Concerning interoperability, along with assuring an accurate communication between different care services throughout the healthcare chain, users need to have their integrity and confidentiality safeguard. Moreover, data coming from self-monitoring devices still lacks clinical appropriateness. Protocols for safety and maintainability need to be incorporated from design stages in order to ensure the safety and protection of personal data from an inappropriate access and use (Czaja, 2016). Moreover, developments in machine learning techniques are likely to promote a wider integration of data into clinical practice by supporting decision-making processes (Baig *et al.*, 2017).

Finally, concerning the issues associated with the sensors themselves, an improper cleaning of devices has been associated with premature deterioration, failure or adverse effects of equipment as top health technology hazards (ERCCI, 2017). Along with body movement, respiration and transpiration, signal's accuracy is disturbed by noises that are hardly filtered by the device itself as it lacks hardware-processing limitations. Such filtering is currently being carried out at the software platform, although is far from being ideally and the results still have an extensive room for improvement (Baig *et al.*, 2017).

Managing the designated challenges and barriers is no one-field effort. As in other contexts where ICT is being successfully implemented, a collaborative partnership comprising overall users, care providers, health care sciences researchers, psychologists and computer scientists is demanded. Moreover, the integration of user-centered approaches from early design stages, to long-term implementation, is highly important towards the development of effective, accurate and user-friendly technology (Czaja, 2016; Nwosu, Quinn, Samuels, Mason, & Payne, 2018). In addition to early involvement in the technology deployment, training of end-users for appropriate use of devices and applications must be ensured continuously (Czaja, 2016).

Using Technology to Increase Older People's Well-Being: A Case Study About Wearable Sensors

Specifically considering the wearable devices, older people can collect their parameters, interpret them, with the support of healthcare professionals, and perform changes that can improve their health status. This enhances their health literacy and leads them to engage in activities that can promote a successful ageing (WHO, 2015).

The ModulEn, financed by FGSIC, Interreg Portugal-Spain, and CENIE, is an example of a project conceived to provide directions for early prevention, by establishing a predictive model of risk of frailty. It aims to help older adults in their health promotion and primary prevention of decline during this stage of life through the use of wearable sensors (Apóstolo et. Al., 2019). It is an Iberian project that involves several partners from Spain and Portugal, including the Institute of Health Carlos III, ISCIII as a coordinator, Chronobiology Laboratory, University of Murcia and Nursing School of Coimbra. In order to accomplish to create the predictive model of frailty, older adults' frailty state and lifestyle are monitored through a technological device - ACM KRONOWISE® 2.0. These sensors, used as wristwatches, allow collecting data concerning the circadian cycle, patterns of physical activity, sleeping patterns, eating habits and exposure to luminosity. The participants are seniors aged 65-80 years, who live in the community and do not present moderate or severe cognitive decline. They are recruited at senior universities, cultural and recreational associations and primary healthcare centers in Portugal and Spain. Each participant uses the sensors for 7- 10 days and then answers eleven questions about usability, functionality, and awareness of healthy habits and usefulness of technologies in health. This wearable sensor allows the health professional to evaluate which behaviors are most likely to be modified towards the promotion of health and prevention of cognitive and physical decline. Older people who participated in this study received an individual health report with personalized recommendations that promote successful ageing. These recommendations were made by a healthcare professional and are based on their own chronotype and health status. The results and the recommendations improve engagement of older people in activities that promote successful ageing, such as: decreased sedentary activities, increased moderate physical activity, and outdoor activities, and improved quantity and quality of sleep. After adopting the suggested changes and healthier lifestyles, older people can use the sensors to monitor the improvement of the health parameters. In addition to active participation and self-responsibility in health, obtaining reliable results through wearable sensors allows the increase of health literacy, well-being and the sense of autonomy of older people.

Considering the probable increase in the use of these technologies, especially in geriatric care (Helbostad et. al., 2017), to understand the perception that seniors have about the utility of wearable sensors in everyday life is highly important. If healthcare professionals wish to increase the potential for older adults and to promote the use of digital technologies to improve the health and well-being of individuals and communities, to fully understand what influences older adults' digital participation is crucial. Such process, should contemplate not only issues associated with the heterogeneity of older adulthood and technology access, but also choice and motivation (George-Walker & Tyler, 2014). The researchers of the ModulEn project reflected about this issue.

Specifically, throughout the ModulEn project most of the participants considered that the sensors were easy to use. Some of them experienced some discomfort, especially at night since they were not used to sleep with wristwatches. In general, the participants were sensitized to adopt healthy lifestyles and the majority considered that the data obtained through sensors was useful to improve their health status and would recommend these sensors to others. Sensors-related data followed by recommendations for maintenance or improvement of health status, were considered the most relevant positive aspect. As negative aspects, the participants of this study indicated sensor design, lack of utility in daily life and time of use. Although preliminary, these results can be used as a set of guidelines in the selection of suitable technological equipment for older adults and can contribute to create innovate wearable sensors that promote healthy lifestyles.

CONCLUSION

Technologies can support older people in the satisfaction of their basic needs, to increase their health literacy and make decisions, to build and maintain relationships, to improve health literacy, the sense of autonomy and well-being and increase a participatory intervention in their own life, enhancing ageing in place. Concretely, robots may assist in daily tasks to enable long-distance communication with family, friends, caregivers and health professionals; IoTs SHAAL and sensors can monitor vital signs and environmental conditions to ensure healthy and safe living; or Apps and other programs that can assist older people in their regular personal care, organization and leisure activities.

Technologies can help older adults to improve their lifestyles. Healthier lifestyles such as daily physical activity and adequate diet are associated with healthy ageing. The healthier lifestyle behaviors adopted, the higher the odds of maintaining a successful ageing. Sensors can be an important tool to control and monitor parameters related with healthy lifestyles, especially because they are a non-invasive electronic device that allows real-time monitoring in a continuously, proactive and accurate way. Through this kind of technologies older people can self-manage their health status and engage themselves in activities that promote the successful ageing, i.e. improve physical activity, eating and drinking habits, sleep patterns and social interaction.

Technology has a great potential to complement person-centered processes both in health and social care, by allowing for highly tailored interventions for older adults at a distance and as a direct response to the monitored data. While attending to the unique characteristics of the older adult, enhancement of self-management of health/

illness events and tailored support by healthcare professionals through technologies, activates older adults towards a more participative and healthier ageing process. The investment in health promotion and the continuous monitoring of older people health status is one of the answers to identify pre-frail or frail people at early states and assist them to improve their lifestyles towards decreasing or reversing frailty states.

Although older people can be reluctant in the adoption of new technologies in their daily living, families, caregivers and health professionals can support them towards a smooth transition. It is important to show the older adults the range of technologies available and they must be able to choose the one they like the most and be able to adapt it to their needs. Technologies can simplify daily routines, monitor health and improve well-being, monitor behaviors and environments, and help older adults feel more empowered and independent. They promote quality of life by facilitating healthy lifestyles, social connections and access to services.

Future studies evaluating physical activity, nutritional and other lifestyle interventions with the use of technology are needed to achieve a better ageing process for these populations.

REFERENCES

American Geriatrics Society Expert Panel on Person-Centered. (2016). Person-Centered Care: A Definition and Essential Elements. *Journal of the American Geriatrics Society*, *64*(1), 15–18. doi:10.1111/jgs.13866 PMID:26626262

Apóstolo, J., Bobrowicz-Campos, E., Moreno-Casbas, T., Teixeira-Santos, L., Sánchez de Madariag, R., Casado-Ramírez, E., ... ModulEn Consortium (2019). A study protocol for development and validation of a clinical prediction model for frailty (modulen): A new European commitment to tackling frailty. *Translational Medicine @ UniSa*, *19*(6), 36-41.

Apóstolo, J., Cooke, R., Bobrowicz-Campos, E., Santana, S., Marcucci, M., Cano, A., ... Holland, C. (2018). Effectiveness of interventions to prevent pre-frailty and frailty progression in older adults: A systematic review. *JBI Database of Systematic Reviews and Implementation Reports*, *16*(1), 140–232. doi:10.11124/JBISRIR-2017-003382 PMID:29324562

Armstrong, D. G., Najafi, B., & Shahinpoorc, M. (2017). Potential Applications of Smart Multifunctional Wearable Materials to Gerontology. *Gerontology*, *63*(3), 287–298. doi:10.1159/000455011 PMID:28076861

Atlam, H., Walters, R., & Wills, G. (2018). Internet of Things: State-of-the-art, Challenges, Applications, and Open Issues. *International Journal of Intelligent Computing Research*, *9*(3), 928–938. doi:10.20533/ijicr.2042.4655.2018.0112

Baig, M. M., GholamHosseini, H., Moqeem, A. A., Mirza, F., & Lindén, M. (2017). A Systematic Review of Wearable Patient Monitoring Systems - Current Challenges and Opportunities for Clinical Adoption. *Journal of Medical Systems*, *41*(7), 115. doi:10.100710916-017-0760-1 PMID:28631139

Barbosa, H., Castro, A. V., & Carrapatoso, E. (2018). Serious Games and Rehabilitation for Elderly Adults. *Global Scientific Journal*, *6*(1), 275–283. Retrieved from http://www.globalscientificjournal.com/researchpaper/Serious-Games-and-Rehabilitation-for-Elderly-Adults.pdf%0Awww.globalscientificjournal.com

Beard, J. R. (2019). Moving Beyond Disease-Based Models of Prevention. In J.-P. Michel (Ed.), *Prevention of Chronic Diseases and Age-Related Disability*. Springer. doi:10.1007/978-3-319-96529-1_20

Blaschke, C. M., Freddolino, P. P., & Mullen, E. E. (2009). Ageing and Technology: A Review of the Research Literature. *British Journal of Social Work*, *39*(4), 641–656. doi:10.1093/bjsw/bcp025

Bonmati-Carrion, M., Arguelles-Prieto, R., Martinez-Madrid, M., Reiter, R., Hardeland, R., Rol, M., & Madrid, J. (2014). Protecting the Melatonin Rhythm through Circadian Healthy Light Exposure. *International Journal of Molecular Sciences*, *15*(12), 23448–23500. doi:10.3390/ijms151223448 PMID:25526564

Brinkman, S., Voortman, T., Kiefte-de Jong, J., van Rooij, F., Ikram, M., Rivadeneira, F., ... Schoufour, J. (2018). The association between lifestyle and overall health, using the frailty index. *Archives of Gerontology and Geriatrics*, *76*, 85–91. doi:10.1016/j.archger.2018.02.006 PMID:29477949

Canham, S., Mauro, P., Kaufmann, C., & Sixsmith, A. (2015). Association of Alcohol Use and Loneliness Frequency Among Middle-Aged and Older Adult Drinkers. *Journal of Aging and Health*, *28*(2), 267–284. doi:10.1177/0898264315589579 PMID:26082130

Center on Technology and Disability. (2018). *Assistive Technology, 101*. Retrieved from https://www.ctdinstitute.org/sites/default/files/file_attachments/CTD-AT101-V4.pdf

Chen, C., Gan, P., & How, C. (2018). Approach to frailty in the elderly in primary care and the community. *Singapore Medical Journal*, *59*(5), 240–245. doi:10.11622medj.2018052 PMID:29799055

Chiauzzi, E., Rodarte, C., & DasMahapatra, P. (2015). Patient-centered activity monitoring in the self-management of chronic health conditions. *BMC Medicine*, *13*(1), 77. doi:10.118612916-015-0319-2 PMID:25889598

Clegg, A., Young, J., Iliffe, S., Rikkert, M., & Rockwood, K. (2013). Frailty in elderly people. *Lancet*, *381*(9868), 752–762. doi:10.1016/S0140-6736(12)62167-9 PMID:23395245

Cosco, T., Prina, A., Perales, J., Stephan, B., & Brayne, C. (2014). Operational definitions of successful ageing: A systematic review. *International Psychogeriatrics*, *26*(03), 373–381. doi:10.1017/S1041610213002287 PMID:24308764

Czaja, S. J. (2016). Long-term care services and support systems for older adults: The role of technology. *The American Psychologist*, *71*(4), 294–301. doi:10.1037/a0040258 PMID:27159436

D'Avanzo, B., Shaw, R., Riva, S., Apostolo, J., Bobrowicz-Campos, E., Kurpas, D., ... Holland, C. (2017). Stakeholders' views and experiences of care and interventions for addressing frailty and pre-frailty: A meta-synthesis of qualitative evidence. *PLoS One*, *12*(7), e0180127. doi:10.1371/journal.pone.0180127 PMID:28723916

Daskalopoulou, C., Stubbs, B., Kralj, C., Koukounari, A., Prince, M., & Prina, A. (2018). Associations of smoking and alcohol consumption with healthy ageing: A systematic review and meta-analysis of longitudinal studies. *BMJ Open*, *8*(4), e019540. doi:10.1136/bmjopen-2017-019540 PMID:29666127

Davis, S., Mirick, D., & Stevens, R. (2001). Night Shift Work, Light at Night, and Risk of Breast Cancer. *Journal of the National Cancer Institute*, *93*(20), 1557–1562. doi:10.1093/jnci/93.20.1557 PMID:11604479

Dent, E., Kowal, P., & Hoogendijk, E. (2016). Frailty measurement in research and clinical practice: A review. *European Journal of Internal Medicine*, *31*, 3–10. doi:10.1016/j.ejim.2016.03.007 PMID:27039014

Dias, D., & Cunha, J. (2018). Wearable health devices - vital sign monitoring, systems and technologies. *Sensors (Basel)*, *18*(8), 2414. doi:10.339018082414 PMID:30044415

ECRI Institution. (2017). *Executive brief: Top 10 Health Technology Hazards for 2018*. A Report from Health Devices. Retrieved from: https://www.ecri.org/Resources/Whitepapers_and_reports/Haz_18.pdf

European Commission. (2014). *Population aging in Europe: Facts, implications and policies*. Retrieved from: https://ec.europa.eu/research/social-sciences/pdf/policy_reviews/kina26426enc.pdf

Feil-Seifer, D., & Mataric, M. (2005). Socially Assistive Robotics. *9th International Conference on Rehabilitation Robotics, 2005. ICORR 2005*. doi:10.1109/icorr.2005.1501143

George-Walker, L., & Tyler, M. (2014). Connected Older Adults: Conceptualising their Digital Participation. *The Journal of Literacy and Technology*, *15*(2), 200–214.

Gerling, K. M. (2011). Exploring the Potential of Gamification Among Frail Elderly Persons. *Ext Abs CHI, 2011*, 1–4.

Gitlow, L. (2014). Technology Use by Older Adults and Barriers to Using Technology. *Physical & Occupational Therapy in Geriatrics*, *32*(3), 271–280. doi:10.3109/02703181.2014.946640

Golinowska, S., Groot, W., Baji, P., & Pavlova, M. (2016). Health promotion targeting older people. *BMC Health Services Research*, *16*(S5), 345. doi:10.118612913-016-1514-3 PMID:27608680

Haghi, M., Thurow, K., & Stoll, R. (2017). Wearable Devices in Medical Internet of Things: Scientific Research and Commercially Available Devices. *Healthcare Informatics Research*, *23*(1), 4–15. doi:10.4258/hir.2017.23.1.4 PMID:28261526

Halse, R., Shoneye, C., Pollard, C., Jancey, J., Scott, J., Pratt, I., ... Kerr, D. (2019). Improving Nutrition and Activity Behaviors Using Digital Technology and Tailored Feedback: Protocol for the LiveLighter Tailored Diet and Activity (ToDAy) Randomized Controlled Trial. *JMIR Research Protocols*, *8*(2), e12782. doi:10.2196/12782 PMID:30801257

Heart, T., & Kalderon, E. (2013). Older adults: Are they ready to adopt health-related ICT? *International Journal of Medical Informatics*, *82*(11), e209–e231. doi:10.1016/j.ijmedinf.2011.03.002 PMID:21481631

Helbostad, J., Vereijken, B., Becker, C., Todd, C., Taraldsen, K., Pijnappels, M., ... Mellone, S. (2017). Mobile Health Applications to Promote Active and Healthy Ageing. *Sensors (Basel)*, *17*(3), 622. doi:10.339017030622 PMID:28335475

Islam, S., Daehan, K., Kabir, M., Hossain, M., & Kyung-Sup, K. (2015). The Internet of Things for Health Care: A Comprehensive Survey. *IEEE Access : Practical Innovations, Open Solutions*, *3*, 678–708. doi:10.1109/ACCESS.2015.2437951

Khosravi, P., Rezvani, A., & Wiewiora, A. (2016). The impact of technology on older adults' social isolation. *Computers in Human Behavior, 63*, 594–603. doi:10.1016/j.chb.2016.05.092

King, N. (2003). Smart Home –A Definition. *Housing Learning & Improvement Network*, 1–6. Retrieved from http://www.housinglin.org.uk/_library/Resources/Housing/Housing_advice/Smart_Home_-_A_definition%5C_September_2003.pdf

Ko, P., Kientz, J., Choe, E., Kay, M., Landis, C., & Watson, N. (2015). Consumer Sleep Technologies: A Review of the Landscape. *Journal of Clinical Sleep Medicine, 11*(12), 1455–1461. doi:10.5664/jcsm.5288 PMID:26156958

Kobayashi, L., & Steptoe, A. (2018). Social Isolation, Loneliness, and Health Behaviors at Older Ages: Longitudinal Cohort Study. *Annals of Behavioral Medicine, 52*(7), 582–593. doi:10.1093/abm/kax033 PMID:29860361

Kuh, D. (2019). A Life Course Approach to Healthy Ageing. In J.-P. Michel (Ed.), *Prevention of Chronic Diseases and Age-Related Disability* (pp. 1–9). Springer. doi:10.1007/978-3-319-96529-1_1

Kuiper, J., Zuidersma, M., Zuidema, S., Burgerhof, J., Stolk, R., Oude Voshaar, R., & Smidt, N. (2016). Social relationships and cognitive decline: A systematic review and meta-analysis of longitudinal cohort studies. *International Journal of Epidemiology*. doi:10.1093/ije/dyw089 PMID:27272181

Kusumastuti, S., Derks, M. G. M., Tellier, S., Di Nucci, E., Lund, R., Mortensen, E. L., & Westendorp, R. G. J. (2016). Successful ageing: A study of the literature using citation network analysis. *Maturitas, 93*, 4–12. doi:10.1016/j.maturitas.2016.04.010 PMID:27156006

Kvaavik, E. (2010). Influence of Individual and Combined Health Behaviors on Total and Cause-Specific Mortality in Men and Women. *Archives of Internal Medicine, 170*(8), 711. doi:10.1001/archinternmed.2010.76 PMID:20421558

Lang, P., Michel, J., & Zekry, D. (2009). Frailty Syndrome: A Transitional State in a Dynamic Process. *Gerontology, 55*(5), 539–549. doi:10.1159/000211949 PMID:19346741

Lesauskaitė, V., Damulevičienė, G., Knašienė, J., Kazanavičius, E., Liutkevičius, A., & Janavičiūtė, A. (2019). Older Adults—Potential Users of Technologies. *Medicina, 55*(6), 253. doi:10.3390/medicina55060253 PMID:31181673

Lowsky, D., Olshansky, S., Bhattacharya, J., & Goldman, D. (2013). Heterogeneity in Healthy Aging. *The Journals of Gerontology. Series A, Biological Sciences and Medical Sciences*, *69*(6), 640–649. doi:10.1093/gerona/glt162 PMID:24249734

Majumder, S., Aghayi, E., Noferesti, M., Memarzadeh-Tehran, H., Mondal, T., Pang, Z., & Deen, M. (2017). Smart Homes for Elderly Healthcare—Recent Advances and Research Challenges. *Sensors (Basel)*, *17*(11), 2496. doi:10.339017112496 PMID:29088123

Majumder, S., Aghayi, E., Noferesti, M., Memarzadeh-Tehran, H., Mondal, T., Pang, Z., & Deen, M. (2017). Smart Homes for Elderly Healthcare—Recent Advances and Research Challenges. *Sensors (Basel)*, *17*(11), 2496. doi:10.339017112496 PMID:29088123

Malcolm, M., Frost, H., & Cowie, J. (2019). Loneliness and social isolation causal association with health-related lifestyle risk in older adults: A systematic review and meta-analysis protocol. *Systematic Reviews*, *8*(1), 48. doi:10.118613643-019-0968-x PMID:30732659

Martinez-Nicolas, A., Madrid, J., García, F., Campos, M., Moreno-Casbas, M., Almaida-Pagán, P., ... Rol, M. (2018). Circadian monitoring as an aging predictor. *Scientific Reports*, *8*(1), 15027. doi:10.103841598-018-33195-3 PMID:30301951

Matias, R., Paixão, V., Bouça, R., & Ferreira, J. (2017). A Perspective on Wearable Sensor Measurements and Data Science for Parkinson's Disease. *Frontiers in Neurology*, *8*, 677. doi:10.3389/fneur.2017.00677 PMID:29312115

McCormack, B. (2004). Person-centredness in gerontological nursing: An overview of the literature. *Journal of Clinical Nursing*, *13*(s13a), 31–38. doi:10.1111/j.1365-2702.2004.00924.x PMID:15028037

Monteserin, R., Brotons, C., Moral, I., Altimir, S., San Jose, A., Santaeugenia, S., ... Padrós, J. (2010). Effectiveness of a geriatric intervention in primary care: A randomized clinical trial. *Family Practice*, *27*(3), 239–245. doi:10.1093/fampra/cmp101 PMID:20053673

Moore, L., Britten, N., Lydahl, D., Naldemirci, O., Elam, M., & Wolf, A. (2017). Barriers and facilitators to the implementation of person-centred care in different healthcare contexts. *Scandinavian Journal of Caring Sciences*, *31*(4), 662–673. doi:10.1111cs.12376 PMID:27859459

Mshali, H., Lemlouma, T., Moloney, M., & Magoni, D. (2018). A survey on health monitoring systems for health smart homes. *International Journal of Industrial Ergonomics*, *66*, 26–56. doi:10.1016/j.ergon.2018.02.002

Ni, Q., Hernando, A., & Cruz, I. (2015). The Elderly's Independent Living in Smart Homes: A Characterization of Activities and Sensing Infrastructure Survey to Facilitate Services Development. *Sensors (Basel)*, *15*(5), 11312–11362. doi:10.3390150511312 PMID:26007717

Nolan, M. R., Davies, S., Brown, J., Keady, J., & Nolan, J. (2004). Beyond 'person-centred' care: A new vision for gerontological nursing. *Journal of Clinical Nursing*, *13*(s1), 45–53. doi:10.1111/j.1365-2702.2004.00926.x PMID:15028039

Nwosu, A. C., Quinn, C., Samuels, J., Mason, S., & Payne, T. R. (2018). Wearable smartwatch technology to monitor symptoms in advanced illness. *BMJ Supportive & Palliative Care*, *8*(2), 237. doi:10.1136/bmjspcare-2017-001445 PMID:29101119

Organization for Economic Co-operation and Development. (2017). *Economic Survey of Portugal*. Available from: https://www.oecd.org/eco/surveys/Portugal-2017-OECD-economic-survey-overview.pdf

Pandi-Perumal, S., Moscovitch, A., Srinivasan, V., Spence, D., Cardinali, D., & Brown, G. (2009). Bidirectional communication between sleep and circadian rhythms and its implications for depression: Lessons from agomelatine. *Progress in Neurobiology*, *88*(4), 264–271. doi:10.1016/j.pneurobio.2009.04.007 PMID:19454302

Peek, C., Higgins, I., Milson-Hawke, S., McMillan, M., & Harper, D. (2007). Towards innovation: The development of a person centred model of care for older people in acute care. *Contemporary Nurse*, *26*(2), 164–176. doi:10.5172/conu.2007.26.2.164 PMID:18041967

Pels, F., & Kleinert, J. (2016). Loneliness and physical activity: A systematic review. *International Review of Sport and Exercise Psychology*, *9*(1), 231–260. doi:10.1080/1750984X.2016.1177849

Robles, R., & Tai-hoon, K. (2010). Applications, Systems and Methods in Smart Home Technology: A Review. *International Journal of Advanced Science and Technology*, *15*, 37–48.

Sadana, R., & Michel, J.-P. (2019). Healthy Ageing: What Is It and How to Describe It? In J.-P. Michel (Ed.), *Prevention of Chronic Diseases and Age-Related Disability* (pp. 11–24). Springer. doi:10.1007/978-3-319-96529-1_2

Smith, J., & Gerstorf, D. (2006). Ageing differently: potential and limits. In S. Daatland & S. Biggs (Eds.), *Ageing and diversity: Multiple pathways and cultural migrations* (pp. 13–28). Policy Press.

Srinidhi, N., Dilip Kumar, S., & Venugopal, K. (2019). Network optimizations in the Internet of Things: A review. *Engineering Science And Technology. International Journal (Toronto, Ont.)*, *22*(1), 1–21. doi:10.1016/j.jestch.2018.09.003

Stenholm, S., Head, J., Kivimäki, M., Kawachi, I., Aalto, V., Zins, M., ... Vahtera, J. (2016). Smoking, physical inactivity and obesity as predictors of healthy and disease-free life expectancy between ages 50 and 75: A multicohort study. *International Journal of Epidemiology*, *45*(4), dyw126. doi:10.1093/ije/dyw126 PMID:27488415

Tanskanen, J., & Anttila, T. (2016). A Prospective Study of Social Isolation, Loneliness, and Mortality in Finland. *American Journal of Public Health*, *106*(11), 2042–2048. doi:10.2105/AJPH.2016.303431 PMID:27631736

Task Force on Research and Development for Technology to Support Aging Adults. (2019). *Emerging Technologies to Support an Aging Population*. Washington, DC: Committee on Technology of the National Science & Technology Council.

Vaportzis, E., Clausen, M. G., & Glow, A. (2017). Older Adults Perceptions of Technology and Barriers to Interacting with Tablet Computers: A Focus Group Study. *Frontiers in Psychology*, *8*, 1687. doi:10.3389/fpsyg.2017.01687 PMID:29071004

Vaportzis, E., Giatsi Clausen, M., & Gow, A. (2017). Older Adults Perceptions of Technology and Barriers to Interacting with Tablet Computers: A Focus Group Study. *Frontiers in Psychology*, *8*, 1687. doi:10.3389/fpsyg.2017.01687 PMID:29071004

Wallace, S., Graham, C., & Saraceno, A. (2013). Older adults' use of technology. *Perspectives on Gerontology*, *18*(2), 50–59. doi:10.1044/gero18.2.50

Wang, Z., Yang, Z., & Dong, T. (2017). A Review of Wearable Technologies for Elderly Care that Can Accurately Track Indoor Position, Recognize Physical Activities and Monitor Vital Signs in Real Time. *Sensors (Basel)*, *17*(2), 341. doi:10.339017020341 PMID:28208620

Wong, R. (2018). A new strategic approach to successful sgeing and healthy ageing. *Geriatrics*, *3*(4), 86. doi:10.3390/geriatrics3040086 PMID:31011121

World Health Organization. (2015). *World Report on Ageing and Health*. Geneva, Switzerland: World Health Organization.

World Health Organization. (2017). *Global strategy and action plan on ageing and health*. Geneva, Switzerland: WHO.

World Health Organization. (2018). *Ageing and health*. Geneva, Switzerland: World Health Organization.

Yusif, S., Soar, J., & Hafeez-Baig, A. (2016). Older people, assistive technologies, and the barriers to adoption: A systematic review. *International Journal of Medical Informatics*, *94*, 112–116. doi:10.1016/j.ijmedinf.2016.07.004 PMID:27573318

Zainab, N., & Naz, H. (2017). Daily living functioning, social engagement and wellness of older adults. *Psychology, Community & Health*, *6*(1), 93–102. doi:10.5964/pch.v6i1.213

Zilidou, V., Douka, S., Ziagkas, E., Romanopoulou, E., & Politopoulos, N. (2018). Technology's Role on Physical Activity for Elderly People. In M. Auer & T. Tsiatsos (Eds.), *Interactive Mobile Communication Technologies and Learning. IMCL 2017. Advances in Intelligent Systems and Computing* (Vol. 725). Cham: Springer. doi:10.1007/978-3-319-75175-7_66

KEY TERMS AND DEFINITIONS

Ageing in Place: The ability of older people to continue living at home and in the community over time, safely and independently.

Chronodisruption: Relevant disturbance of orderly biological rhythms, has been related to the inadequate exposure to environmental synchronizers and unhealthy behaviors.

Chronotype: Body's biological clock. When people work against their natural inner schedule, their circadian rhythms enter in chronodisruption.

Frailty: Transitional phase between successful ageing and disability characterized by a state of increased vulnerability that entails a high risk of adverse outcomes closely associated with loss of independence and quality of life.

Gerontechnology: Technological solutions for innovative and independent living and social participation of older adults in good health, comfort, and safety. Defined as implementing successful aging and assisting older adults in meeting the domains of housing, communication, health, safety, comfort, mobility, and leisure.

Person-Centered Care: A type of care where the patients actively participate in their own medical treatment in close cooperation with the healthcare professionals, informal/formal caregivers or stakeholders, in accordance with their preferences, needs, wishes, and values.

Successful Ageing: Implies the active and continuous participation of the older adult both in health promotion and in the search for answers in preventing associated physical and cognitive declines; coping with age-related stressors in a purposeful way, and finding ways to maintain quality of life.

Chapter 6
Factors Determining E-Health Readiness by Higher Education Institution Students in an Emerging Country

Onneile Juliet Ntseme
North-West University, South Africa

Osden Jokonya
University of the Western Cape, South Africa

Joshua Ebere Chukwuere
https://orcid.org/0000-0001-8366-4328
North-West University, South Africa

ABSTRACT

Information and communication technologies (ICTs) are important for improving healthcare services worldwide. Using tools related to ICTs such as smartphones (cell phones), video conferencing, computers enhances the delivery of health services as well as electronic health (e-health). Therefore, this study's main objective is to investigate the e-health readiness for higher education institution students in an emerging country (Botswana). The study achieved this by identifying the readiness factors that affect the adoption of e-health using the conceptual framework (technology readiness and acceptance model for e-health). The study established that students' optimism, innovativeness, discomfort, and insecurity influence e-health perceived ease of use. However, only optimism and discomfort influence e-health perceived usefulness whereas innovativeness and insecurity did not influence e-health perceived usefulness. Additionally, the study found out that e-health perceived usefulness and e-health perceived ease of use have an influence on e-health adoption.

DOI: 10.4018/978-1-7998-1937-0.ch006

INTRODUCTION

Information and communication technologies (ICTs) have been used in many sectors such as the commerce and the banking sector to solve problems around the world. While the prior observation is the case, ICTs are also important in the provision of tools and knowledge needed for improving healthcare services delivery in both private and public sectors thereby transforming health operations and processes in developing nations through the use of electronic health (Kgasi & Kalema, 2014).

By tradition, the most reliable source of health-related information to patients are healthcare professionals (De Rosis & Barsanti, 2016; Xiang & Stanley, 2017). Moreover, the recording of patients' health information has been done and is still being done on paper in most countries. The use of paper to record patients' information comes with its limitation of poor availability, incomplete data and data that has been fragmented. However, greater accessibility to the internet makes it possible for the broad accessibility of online health-related information that provides people with a new source of health knowledge (Xiang & Stanley, 2017).

Many countries have introduced and implemented e-health. Developed countries are at an advanced level of implementation and adoption of e-health as compared to developing countries. Adding on, it is important in any country to understand the compound processes of change and learning that come with the implementation of e-health at the levels of medical professionals, patients and healthcare organizations (Faber, van Geenhuizen & de Reuver, 2017; Lee, Cain, Young, Chockley & Burstin, 2005) because knowledge is still limited and uncertain on the adoption processes of e-health. Moreover, it is also vital to understand the readiness of stakeholders that are affected by the implementation of e-health as it may assist in determining whether the technology is likely to be adopted.

In terms of where this study has been carried, Botswana, the country has an enabling environment that supports and funds information and communication technology (ICT) from the private and public sector (World Health Organization Regional Office for Africa, 2014). This enabling environment that supports and funds ICT from the private and public sector has been put in place since 1997 (World Health Organization Regional Office for Africa, 2014). Nonetheless, Botswana has also developed a national ICT policy aimed at guiding, integrating and coordinating all the ICT initiatives (Government of Botswana, 2004). This was developed after the health electronic readiness (e-readiness) assessment was conducted (World Health Organization Regional Office for Africa, 2014). According to the Government of Botswana (2004), the country is still behind in enjoying the full benefits of ICT when compared to other developing countries. One of the areas addressed in the national ICT policy included the use of ICT in the health sector.

In the health sector, Botswana as a developing country established an integrated health service plan for 2010-2020. In the ten-year strategic plan, the strategic information management area has the main strategic objective of strengthening the information management system of the national response, which would allow information sharing, and its use for evidence-based planning (Ministry of Health,Government of Botswana, 2010). Additionally, the main strategic objective was followed by the strategic objective that focuses on e-health whereby the health information system is strengthened to enhance the generation of data that could be further used for evidence-based planning (Ministry of Health,Government of Botswana, 2010). With the strategies on e-health put in place in Botswana, e-health initiatives are still in their infancy. However, the government of Botswana collaborated with developed countries to get support on e-health since it requires substantial financial and human capital investments (Nkwe, 2012). The partnership with other developed countries helped Botswana to get e-health machines from the government of India that enabled projects such as telemedicine and the integrated systems for patient management and health workers being commissioned (Nkwe, 2011).

E-health initiatives already in place in Botswana and those that are to come in later years are used by several stakeholders, including higher education institution students. According to The Enterprise of HealthCare Magazine (2010) Bokamoso Private Hospital which is located in the capital of Botswana, Gaborone, has a progressive information technology department which supports the use of electronic medical records and the telemedicine capability that has satellite connectivity.

PROBLEM STATEMENT

Despite the well documented benefits on e-health such as the increase in the quality of data, reduced errors and costs in the health sector, most developing countries find it challenging to adopt e-health (Mugo & Nzuki, 2014). Some of these challenges faced by the health system in Botswana include the use of paper-based patient health records, which makes it difficult to track patient's health problems and the long queues at hospitals and clinics caused by patients who seek medical assistance. With the prior statement said, most developing countries find it challenging to adopt e-health (Mugo & Nzuki, 2014). Although that is the case, before the implementation of any e-health system, the readiness and the preparedness must be established to avoid failure to innovate (Chattopadhyay, Li, Land & Ray, 2008; Kiberu, 2016; Li, Ray, Seale & MacIntyre, 2012). Several studies have been done on e-health as demonstrated by several authors (Coleman, Helselman & Potass, 2012; Hoque, Bao & Sorwar, 2016; Lee, Cain, Young, Chockley & Burstin, 2005; Partnaik & Partnaik,

2015; Lee et al., 2005; Yusif & Soar, 2014). However, research in e-health seems to be disjointed in developing countries (Mugo & Nzuki, 2014).

Literature shows that several studies have been conducted on the readiness to adopt e-health by developing countries with most studies focusing on the readiness of practitioners or healthcare providers (Abdullrahim & Coster, 2016; Coleman et al., 2012; Kiberu, 2016; Lee *et al.*, 2005; Li *et al.*, 2012; Partnaik & Partnaik, 2015; Rezai-Rad, Vaezi & Nattagh, 2012; Saleh, Khodor, Alameddine & Baroud, 2016; Yusif & Soar, 2014) and a few studies focusing on the patients readiness to adopt e-health in developing countries (Heart & Kalderon, 2013; Khatun, Heywood, Ray, Hanifi, Bhuiya & Liawa, 2015; Khatun, Heywood, Ray, Bhuiya & Liawa, 2016). Chattopadhyay *et al.* (2008) states that the analysis of e-health readiness is still limited to its broader perspective. In addition, the existing literature has failed to neither capture, determine nor recognise the factors affecting the e-health readiness of students (higher education institution students) who are also the significant recipients of health services. This study therefore seeks to address the gaps identified by the literature through investigating the e-health readiness of higher education institution students in Botswana.

RESEARCH OBJECTIVES

Based on the problem statement, the overall objective of this study was to investigate readiness factors that affect adoption of e-health by higher education institution students at the University of Botswana. In order to achieve this, the study specifically seeks: To investigate technology readiness factors affecting e-health adoption among students in a higher education institution; To investigate perceived usefulness as a factor that affect e-health adoption by students in a higher education institution; and to finally investigate perceived ease of use as a factor that affect e-health adoption by students in a higher education institution.

LITERATURE REVIEW

The interest of this study is to find out the readiness factors that affect e-health adoption by higher education institution students at the University of Botswana, something that must done before the implementation of any e-health system to avoid failure to innovate. The study is based on the conceptual framework (technology readiness and acceptance model for e-health) which was developed by integrating the technology readiness index model and the technology acceptance model. This section dwells much on e-health readiness and higher education institution students' e-health readiness, healthcare and e-health in Botswana. The section goes on to also discussion the conceptual framework of the study and hypotheses.

E-Health Readiness and Higher Education Institution Students' e-Health Readiness

The use and adoption of any technology involves users' readiness at all times. This section provides a detailed explanation of e-health readiness as well as higher education institution students' e-health readiness.

According to Kgasi (2014) e-health readiness is defined as the extent of preparedness to participate and succeed in implementing e-health by healthcare institutions, users, and the healthcare system as a whole. Similarly, Ojo, Olugbara, Ditsa, Adigun and Xulu (2007) state that e-health readiness is the extent of readiness for a community to participate and succeed in adopting e-health. It is also related to the level of preparedness of technological innovation and the willingness to adapt to these new technologies. Any implementation of a new technology brings disruptions, as people have to adapt to the changes brought by the new technology innovation. With this said, the healthcare system is affected by the implementation of e-health. Hence Ojo *et al.* (2007) states that due to the anticipated resistant to accepting and adopting e-health, the e-health readiness assessment important.

The problem statement recognises that there have been several studies focusing on the readiness of practitioners or healthcare providers and a few studies focusing on the patients' readiness to adopt e-health in developing countries. This shows there is a gap to cover higher education institution students' (recipients of health services) e-health readiness. In this study e-health, readiness means the preparedness of higher education students to participate and adopt the new technological innovations brought about by the concept of e-health. The level of preparedness is confirmed by investigating the readiness factors that affect the adoption of e-health by higher education institution students. Understanding the students' e-health readiness through the readiness factors that affect the adoption will aid in knowing whether the students will adapt to the introduction of the technology and adopt it in their daily lives hence this study title.

Healthcare in Botswana

Healthcare differs around the world and it is a concern for all developing and developed countries (Bantom, 2016). Developed countries are well resourced and with good infrastructure (Bantom, 2016). In this section, Botswana's healthcare in general is examined as well as the current state of e-health implementation in the country.

There is a variety of health service delivery in Botswana such as public, profit and nonprofit private and traditional medicine practices (Ministry of Health, Government of Botswana, 2010). Higher education institutions (Universities) are not left behind as they also have clinics on campuses aimed at giving health assistance to staff and students. Although that is the case, the Ministry of Health (MOH) has the sole responsibility of formulating policies, regulations, norms, standards and guidelines for the entire health services (Ministry of Health, Government of Botswana, 2010). Furthermore, the MOH is the main healthcare provider in the public sector. The government of Botswana managed to contribute 15% of its expenditure to the health sector (Ministry of Health, Government of Botswana, 2010). However, the sector is still faced by several challenges such as a shortage of qualified and trained staff, staff turnover that leads to more shortage of staff members and weak supply chain management systems that result in inadequate availability of stock and regular stock out of important drugs (Ministry of Health, Government of Botswana, 2010). Another challenge is that of weak health management information which leads to data collection that is untimely, leading to weaker or impossible analysis, interpretation, dissemination of information and inability to attend to patients on time which leads to them spending hours in queues. The situation is worsened by the existence of parallel several databases such as the human resource, finance, information technology, and epidemiology databases. Because of the parallel databases, monitoring and evaluation is fragmented and ultimately compromises the tracking of health outcomes and the measurement of specific interventions (Government of Botswana, Ministry of Health, 2010).

In terms of the shortage of staff, statistics show that per 10,000 (ten thousand) population there were four doctors, 26 nurses and midwives as well as two pharmacists (Government of Botswana, Ministry of Health, 2010). However, the Ministry of Health tried to intervene to meet the shortage of staff and staff turnover by using appropriate measures for division of labour (Government of Botswana, Ministry of Health, 2010). There is also training of healthcare professionals both in the country and outside the country with heavy reliance on in-the-country-training. Eight training institutions are used mainly to train nurses and there is a limited number of nurses focusing on health technologies and pharmacy. The medical school has also been established and a few graduates are now deployed to the workplaces. However, due to a limited number of native trained and skilled health professionals, the sector still employs more expatriates (Government of Botswana, Ministry of Health, 2010).

With regards to shortage of drugs there has been the Botswana national drug policy (BNDP) that was put in place in 2002 to help deal with the challenge (Government of Botswana, Ministry of Health, 2010). Nevertheless, there has been another major challenge in the regulation of medicines where there was staff shortage at the drugs regulatory unit responsible for registering medicines and conducting drug control activities (Government of Botswana, Ministry of Health, 2010). Adding onto it is the challenges of insufficient legislation to deal with the importation and distribution of fake medicines; the prescription and dispensing of drugs by unqualified staff contrary to provision of the drugs and related substances act of 1992 (DRSA); and inadequate regulation and control of traditional medicines. Supply chains in clinics and hospitals are also weak, thereby resulting in inconsistent availability and shortage of necessary drugs (Government of Botswana, Ministry of Health, 2010). However, there has been an ongoing reform at the central medical stores that was aimed at improving its performance and ensuring future universal access to necessary medicines.

With regards weak health management information, there is a current limitation to the use of data for purposes of planning and programme improvement, something that reduces the quality of information. There is poor compatibility and coordination of dissimilar information systems such as epidemiological, human resources, logistics, health statistics as well as finance. The present monitoring and evaluation processes is therefore disjointed hence affecting the tracking of outcomes, the impact on health status, and the programme interventions.

E-Health in Botswana

Health information management (HIM) is regarded as weak in Botswana's public healthcare provision system (Sebina & Grand, 2017). This weak HIM also affects higher education institution students as they are also clients in the health services. The weak HIM is attributed to the fact that there is no central database, something which makes it difficult to collect, use, disseminate and share data (Government of Botswana, Ministry of Health, 2010). Furthermore, Moloi and Mutula (2007) argue that managing electronic records (e-record) in Botswana is in its initial stages and fairly new. Although the point is valid in this case, the government of Botswana continues to implement their "integrated health service plan: a strategy for changing the health sector for a healthy Botswana 2010-2020" by getting involved in several e-health systems and initiatives. These include types of e-health systems used to collect health data such as integrated patient management system (IPMS) that collects data from hospitals on patient diagnostic information, the patient management system is used by the maternity sector in clinics as well as the district health information systems 2 (DHIS2) that is used for the aggregation of health data from all the health facilities found within Botswana (MEASURE Evaluation, 2018). These majors are aimed to facilitate data, content sharing and storage in the health sector. Private healthcare practitioners in Botswana are also not left behind in implementing e-health initiatives. Diagnofirm medical laboratories (DML) in Botswana also reported the implementation of a DML mobile app which provides the status of patients' (including higher education institution students) samples as it happens (Diagnostics, 2017). With this app, doctors, referrers and patients can also view the sample action in each stage of processing (Diagnostics, 2017).

E-Health Systems and Initiatives in Botswana

This section discusses several e-health systems and initiatives that have been undertaken by the Botswana government with an effort to appreciate e-health initiatives and the benefits.

Integrated Patient Management System (IPMS)

Botswana uses the IPMS to enhance the sharing of information between healthcare providers in various healthcare sites in the country (Ndlovu, Mauco & Littman-Quinn, 2017). The IPMS houses patients' electronic records for the rest of their lives and the record can be accessed over a portal in any health facility, throughout the country as long as the patient is alive (Ndlovu, *et al.*, 2017). The IPMS therefore allows patients to seek medical help from hospital to hospital since their medical records are available for retrieval in the systems by authorised providers (Ndlovu, et al., 2017). An example of the IPMS include the medical practice management module which is used for managing human immunodeficiency virus (HIV).

Multi Drug Resistant Tuberculosis (MDR-TB) M-Health Clinical Support

Facilitation of sharing knowledge between tuberculosis (TB) clinicians and medical officers is very important in managing and providing quality healthcare services to the patients. Botswana provided its medical practitioners with tablets loaded with multi drug resistant Tuberculosis (TB) (MDR-TB) resources (Moahi & Bwalya, 2017). The resources include guidelines for preventing, monitoring and treating Tuberculosis. However, the MDR-TB pilot study was conducted partially and never concluded or assessed due to budget constraints as well as some technical delays.

Mobile health (M-Health) Pilot Projects

Botswana also piloted its first mobile health projects. They include Tuberculosis (TB) Contact Tracing which replaced the paper-based TB tracing for a period of six months (Ndlovu, *et al.*, 2017). The project was done by the Ministry of Health together with the Botswana-UPenn Partnership. The m-health projects showed a good reception and good results when evaluated as compared to the paper-based

TB tracing (Ndlovu, *et al.*, 2017). On the whole, the m-health approach also had higher favourable ratings score in terms of the usefulness of the system, quality of information and interface quality.

Television White-Space (TVWS) Pilot Project

The TVWS pilot project was done to help deliver telemedicine services to clinics and health posts that are outside Botswana's capital city and other towns where there is a limited number of medical specialists (Ndlovu, *et al.*, 2017). Phase 1 of the project was launched in March 2015. Phase 2 of the project were consultations that were supported through the use of the normal skype application. To make sure that confidentiality of patients was guaranteed, patients' identifiers were not available on pictures that were discussed during the skype sessions. Phase 3 of the project that was earlier envisioned streamlined some of the clinical consultations (Ndlovu, et al., 2017). This was due to the complexity of having different stakeholders at time zones that are different within a health system that was dynamic, something that affected the speed of the implementation.

Portable Eye Examination Kit (Peek) Botswana Project

The Peek Botswana started its phase 1 in July 2016. It is the Peek vision technology which provides access to eye tests that are clinically approved to people at rural areas with the aim to fight blindness in developing countries (Ndlovu, *et al.*, 2017). Furthermore, the PEEK project allows the use of cheaper devices to manage and monitor patients eye treatments. In carrying out this project, several school children were tested, and some were provided with the necessary medication and ophthalmic services (Ndlovu, *et al.*, 2017). The challenges faced when implementing this project was participants' incompetency when using smartphones because most of them were first time users. Additionally, mobile data bundles were also finishing quickly, and it was difficult to get the participants on the training site on schedule.

CONCEPTUAL FRAMEWORK OF THE STUDY AND HYPOTHESES

Hypotheses for the study

The hypotheses below were incorporated from the components of technology readiness index (TRI 1.0) (Parasuraman, 2000). As well as two components from technology acceptance model (TAM) - perceived usefulness and perceived ease of use (Davis, 1989).

H1a: Higher education institution students perceive that optimism has an influence on e-health perceived ease of use.
H1b: Higher education institution students perceive that optimism has an influence on e-health perceived usefulness.
H2a: Higher education institution students perceive that innovativeness has an influence on e-health perceived ease of use.
H2b: Higher education institution students perceive that innovativeness has an influence on e-health perceived usefulness.
H3a: Higher education institution students perceive that discomfort has an influence on e-health perceived ease of use.
H3b: Higher education institution students perceive that discomfort has an influence on e-health perceived usefulness.
H4a: Higher education institution students perceive that insecurity has an influence on e-health perceived ease of use.
H4b: Higher education institution students perceive that insecurity has an influence on e-health perceived usefulness.
H5: Higher education institution students perceive that e-health usefulness has an influence on e-health adoption.
H6: Higher education institution students perceive that e-health ease of use influence e-health adoption.

RESEARCH METHODOLOGY

This study used a quantitative research with the collection of data from the University of Botswana to get students' insight on e-health readiness. Because of a larger population of students at the University of Botswana (13835 students), the sample size used for this study was 372 participants coming from various faculties in the university. The sample size was based on the sample size determination table of Krejcie and Morgan's (1970). Convenience sampling was used due to the fact that it allows a researcher to "collect information from members in a population who are conveniently available to provide it" (Serakan & Bougie, 2013: 252). Time contraints did not allow the researcher to use random sampling. Therefore, to achieve the goals of this research, the study adopted a survey strategy whereby students were administered a close ended questionnaire based on convenience of whether lecturers allowed accessibility to them after lectures. Additionally, they were also

Figure 1. e-health TRAM with hypotheses

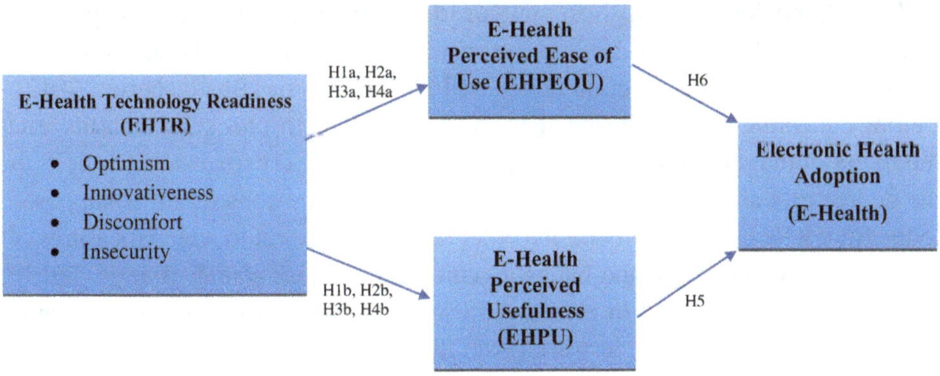

administered the questionnaire as to when the students were available and willing to partake in the study anywhere around the University of Botswana. Convenience sampling however leads to bias and the inability to generalize the results to the studied population (Teddlie & Yu, 2007; Serakan & Bougie, 2013). Saunders, Lewis and Thornhill (2016) also adds that the likelihood of the sample being a representative of the population in convenience sampling is very low and often lacks credibility. Therefore, the results obtained in this study may not be entirely generalised to the student population of University of Botswana. As a close ended questionnaire was used to collect data from students, it was relevant for this study because its more positivist-oriented in nature, carefully designed and structured questionnaires are often favoured to collect information (Thomas & Hodges, 2010). Additionally, data inflow in questionnaires is faster and interview bias is also avoided (Gray, 2013). Moreover, with the use of questionnaire time and money are less consumed (Gray, 2013). The questionnaire used in this study contained questions on demographics, internet access, e-health knowledge, benefits and challenges as well as questions covering TRI 1.0 and some technology acceptance model constructs. To ensure a higher response rate, the questionnaire was kept short.

DATA ANALYSIS

In this study, the data collected was coded and analysed using the Statistical Package for Social Science (SPSS) and Microsoft Excel. Each questionnaire was checked thoroughly to see whether it qualified to be used in the study and empty questionnaires were removed. 385 questionnaires were handed out to the students but only 372 qualified for analysis. The questionnaires that qualified to be used for analysis were then sorted according to the faculty the respondent belonged to. Then each questionnaire was then given a unique identifier so that if anything happens the researcher could always go back to the specific questionnaire. The data collected was then coded in the form of numbers in SPSS for analysis (Bhattacherjee, 2012). Before collecting and analysing data, it is important to check for validity and reliability of the research instrument. Bhattacherjee (2012) explains that validity is the degree to which a measure represents adequately the construct it is supposed to measure whereas reliability on the other hand is the extent to which measures of a construct are consistent and hangs together as a set (Serakan & Bougie, 2013). Content validity was used to measure the validity of the research questionnaire. In this study, different people were given the questionnaire to check if questions in the questionnaire were essential, useful but not essential or not necessary at all. In terms of reliability, Cronbach's alpha was used in this study to test the internal consistency of the constructs in the questionnaire. Cronbach's alpha values above 0.70 indicates that the questions combined in a construct measures the same thing (Saunders, *et al.*, 2016). Therefore, in this study, only constructs with alpha values above 0.70 were accepted otherwise questions lowering the constructs alpha values were removed as it indicated that the question was not measuring what other questions in the constructs measured.

This study tested the reliability of the questionnaire and it was found to be alpha of 0.882 as shown by Table 1. The reliability analysis statistics of this research questionnaire is therefore good as it is above 0.70.

Table 1. Reliability analysis of the research questionnaire

Reliability Statistics	
Cronbach's Alpha	**N of Items**
.882	65

Table 2 shows the reliability analysis of the constructs which are all above the accepted level of 0.70. However, with the case of insecurity, the alpha value was lower that 0.70 when computed with the 5 items. To raise the alpha value, the statement that lowered the alpha value was removed and the new Cronbach's alpha value based of the 4 items than the original 5 items was re-computed. This was done based on Serakan and Bougie (2013) argument that items can be removed to raise the alpha value if it is low although this can affect the validity of a measure.

In this study, descriptive and inferential statistics were also used to analyse the data. Descriptive statistics "describe a body of data" (Leedy & Ormrod, 2010: 265).

Table 2. Reliability analysis of the conceptual framework constructs

Construct	Cronbach's Alpha	N of items	N of Items deleted
Optimism (OPT)	0.804	5	0
Innovativeness (INN)	0.837	5	0
Discomfort (DIS)	0.716	4	0
Insecurity (INS)	0.706	4	1
E-health Perceived Usefulness (EPU)	0.819	6	0
E-health Perceived Ease of Use (EPEU)	0.782	7	0
E-health Adoption (EA)	0.819	3	0

On the other hand, inferential statistics allow a researcher to make inferences about a large population from small samples. It has two main functions of estimating a population parameter from a random sample and to test statistically based hypotheses (Leedy & Ormrod, 2010).

Multiple regression analysis was used to test the hypotheses in Figure 1 to see if one independent variable affected one dependent variable (Serakan & Bougie, 2013). An independent variable is a variable that the researcher manipulates because it is a possible cause of something while a dependent variable is a variable that is influenced by the independent variable (Leedy & Ormrod, 2010). The coefficient of determination R^2 provides the goodness of fit of a regression model. R^2 is a percentage of the variance in the dependent variable which is explained by variation in the independent variable (Serakan & Bougie, 2013). When R^2 is 1 the regression model fits the data perfectly and when R^2 is 0 none of the variation to the dependent variable cannot be attributed to the variation in the independent variable (Serakan & Bougie, 2013). For example, if R^2 is 0.619 it means that almost 62% of the variation in the dependent variable is explained by the variation in the independent variable. The hypotheses were accepted at a significance value below 0.05 and those above significance value 0.05 were rejected.

Regression analysis for H1a, H2a, H3a and H4a

Table 3 shows the model summary for H1a, H2a, H3a and H4a. The R^2 of the model is 0.395 meaning that in this study 39.5% of the variation on the dependent variable e-health perceived ease of use is explained by the variation in the independent variables: insecurity, optimism, innovativeness and discomfort. The model is also significant because of its p-value of 0.000.

Table 3. Model Summary 1

Model	R	R Square	Adjusted R Square	Std. Error of the Estimate	Change Statistics				
					R Square Change	F Change	df1	df2	Sig. F Change
1	.629[a]	.395	.389	.55577	.395	59.980	4	367	.000
a. Predictors: (Constant), Insecurity, Optimism, Innovativeness, Discomfort									

Table 4 shows the regression analysis between the dependent variable e-health perceived ease of use and the independent variables optimism, innovativeness, discomfort and insecurity. All the hypotheses H1a, H2a, H3a and H4a are accepted as they have p-values below 0.05. These findings mean that in this study optimism, innovativeness, discomfort and insecurity influences e-health perceived ease of use.

Table 4. Regression analysis 1

Coefficients[a]							
Model		Unstandardized Coefficients		Standardized Coefficients	t	Sig.	Results
		B	Std. Error	Beta			
1	(Constant)	.888	.161		5.497	.000	
	Optimism	.218	.039	.249	5.600	.000	Accepted
	Innovativeness	.083	.033	.111	2.506	.013	Accepted
	Discomfort	.310	.042	.343	7.394	.000	Accepted
	Insecurity	.170	.035	.203	4.806	.000	Accepted
a. Dependent Variable: E-Health Perceived Ease Of Use							

Regression Analysis for H1b, H2b, H3b and H4b

Table 5 shows the model summary for H1b, H2b, H3b and H4b. The R^2 of the model is 0.322 meaning that 32.2% of the variation on the dependent variable e-health perceived usefulness is explained by the variation in the independent variables: insecurity, optimism, innovativeness and discomfort. The model is also significant because of its p-value of 0.000.

Table 6 shows the regression analysis between the dependent variable e-health perceived usefulness and the independent variables optimism, innovativeness, discomfort and insecurity. Hypotheses H1b and H3b are accepted because they

Table 5. Model summary 2

Model	R	R Square	Adjusted R Square	Std. Error of the Estimate	Change Statistics				
					R Square Change	F Change	df1	df2	Sig. F Change
1	.574[a]	.329	.322	.62132	.329	44.986	4	367	.000
a. Predictors: (Constant), Insecurity, Optimism, Innovativeness, Discomfort									

Table 6. Regression analysis 2

Coefficients[a]							
Model		Unstandardized Coefficients		Standardized Coefficients	t	Sig.	Results
		B	Std. Error	Beta			
1	(Constant)	1.258	.181		6.967	.000	
	Optimism	.326	.044	.351	7.491	.000	Accepted
	Innovativeness	.059	.037	.075	1.599	.111	Rejected
	Discomfort	.262	.047	.273	5.577	.000	Accepted
	Insecurity	.065	.040	.073	1.642	.101	Rejected
a. Dependent Variable: E-Health Perceived Usefulness							

had p-values below 0.05 whilst hypotheses H2b and H4b were rejected as they had p-values above 0.05.

These findings mean that in this study optimism and discomfort influences e-health perceived usefulness whereas innovativeness and insecurity do not influence e-health perceived usefulness.

Table 7. Model summary 3

Model	R	R Square	Adjusted R Square	Std. Error of the Estimate	Change Statistics				
					R Square Change	F Change	df1	df2	Sig. F Change
1	.699[a]	.488	.486	.57908	.488	176.152	2	369	.000
a. Predictors: (Constant), E-Health Perceived Ease Of Use, E-Health Perceived Usefulness									

Regression Analysis for H5 and H6

Table 7 shows the model summary for H5 and H6. The R^2 of the model is 0.488 meaning that 48.8% of the variation on the dependent variable e-health adoption is explained by the variation in the independent variables e-health perceived usefulness and e-health perceived ease of use. The model is also significant because of its p-value of 0.000.

Table 8 shows the regression analysis between the dependent variable e-health adoption and the independent variables e-health perceived usefulness and e-health perceived ease of use. Both hypotheses H5 and H6 are accepted because they had p-values below 0.05.

Table 8. Regression analysis 3

Coefficients[a]								
Model		Unstandardized Coefficients		Standardized Coefficients	t	Sig.	
		B	Std. Error	Beta			Results
1	(Constant)	.566	.165		3.423	.001	
	E-Health Perceived Usefulness	.442	.046	.413	9.565	.000	Accepted
	E-Health Perceived Ease Of Use	.445	.049	.392	9.063	.000	Accepted
a. Dependent Variable: E-Health Adoption							

These findings mean that in this study e-health perceived usefulness and e-health perceived ease of use influence e-health adoption.

DISCUSSION OF THE FINDINGS

Discussion and Implications of the Findings in Relation to Sub-Objective 1

H1a: Higher education institution students perceive that optimism has an influence on e-health perceived ease of use – **Accepted**

The results of this study confirmed that students perceive that optimism has an influence on e-health perceived ease of use. The results of this study correspond with the findings by Esen & Erdogmus, (2014); Rahman, Taghizadeh, Ramayah & Alam (2017) that optimism influences perceived ease of use. Furthermore, the findings match the findings of Kuo, Liu & Ma (2013) where he identifies that optimism had a notable impact on perceived ease of use.

H2a: Higher education institution students perceive that innovativeness has an influence on e-health perceived ease of use – **Accepted**

The results of this study found that students perceive that innovativeness has an influence on e-health perceived ease of use. The results of this study correspond with the findings by Esen & Erdogmus, (2014); Rahman, *et al.* (2017) that innovativeness influences perceived ease of use. Furthermore, the findings confirm the findings of Kuo, *et al.* (2013) that innovativeness had a notable impact on perceived ease of use.

H3a: Higher education institution students perceive that discomfort has an influence on e-health perceived ease of use – **Accepted**

The results of this study found that students perceive that discomfort has an influence on e-health perceived ease of use. The results of this study agree with the findings of Kuo, *et al.* (2013) who identify that discomfort had a notable impact on perceived ease of use. On the other hand, the findings of this study disagree with Esen & Erdogmus, (2014); Rahman, *et al.* (2017) findings that discomfort does not have an effect on perceived ease of use.

H4a: Higher education institution students perceive that insecurity when has an influence on e-health perceived ease of use – **Accepted**

The results of this study found that students perceive that insecurity has an influence on e-health perceived ease of use. The results of this study validate the findings of Kuo, *et al.* (2013) wherein insecurity had a notable impact on perceived ease of use. On the other hand, the findings of this study disagree with Esen & Erdogmus, (2014); Rahman, *et al.* (2017) findings that insecurity does not have an effect on perceived ease of use.

H1b: Higher education institution students perceive that optimism has an influence on e-health perceived usefulness – **Accepted**

The results of this study found that students perceive that optimism has an influence on e-health perceived usefulness. The results of this study agree with the findings of Kuo, *et al.* (2013); Esen & Erdogmus, (2014); Rahman, *et al.* (2017) who also reached the conclusion that optimism had a notable impact on perceived usefulness.

H2b: Higher education institution students perceive that innovativeness has an influence on e-health perceived usefulness – **Rejected**

The results of this study found that students perceive that innovativeness does not have an influence on e-health perceived usefulness. The results of this study agree with the findings of Kuo, *et al.* (2013) that innovativeness does not have any impact on perceived usefulness. However, it differs with Esen & Erdogmus, (2014); Rahman, *et al.* (2017) that innovativeness had a notable impact on perceived usefulness.

H3b: Higher education institution students perceive that discomfort has an influence on e-health perceived usefulness – **Accepted**

The results of this study found that students perceive that discomfort has an influence on e-health perceived usefulness. The results of this study disagree with the findings of Kuo, *et al.* (2013); Esen & Erdogmus, (2014); Rahman, *et al.* (2017) that discomfort does not have a notable impact on perceived usefulness.

H4b: Higher education institution students perceive that insecurity has an influence on e-health perceived usefulness – **Rejected**

The results of this study found that students perceive that insecurity has no influence on e-health perceived usefulness. The results of this study agree with the findings of Kuo, *et al.* (2013); Esen & Erdogmus, (2014); Rahman, *et al.* (2017) that insecurity does not have a notable impact on perceived usefulness.

Discussion and Implications of the Findings in Relation to Sub-Objective 2

H5: Higher education institution students perceive that e-health usefulness has an influence on e-health adoption – **Accepted**

The results of this study found that students perceive that e-health usefulness has an influence on e-health adoption. The results of this study similarly agree with the findings of Wook, Yusuf & Nazri (2017) that perceived usefulness influences the acceptance of a technology although this study focused on adoption of a technology.

Discussion and Implication of the Findings in Relation to Sub-Objective 3

H6: Higher education institution students perceive that e-health ease of use influence e-health adoption – **Accepted**

The results of this study found that students perceive that e-health ease of use has an influence on e-health adoption. The results of this study similarly agree with the findings of Wook, *et al.* (2017) that perceived ease of use influences the acceptance of a technology although this study focused on adoption of a technology.

RECOMMENDATION AND FUTURE STUDY

In future, similar studies may use a combination of quantitative and qualitative methods to investigate the e-health readiness of higher education institution students. Other sampling techniques other than convenience sampling could be used in carrying a similar study. Other sets of respondents from other universities or institutions may also be investigated of the readiness factors that influence their e-health readiness. Furthermore, other studies can discuss the technical, infrastructural or managerial requirements for the effective implementation of an e-health programme. Additionally e-health readiness frameworks that can measure the patients readiness to adopt e-health should be developed.

CONCLUSION

To enhance the understanding of the e-health readiness of higher education institution students, this study used an integrated conceptual framework for e-health (technology readiness and acceptance model) which was tested by hypotheses. For this study, it is concluded that optimism, innovativeness, discomfort and insecurity influence e-health perceived ease of use. However, only optimism and discomfort influence e-health perceived usefulness whereas innovativeness and insecurity did not influence e-health perceived usefulness. Additionally, e-health perceived usefulness and e-health perceived ease of use have an influence on e-health adoption.

REFERENCES

Abdullrahim, A., & De Coster, R. 2016. *A Framework of E-Health Systems Adoption and Telemedicine Readiness in Developing Countries.* International Conference on Information Society (i-Society). 10.1109/i-Society.2016.7854188

Bantom, S. A. (2016). *Accessibility to patients' own health information: A case in rural Eastern Cape, South Africa.* Cape Town: Cape Peninsula University of Technology. doi:10.1145/2987491.2987505

Bhattacherjee, A. (2012). Social Science Research: Principles, Methods, and Practices (2nd ed.). Tampa: Creative Commons Attribution-NonCommercial-ShareAlike 3.0 Unported License.

Chang, A.-M., & Kannan, P. K. (2006). Employee Technology Readiness and Adoption of Wireless Technology and Services. *39th Hawaii International Conference on System Sciences.*

Chattopadhyay, S., Li, J., Land, L., & Ray, P. (2008). A Framework for Assessing ICT Preparedness for e-Health Implementations. *10th IEEE International Conference on e-Health Networking, Applications and Service (HEALTHCOM 2008).* 10.1109/HEALTH.2008.4600122

Coleman, A., Herselman, M. E., & Potass, D. (2012). *E-Health Readiness Assessment for E-Health Framework for Africa: A Case Study of Hospitals in South Africa.* Malaga: Institute for Computer Sciences, Social Informatics and Telecommunications Engineering.

Davis, F. D. (1989). Perceived Usefulness, Perceived Ease Of Use, and User Acceptance Of Information Technology. *MIS Quartely, 13*(3), 319–339. doi:10.2307/249008

De Rosis, S., & Barsanti, S. (2016). Patient satisfaction, e-health and the evolution of the patient-general practitioner relationship: Evidence from Italian survey. *Health Policy (Amsterdam), 120*(11), 1279–1292. doi:10.1016/j.healthpol.2016.09.012 PMID:27836231

Diagnostics. (2017). iBreast Exam. *Botswana's Premier Health Journal, 16*, 1-15.

Esen, M. & Erdogmus, N. (2014). The Effects Of Technology Readiness On Technology Acceptance In E-HRM: Mediating Role Of Perceived Usefulness. *Bilgi Ekonomisi ve Yönetimi Dergisi, 9*(1).

Faber, S., van Geenhuizen, M., & de Reuver, M. (2017). eHealth adoption factors in medical hospitals: A focus on theNetherlands. *International Journal of Medical Informatics, 100*, 77–89. doi:10.1016/j.ijmedinf.2017.01.009 PMID:28241940

Government of Botswana. (2004). *Maitlamo: Botswana's National ICT Policy*. Gaborone: Government of Botswana.

Government of Botswana. Ministry of Health, 2010. Integrated health service plan: A strategy for changing the health sector for a healthy Botswana 2010-2020, Gaborone: Government of Botswana, Ministry of Health.

Gray, D. E. (2013). *Doing Research in the Real World* (3rd ed.). London: Sage Publications.

Heart, T., & Kalderon, E. (2013). Older adults: Are they ready to adopt health-related ICT? *International Journal of Medical Informatics*, *82*, e209–e231.

Hoque, R. M., Bao, Y., & Sorwar, G. (2016). Investigating factors influencing the adoption of e-Health in developing countries: A patient's perspective. *Informatics for Health & Social Care*, *§§§*, 1–17. PMID:26865037

Kgasi, M. R. (2014). *Assessment of e-health readiness in rural South Africa*. Pretoria: Tshwane University Of Technology.

Kgasi, M. R., & Kalema, B. M. (2014). Assessment E-health Readiness for Rural South African Areas. *Journal of Industrial and Intelligent Information*, *2*(2), 131–135. doi:10.12720/jiii.2.2.131-135

Khatun, F., Heywood, A. E., Ray, P. K., Bhuiya, A., & Liawa, S.-T. (2016). Community readiness for adopting mHealth in rural Bangladesh: Aqualitative exploration. *International Journal of Medical Informatics*, *93*, 49–56.

Khatun, F., Heywood, A. E., Ray, P. K., Hanifi, S., Bhuiya, A., & Liawa, S.-T. (2015). Determinants of readiness to adopt mHealth in a rural community of Bangladesh. *International Journal of Medical Informatics*, *84*, 847–856.

Kiberu, V. M. (2016). E-Health Readiness Assessment in Uganda: Integration of Telemedicine services into Public Healthcare System. IEEE Computer Society.

Krejcie, R. V., & Morgan, D. W. (1970). Determining sample size for research activities. *Educational and Psychological Measurement*, *30*(3), 607–610.

Kuo, K. M., Liu, C. F., & Ma, C. C. (2013). An investigation of the effect of nurses' technology readiness on the acceptance of mobile electronic medical record systems. *Medical Informatics and Decision Making*, *13*(1), 88. doi:10.1186/1472-6947-13-88 PMID:23938040

Lee, J. (2005). *The Adoption Gap: Health Information Technology In Small Physician Practices*. The People to People Health Foundation.

Lee, J., Cain, C., Young, S., Chockley, N., & Burstin, H. (2005). The Adoption Gap: Health Information Technology In Small Physician Practices. The People toPeople Health Foundation.

Leedy, P. D., & Ormrod, J. E. (2010). *Practical Research: Planning and Design* (9th ed.). Boston: Pearson Education International.

Li, J., Ray, P., Seale, H., & MacIntyre, R. (2012). An E-Health Readiness Framework For Public Health Services-Pandemic Perspective. In *System Science (HICSS), 2012 45th Hawaii International Conference*. IEEE. 10.1109/HICSS.2012.95

MEASURE Evaluation. (2018). MEASURE Evaluation Organisation. Retrieved 05 22, 2018, from https://www.measureevaluation.org/his-strengthening-resource-center/country-profiles/botswana

Ministry of Health, Government of Botswana. (2010). Integrated Health Service Plan: A Strategy for Changing the Health Sector For Healthy Botswana 2010-2020. Gaborone: Government of Botswana.

Moahi, K. H., & Bwalya, K. J. (2017). Knowledge Sharing for Healthcare and Medicine in Developing Countries: Opportunities, Issues, and Experiences. In K. H. Moahi, K. J. Bwalya, & P. M. I. Sebina (Eds.), *Health Information Systems and the Advancement of Medical Practice in Developing Countries* (pp. 60–77). Hershey, PA: IGI Global. doi:10.4018/978-1-5225-2262-1.ch004

Moloi, J., & Mutula, S. (2007). E-records management in an e-government setting in Botswana. *Information Development*, *23*(4), 290–306.

Mugo, D. M., & Nzuki, D. (2014). Determinants of Electronic Health in Developing Countries. *International Journal of Arts and Commerce*, *3*(3), 49–60.

Ndlovu, K., Mauco, K. L., & Littman-Quinn, R. (2017). Telemedicine in Low Resource Settings: A Case for Botswana. In K. H. Moahi, K. J. Bwalya, & P. M. I. Sebina (Eds.), *Health Information Systems and the Advancement of Medical Practice in Developing Countries* (pp. 129–148). Hershey, PA: IGI Global. doi:10.4018/978-1-5225-2262-1.ch008

Nkwe, N. (2011). State of Information Technology Auditing in Botswana. *Asian Journal of Finance & Accounting*, *3*(1), 125–137. doi:10.5296/ajfa.v3i1.894

Nkwe, N. (2012). E-Government: Challenges and Opportunities in Botswana. *International Journal of Humanities and Social Science*, *2*(17), 39–48.

Ojo, S. O., Olugbara, O. O., Ditsa, G., Adigun, M. O., & Xulu, S. S. (2007). Formal Model for e-Healthcare Readiness Assessment in Developing Country Context. Dubai: 4th International Conference in Innovations in Information Technology, 2007. IIT '07.IEEE.

Parasuraman, A. (2000). Technology Readiness Index (TRI): A Multiple Item Scale to Measure Readiness to Embrace New Technologies. *Service Research*, *2*(4), 307–320. doi:10.1177/109467050024001

Patnaik, S., & Patnaik, A. N. (2015). E-Health For All - Is India Ready? *National Journal of Community Medicine*, *6*(4), 633–638.

Rahman, S. A., Taghizadeh, S. K., Ramayah, T., & Alam, M. M. D. (2017). Technology acceptance among micro-entrepreneurs in marginalized social strata: The case of social innovation in Bangladesh. *Technological Forecasting and Social Change*, *118*, 236–245. doi:10.1016/j.techfore.2017.01.027

Rezai-Rad, M., Vaezi, R., & Nattagh, F. (2012). E-Health Readiness Assessment Framework in Iran. *Iranian Journal of Public Health*, *41*(10), 43–51. PMID:23304661

Saleh, S., Khodor, R., Alameddine, M., & Baroud, M. (2016). Readiness of healthcare providers for eHealth: The case from primary healthcare centers in Lebanon. *BMC Health Services Research*, *16*(644), 1–11. doi:10.118612913-016-1896-2 PMID:27832788

Saunders, M., Lewis, P., & Thornhill, A. (2016). *Research Methods For Business Students* (7th ed.). Harlow: Pearson.

Sebina, P. M., & Grand, B. (2017). Records Management and Open Data in Healthcare Provision in Africa: Reflections and Lessons for Botswana. In K. H. Moahi, K. J. Bwalya, & P. M. Sebina (Eds.), *Health Information Systems and the Advancement of Medical Practice in Developing Countries* (pp. 1–13). Hershey: IGI Global.

Serakan, U., & Bougie, R. (2013). *Research Methods for Business:A Skill-Building Approach* (6th ed.). West Sussex: Wiley and sons.

Son, M., & Han, K. (2011). Beyond the technology adoption: Technology readiness effects on post-adoption behavior. *Journal of Business Research*, *64*(11), 1178–1182. doi:10.1016/j.jbusres.2011.06.019

Teddlie, C., & Yu, F. (2007). Mixed methods sampling: A typology with examples. *Journal of Mixed Methods Research*, *1*(1), 77–100. doi:10.1177/1558689806292430

The Enterprice Of Healthcare Magazine. (2010). *e-Health,The Enterprice Of HealthCare*. Available at: https://ehealth.eletsonline.com/2010/04/paperless-hospital-in-africa-offers-prototype-for-new-model-of-care/

Thomas, D. R., & Hodges, I. D. (2010). *Designing and managing your research project: core skills for social and health research.* Sage Publications. doi:10.4135/9781446289044

Tsikriktsis, N. (2004). A Technology Readiness–Based Taxonomy of Customers:A Replication and Extension. *Journal of Service Research*, *7*(1), 42–52. doi:10.1177/1094670504266132

Walczuch, R., Lemmink, J., & Streukens, S. (2007). The effect of service employees' technology readiness on technology acceptance. *Information & Management*, *44*(2), 206–215. doi:10.1016/j.im.2006.12.005

Wook, M., Yusof, Z. M., & Nazri, M. Z. A. (2017). Educational data mining acceptance among undergraduate students. *Education and Information Technologies*, *22*(3), 1195–1216. doi:10.100710639-016-9485-x

World Health Organization Regional Office for Africa. (2014). *World Health Organization Regional Office for Africa.* Available at. http://www.aho.afro.who.int/profiles_information/index.php/Botswana:Health_information,_research,_evidence_and_knowledge

Xiang, J., & Stanley, S. J. (2017). From online to offline: Exploring the role of e-health consumption,patient involvement, and patient-centered communication on perceptions of health care quality. *Computers in Human Behavior*, *70*, 446–452. doi:10.1016/j.chb.2016.12.072

Yusif, S., & Soar, J. (2014). Preparedness for e-Health in developing countries: The case of Ghana. *Journal of Health Informatics in Developing Countries*, *8*(2), 18–37.

Section 3

Systemic Approaches of Current ICT Trends and Technology Supporting the Model

In this last section we develop and explore the subtleties and intricacies of deploying a system as complex as this one to a wider public. Different angles of impacts both in the targeted population (co-morbid conditions elderly), in their closest environment (family and neighbors, the informal caregivers) and in the professional healthcare professionals that are responsible for the lifelong process of health and care. The most recent, although stable, technological trends are considered and weighed trying to come as close as possible to a proposal that is simultaneously the most economically viable and appealing to the professionals, trying to relief their heavy burden and burnout.

Chapter 7
Frailty in the Elderly and Interventions Supported by Information and Communication Technologies: A Systematic Review

Gorete Mendonça Reis
Comprehensive Health Research Center, Universidade de Évora, Portugal

Luís Manuel Mota Sousa
https://orcid.org/0000-0002-9708-5690
Comprehensive Health Research Center, Universidade de Évora, Portugal

Paulo Silva
Unidade Local de Saúde do Baixo Alentejo, Portugal

Patricia Pereira
Hospital Espírito Santo de Évora, Portugal

Margarida Sim-Sim
https://orcid.org/0000-0002-0028-2664
Comprehensive Health Research Center, Universidade de Évora, Portugal

ABSTRACT

Fragility affects the ability to recover from stress conditions as the use of information and communication technologies in health care grows. The objective of this chapter is to identify evidence on interventions using ICT technology to prevent or delay frailty. A systematic review of the literature was used. Search was performed in April 2019

DOI: 10.4018/978-1-7998-1937-0.ch007

through B-on and EBSCO host, in databases Academic Search Complet, with Full Test in MEDLINE, CINAHL Plus®, and MedicLatina. Boolean equation ((Telemedicine) OR (mobile health) OR (computer reality) OR (virtual reality)) AND (Frail Elderly) AND (randomized controlled trial), from 2013 to 2017. Articles followed PRISMA flowchart. Results show that 2946 articles were selected, and 17 met the criteria. The used ICT were virtual-augmented reality, multidisciplinary home-telehealth and telemonitoring, nurse home visits, Wii Fit, and other interactive video games. The chapter conclude that the implementation of ICT to manage self-care at home requires an interdisciplinary, collaborative, and user-centered approach to improve the viability, acceptability, and usability of innovations.

INTRODUCTION

Population aging is an inexorable change. The elderly, the result of physiological and psychosocial processes, become vulnerable, with their multidimensional fragility becoming visible. Elderly frailty challenges governments and societies in developed countries (Chen & Schulz, 2016), and lacks the implementation of policies, prevention programs, or assistance and support to a significant portion of the population and their caregivers (Andrew et al., 2018; Magalhães, Giacomin, dos Santos, & Firmo, 2015).

Frailty is theoretically defined as a clinically recognizable state of increased vulnerability, resulting from the decline associated with aging, loss of functional reserve and changes in functions and multiple physiological mechanisms that compromise the ability to cope with daily or acute stressors. The original approach to frailty focused on the physiological elements, often translated into medical attention focus points such as multimorbidity and chronic disease (Rockwood, Fox, Stolee, Robertson, & Beattie, 1994) . Subsequently, the understanding of the concept was broadened. Currently, a multidimensional vision is proposed, characterized by a dynamic state, affecting individuals who experience losses in the physical, psychological and social domains (Gobbens, Luijkx, Wijnen-Sponselee, & Schols, 2010).

Seen from a holistic point of view, frailty affects the ability of older adults to recover from acute illness, injury and other stress conditions (Puts et al., 2017). Dependence is one of the consequences of frailty that must be minimized to allow the person to be kept in a space familiar to them. The supports can be different according to the dimensions that are precariously balanced. The intervention will preferably cover altered dimensions, which intersect with systemic effect, in order to reduce vulnerability and improve the dynamic state.

Problems associated with reduced balance and mobility call for an effective and engaging rehabilitation regime. This is essential for reducing deficits, for recovery and for preventing motor skills degradation (Strum, Better, Mousse, Desai, & Goodman, 2011). Physical activity of all types and combinations, and rehabilitation significantly reduce the number or prevalence of frailty markers (Puts et al., 2017). A connection with psychological and social aspects is recognized in this context.

The elderly also shows noticeable frailty with regard to the social domain. The most prevalent manifestation is social isolation, with negative consequences on physical and psychological health. Segmenting social isolation has become a focus area, whereas the need for professional policies and practices emerges (Chen & Schulz, 2016). In this sense, the *Aging in Place* concept reflects societal concerns (Fonseca, 2018; WHO, 2015). The concept, whose substratum is the elderly resident in the community and in the family space, emerges as a recognition of the elderly person's skills, supported by the surroundings, as far as their needs are concerned. These needs have a significant economic burden, perhaps alleviated when other measures, such as remote care, are introduced into care as recognized by WHO (WHO, 2015) and recommended by the European Commission (e.g. e-health app guidelines developed to improve elderly carehttps://cordis.europa.eu/news/rcn/124486/en).

Information and communication technologies (ICTs) are recognized as an effective tool to combat the social isolation of seniors, although they are not appropriate for all (Chen & Schulz, 2016). However, it is possible to apply them with the support of a proximity mediator and with strategies designed for the situation at hand. The use of mHealth technologies in health care for community-dwelling seniors is increasing (Matthew-Maich et al., 2016). At the same time, the number of studies on the use of virtual reality (VR) and game technology has grown. These new resources are currently complementary tools for the maintenance and rehabilitation of the elderly population (Skjaeret et al., 2016). ICTs require an interdisciplinary, collaborative and beneficiary-centered approach to improve viability, acceptability and usability. (Greenhalgh et al., 2015; Matthew-Maich et al., 2016).

Although difficulties are anticipated, there are elderly people who are able to use ICTs with a playful purpose, in managing daily tasks and in controlling the situation of health-diseases. The implementation of ICT in home care for the elderly and self-management of chronic disease are important areas for future research (Matthew-Maich et al., 2016). Thus, the objective of this systematic literature review is to identify evidence on ICT interventions aimed at preventing and/or delaying frailty in the elderly people of the community.

MATERIAL AND METHODS

Study Design

The methodology of systematic literature review (SLR) was chosen because it allows the identification, selection, inclusion and analysis of experimental articles on the subject under study. This type of review is characterized by being focused on a clearly formulated question that uses systematic, explicit and reproducible methods to identify, evaluate and synthesize studies with relevant evidence. (Sousa, Firmino, Marques-Vieira, Severino, & Pestana, 2018) .

Research Question

Joanna Briggs Institute [JBI] recommendations were followed (JBI, 2011) which resulted in the research question. The research question was formulated based on the PICO strategy: "What are the results (O) of applying ICTs aimed at preventing and reducing frailty (I) in community-dwelling seniors (P) compared to community-living seniors receiving conventional care (C)?"

Data Source and Research Strategy

The survey was conducted in April 2019 through the B-on and EBSCO host, considering the databases 1) Academic Search Complet, 2) MEDLINE with Full Text, 3) CINAHL Plus® with Full Text, 4) MedicLatina, via the browser of University of Evora, Portugal.

The research exact descriptors in the Virtual Health Library, Health Sciences Descriptors (i.e., DeCS), were combined with Boolean operators in the following equations:

1. ((Telemedicine) OR (Mobile health) OR (computer) OR (virtual reality)) AND ((Aged) OR (elderly) OR (Community Dwelling) OR (Frail Elderly) OR (Older Adults)) AND (randomized controlled trial)
2. ((Telemedicine) OR (Mobile health) OR (computer) OR (virtual reality)) AND (Frail Elderly) AND (randomized controlled trial)

The references of the included studies were also researched manually.

Study Selection

The dimensions of the acronym PICO contributed to define the inclusion criteria: Population (P) - people over 65 living in the community; Intervention (I) - ICT-based interventions aimed at preventing and reducing frailty; Comparison (C) - conventional interventions in the context of prevention and reduction of frailty; Results (O) - reduction/prevention of frailty and its consequences.

Inclusion criteria were: a) quantitative studies of experimental or quasi-experimental design; b) by a trilingual access Portuguese, English and Spanish, c) with accessible full text, d) published in the last 6 years (2013-2019) given the time-frame of research on the economic evaluation of "*Aging in Place*" (Marek, Stetzer, Adams, Popejoy, & Rantz, 2012)

Frailty was defined by validated criteria of a multifactorial nature (i.e., physical frailty (i.e., decline in nutrition, mobility, physical activity, strength, balance), social frailty (i.e., decline in relationships and social support) and psychological fragility (i.e., cognitive decline, mood and coping) (Gobbens et al., 2010)

Exclusion criteria were: a) studies in gray literature, b) observational studies (cohort and cross-sectional), c) qualitative studies, d) letters to the editor, e) methodological studies, f) meta-synthesis, g) meta-analysis and h) umbrella reviews

The selection of articles followed the PRISMA flowchart. It began by two researchers reading the title and *abstract* independently (LS; GR). Disagreements were resolved by consensus, with no need for third-party intervention. An independent reading of the full text followed (LS; GR). The review of the entire process and preparation of the manuscript prior to submission was performed by the remaining three members of the research team.

Data Extraction

Grids were applied for JBI experimental studies (i.e., Critical appraisal criteria for a randomized controlled trial/pseudo randomized trial). The data collected from each included article were: type of study (experimental or quasi-experimental), first author, year of publication, country, sample size, age, frailty criteria, assessment tools, intervention data (i.e., modality, frequency, intensity, volume, duration and progression) and relevant results. The classification of evidence levels of the included studies was based on the criteria of the Registered Nurses Association of Ontario (RNAO, 2007).

Figure 1. Study identification and inclusion flowchart

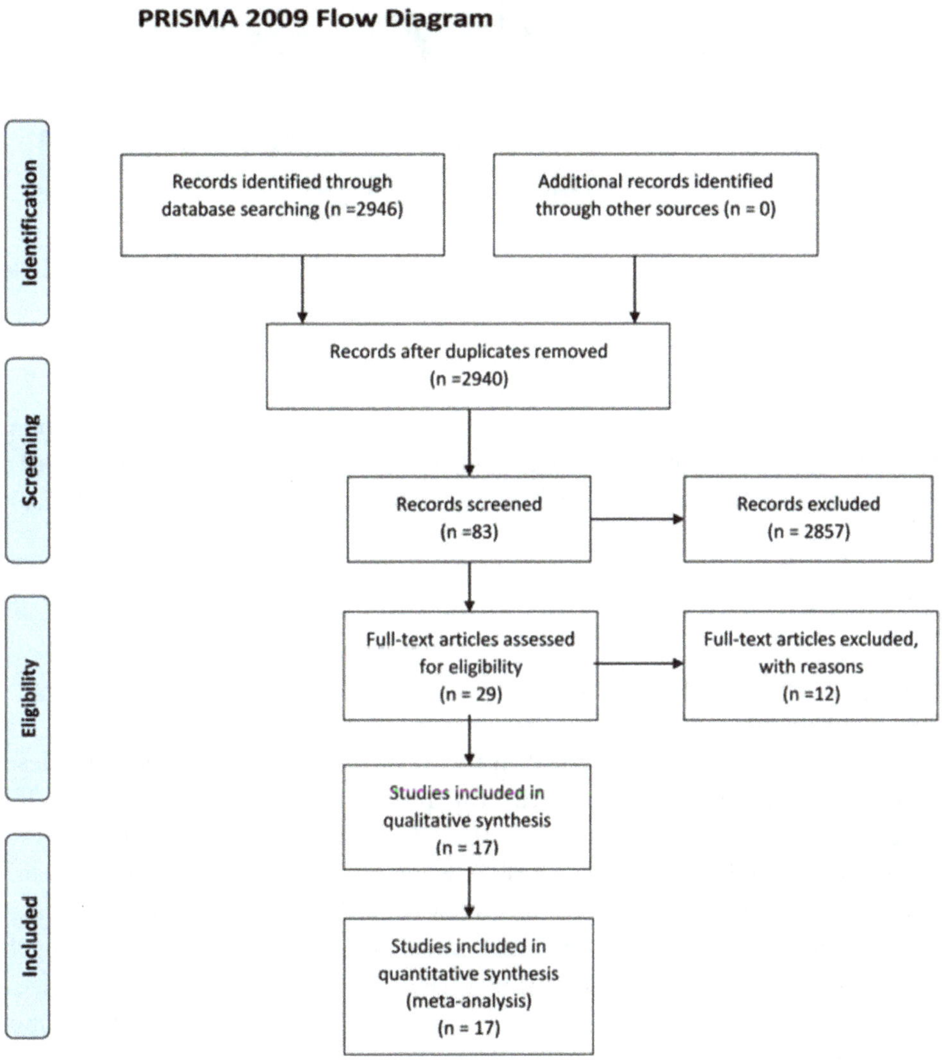

Methodological Quality Assessment

Experimental and quasi-experimental studies considered eligible for systematic review (SR) were subsequently evaluated for methodological quality according to criteria proposed by the JBI. (JBI, 2011) (i.e., Critical appraisal criteria for a randomized controlled trial/pseudo randomized trial). The methodology of each study was considered adequate for inclusion if the articles presented more than 75% of the criteria (Vilelas, 2017). Bias risk assessment is based on five criteria for

Figure 2. Bias analysis chart

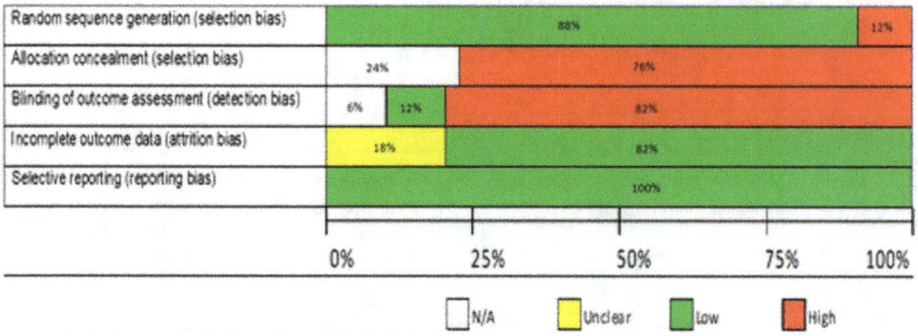

randomized trials: a) Random sequence generation (selection bias), b) Allocation concealment (selection bias), c) Blinding of outcome assessment (detection bias), d) Incomplete outcome data (attrition bias) and e) Selective reporting (reporting bias)

RESULTS

Descriptive results are presented, illustrated by a Prisma flowchart and other images for better data exposure.

Seventeen studies were included in this review, published in nine countries. Namely: Germany (Golla et al., 2018), Brazil (Gomes et al., 2018; Santos, Wolf, Silva, Rodacki, & Pereira, 2019), China (E. S. Hung et al., 2019; Hung et al., 2016; Yang, Wang, Wu, Lo, & Lin, 2016), Hong Kong (Fu, Gao, Tung, Tsang, & Kwan, 2015), Italy (Bernocchi et al., 2019; Straudi et al., 2017), Mexico (Favela et al., 2013), Poland (Kamińska, Miller, Rotter, Szylińska, & Grochans, 2018), Portugal (Gouveia et al., 2018), Republic of Korea (Hong, Kim, Kim, & Kong, 2017; Lee, Kim, & Lee, 2014) and USA (Henry & Moore, 2016; Padala et al., 2017; Upatising et al., 2013).

Regarding the year of publication, we identified the following: 2013 (Favela et al., 2013; Upatising et al., 2013), 2014 (Lee et al., 2014), 2015 (Fu et al., 2015), 2016 (Henry & Moore, 2016; Hung et al., 2016; Yang et al., 2016), 2017 (Hong et al., 2017; Padala et al., 2017; Straudi et al., 2017), 2018 (Golla et al., 2018; Gomes et al., 2018; Gouveia et al., 2018; Kamińska et al., 2018) and 2019 (Bernocchi et al., 2019; E. S. Hung et al., 2019; Santos et al., 2019).

All studies have a level of evidence Ib, except one that had level of evidence IIb. (Kamińska et al., 2018) . The image documents the five criteria (Higgins & Green, 2008), noting that all meet the last criterion (i.e., Selective reporting (reporting bias)). The highest risk of bias is associated with the second (i.e., allocation concealment (selection bias)) and third criteria (i.e., blinding of outcome assessment (detection bias)).

The sample size ranged from 14 to (Golla et al., 2018) 283 participants (Bernocchi et al., 2019) in 1000 seniors. Heterogeneous samples from seniors with the following conditions were included: (Fu et al., 2015; Gouveia et al., 2018; Hong et al., 2017; Kamińska et al., 2018; Padala et al., 2017; Santos et al., 2019; Upatising et al., 2013) with chronic disease (Bernocchi et al., 2019), with frailty (Favela et al., 2013; Gomes et al., 2018), with cerebrovascular accident (stroke) (Golla et al., 2018; Hung et al., 2016; Lee et al., 2014), with human cognitive impairment associated with Human Immunodeficiency Virus (HIV) (Henry & Moore, 2016), with diabetic neuropathy (E. S. Hung et al., 2019), with chronic brain injury (Straudi et al., 2017) and with Parkinson's disease (Yang et al., 2016).

The interventions on prevention/reduction in community-dwelling elderly people with fragility identified in the studies were: Virtual reality / Augmented reality (Kamińska et al., 2018; Lee et al., 2014; Straudi et al., 2017; Yang et al., 2016); Yang et al., 2016); Multidisciplinary Home-Telehealth Program to Prevent Falls (Bernocchi et al., 2019); Nurse home visits with or without alert buttons (Favela et al., 2013); Balance training using Wii Fit (Fu et al., 2015; Golla et al., 2018; Gomes et al., 2018; Padala et al., 2017); Interactive Video Game-Based Exercise on Balance (Gouveia et al., 2018; E. S. Hung et al., 2019; Hung et al., 2016; Santos et al., 2019) and Home Telemonitoring (Henry & Moore, 2016; Hong et al., 2017; Upatising et al., 2013).

A summary of the data extraction can be found in Table 1.

DISCUSSION

The included studies refer to very different interventions carried out in populations within the frail elderly. The samples were, however, heterogeneous, making comparison difficult. The greatest weaknesses of the 17 studies lie in the blinding process. Bias analysis suggests that the elements that apply the intervention and evaluate results have access to the identification of the experimental and control group. The blinding process in such interventions is difficult to ensure.

The analysis by modality of interventions on prevention/reduction in community-dwelling elderly people with frailty was performed, listing the respective results, to be described below. These include: a) frequency of ICT application b) gains from intervention c) duration of application d) type of interaction.

Results with Virtual/Augmented reality, either in balance or decreased risk of falling(Kamińska et al., 2018), as well as body posture or gait of people with stroke (Lee et al., 2014), or even in the balance of those with chronic brain trauma (Straudi

Table 1. Summary of extracted data

Author, Year, Country	Sample	Objective	Intervention	Results	Evidence Level
Bernocchi et al., 2019, Italy (C4)	Elderly with chronic disease intervention group, n = 141 and conventional care group, control group, n = 142.	To determine the feasibility and effectiveness of a 6-month home telerehabilitation program to prevent falls in the elderly with 1 or more chronic diseases (heart, respiratory, neuromuscular or neurological) after hospital rehabilitation for their chronic disease.	The telerehabilitation consisted of a fall prevention program involving individual home exercises (strength, balance and walking) and a structured telephone call made by a nurse asking about the disease status and symptoms, providing support to the elderly.	At the end, the intervention group had lower risk and fewer falls. A 6-month home telerehabilitation program integrated with medical and nursing tele monitoring is feasible and effective in preventing falls in seniors with chronic diseases at high risk of falling.	Ib
Favela et al., 2013, México (C15)	133 People over the age of 60, with a frailty index greater than 0.14. Groups NV + AB - nursing home visits, including alert buttons (n = 45) NV only group - nursing home visits (n = 44) and control group - usual care (n = 44)	To assess whether an intervention based on home visits by nurses, including alert buttons, is effective in reducing frailty compared to home nursing visits alone and usual care for the elderly.	Home visit for 9 months. They could contact their nurses whenever they felt the need by pressing the alert button. The nurses immediately answered the call using a mobile phone and used the screening protocol application installed on an iPod Touch to resolve the telephone call, including clinical emergencies.	At the end of follow-up, the adjusted prevalence of frailty in the NV + AB group was 23.3% versus 58.3% in the control group. **Conclusion:** An intervention based on NV + AB seems to have a positive effect on frailty scores.	Ib
Fu et al., 2015, Hong Kong (C16)	Sixty seniors over 65 years old Wii Fit® balance training intervention group (n = 30) Control group - conventional balance training (n = 30)	Use Nintendo's Wii Fit® balance board to determine the effectiveness of exergaming training in reducing the risk and incidence of falls in seniors with a history of falls.	Wii Fit balance training lasted one hour per session, three sessions per week for six weeks. Since all participants had a history of falls, a rehabilitation assistant who provided immediate manual support when needed, both during Wii Fit and during conventional balance training, monitored them.	Wii Fit balance training was more effective than conventional balance training in reducing risk and incidence of falls.	Ib
Golla et al., 2018, Germany (C19)	14 Stroke survivors over 60 Wii Fit™ intervention group (n = 6) Conventional control group (n = 8)	Investigate the feasibility of a Wii™ balance home workout for people after stroke	12 weeks after hospital discharge, participants received a 6-week supervised balance training (once a week) at the study center, followed by a 6-week (three times per week) unsupervised balance training at home. The intervention group used the Nintendo Wii™ Balance Board and the control group did conventional balance exercises.	Participants in both groups evaluated the unsupervised and supervised training as positive and feasible for self-application. No falls or injuries occurred during the intervention period. Both home balance-training interventions were viable for elderly stroke survivors with low functional limitations.	Ib
Gouveia et al., 2018, Portugal (C22)	46 elderly residents in the community aged 65 to 85 years, with altered balance. Intervention (n=26) Control (n=20)	To evaluate the effectiveness of the ProBalance rehabilitation program on the quality of life of community-dwelling older adults with impaired balance.	The rehabilitation program included gait, balance, functional training, strengthening, flexibility and 3D training for 12 weeks (90 min sessions, 2 days per week).	The ProBalance program had a beneficial effect on the quality of life of community-dwelling seniors, involved young and old adults, both in the physical and mental domain.	Ib
Henry et al., 2016, United States of America (C24)	21 people with HIV-related cognitive impairment (executive function, attention and memory) Intervention (n=11) Control (n=10)	Evaluate a 16-week short message service/multimedia messaging service (SMS/MMS) intervention (iSTEP), designed to increase moderate physical activity and improve neuro-cognition.	Use of text messaging to monitor and encourage physical activity	All iSTEP participants (100%) and 70% of control participants indicated that they would recommend the study to other people living with HIV. Results indicate that an SMS/MMS physical activity intervention can be administered to people with HIV-associated neurocognitive impairment.	Ib
Hong et al., 2017, Republic of Korea (C27)	23 seniors, aged between 69 and 93 years. Tele-exercise group (n = 11) control group (n = 12)	To investigate the effects of a tele-exercise intervention on improving sarcopenia-related factors of body composition and functional fitness in community-dwelling older adults	The tele-exercise program implemented via videoconferencing (Skype™), with connectivity. The tele-exercise group performed supervised resistance exercises at home for 20 to 40 minutes a day, three times a week for 12 weeks.	Tele-exercise may be a new and effective intervention method to increase skeletal muscle mass and lower limb physical functioning with a view to improving sarcopenia in community-dwelling seniors.	Ib
Hung et al., 2019, China (C30)	Twenty-four people with peripheral diabetic neuropathy 2 Groups (n = 12 and n = 12) received an interactive video game based exercise program (EBVI)	To evaluate the effects of EBVI on balance in people with peripheral diabetic neuropathy.	Group A received EBVI training for the first 6 weeks without exercise for the next 6 weeks. Group B did not exercise for the first 6 weeks and then underwent EBVI training for the next 6 weeks.	The 6-week interactive video game exercise program had a positive effect on functional balance in people with peripheral diabetic neuropathy.	Cross Ib

continued on following page

Table 1. Continued

Author, Year, Country	Sample	Objective	Intervention	Results	Evidence Level
Hung et al., 2016, China (C31)	23 people with stroke hemiplegia for at least 6 months but were still able to stand independently for more than 5 minutes. intervention group (n = 12) control group (n = 11)	To investigate the viability and potential efficacy of the Tetrax biofeedback system for balance training in people with chronic hemiplegia.	All participants received conventional rehabilitation training. The intervention group underwent 20 minutes of Tetrax biofeedback games controlled by the change in pressure center 3 times a week, for 6 weeks.	The intervention group showed a significant improvement in reaction time (p = 0.002), proprioception (p <0.001), symmetrical rolling weight (p = 0.027), Timed Up and Go (p <0.001) and Forward Reach (p <0.001) compared to the control group. The use of Tetrax biofeedback video games for balance training is a viable adjunct program that can enhance conventional therapy in people with chronic hemiplegia.	Ib
Kamińska et al., 2018, Poland (C35)	23 people, 19 women and 4 men (average 75.74 ± 8.09 years).	To evaluate the effectiveness of Virtual Reality (VR) training using the Xbox 360 Kinect in people over 60 years of age.	30-day VR training using an Xbox 360 Kinect 3 times per week with 30-minute training sessions.	RV-based training increases motor training possibilities and can help reduce the risk of falls by improving static and dynamic balance.	IIb
Lee et al., 2014, Republic of Korea (C43)	Twenty-one people with stroke experimental group (n = 10) control group (n=11).	To determine the effects of augmented reality-based postural control (AR) training on balance and gait function in people with stroke	Both groups received a general physiotherapy program for a period of 30 minutes per session, 5 days a week for 4 weeks. Participants in the experimental group received additional AR-based postural control training for 30 minutes per day, 3 days per week for 4 weeks.	There was a significant main effect of time on the Timed up-and-go test, Berg Balance Scale, speed, cadence, stride length and stride length on the paretic and non-paretic sides. The results of this study provide evidence on the use of an AR environment in postural control training to improve gait in people with stroke.	Ib
Padala et al., 2017, United States of America (C51)	Thirty community-resident veterans with 68 years of age (± 6.7). Intervention (n=15) Control (n=15)	To evaluate the effectiveness of an exercise program through Wii-Fit interactive video game to improve balance in elderly veterans	The intervention group completed the Wii-Fit program while the control group performed a computer-based cognitive program for 45 minutes, three days a week for 8 weeks.	There were no adverse events related to the study. Significant effects were found. Namely, a higher BBS score in the exercise group (6.0; 95% CI, 5.1-6.9) compared to the control group (0.5; 95% CI, −0.3 −1.3) at 8 weeks (mean intergroup difference (95% CI), 5.5 (4.3-6.7), p <0.001). Conclusion: The Wii-Fit exercise program is effective for improving balance in community-dwelling senior veterans.	Ib
Santos et al, 2019, Brazil (C63)	Thirty-four women (69.5 ± 5.4 years) Intensity group (GM: 11-13 perceived effort) Vigorous exercise intensity group (GV: 14-16 perceived effort).	To compare the effects of two exercise intensities in the exergame training program on muscle strength, functional capacity and perceptual parameters in pre-frail elderly women.	The exercise training included 3 sessions per week for 12 weeks using the Xbox 360 (Microsoft Inc., Redmond, WA, USA) with the Microsoft® Console and Kinetic.	Regardless of the intensity of exercise, exergame training improved muscle strength and functional capacity in pre-frail elderly women. However, positive affection and pleasure were reported only when elderly women practiced moderate intensity exergam exercises.	Ib
Straudi et al., 2017, Italy (C69)	21 People with Chronic Brain Injury video game therapy (VGT) (n = 12) balance platform therapy (BPT) (n = 8)	Test the effects of VGT compared to BPT on balance, mobility, and selective attention in people with chronic head injury.	VGT or BPT 3 sessions per week for 6 weeks.	Both groups improved Community Balance & Mobility Scale scores, but only the VGT group increased in Unified Balance Scale and TUG (p <0.05). Selective attention significantly improved in the VGT group (p <0.01). Conclusions: Video game therapy is an option for treating people with chronic head injury to improve balance and attention deficits.	Ib

continued on following page

Table 1. Continued

Author, Year, Country	Sample	Objective	Intervention	Results	Evidence Level
Upatising et al., 2013, United States of America (C72)	Adults over 60 at high risk of hospitalization and emergency room visits. Telemonitoring group (n = 97) Control group (n = 97)	To evaluate the effect of home telemonitoring on reducing the rate of deterioration in frailty and death in elderly with comorbidity problems.	For 12 months, the intervention group received usual medical care and telemonitoring case management, and the control group received usual care.	During the first 6 months, 19 (25%) telemonitoring participants decreased in frailty or died, compared with 17 (19%) under normal treatment (odds ratio of 1.41, 95% confidence interval [CI]). 0.65–3.06, P = 0.38). Over the next 6 months, there was no transition to a state of frailty, but seven (7%) telemonitoring participants and one (1%) of the usual care group died (odds ratio 5.94, 95% CI 0.52–68), 48, P = 0.15). Gait speed (hazard ratio 3.49, 95% CI 1.42-8.58) and low activity (hazard ratio 3.10, 95% CI 1.25–7.71) allowed the prediction of mortality.	Ib
Vieira Gomes et al, 2018, Brazil (C86)	30 frail seniors Experimental group (EG, n = 15) or control group (CG, n = 15).	To evaluate the feasibility, safety, and acceptability of interactive Nintendo Wii Fit Plus™ (NWFP) video games and functional outcomes (postural control, gait, cognition, mood, and fear of falling) in frail elderly people and elderlies in general.	The EG participants performed 14 training sessions, lasting 50 min each, twice a week. In each training session, participants played five of the 10 selected games, with two attempts in each game. CG participants received general advice on the importance of physical activity	The use of NWFP was feasible, acceptable and safe for frail seniors and improved postural control and gait. There were no effects on cognition, mood or fear of falling.	Ib
Yang et al., 2016, China, (C88)	20 people with Parkinson's Experimental group (EG, n = 10) or control group (CG, n = 10).	To test whether virtual reality balance training at home is more effective than conventional home balance training to improve balance, gait, and quality of life in people with Parkinson's disease (PD).	In the experimental group, the training was performed with the VR Balance Training System. In each session, the participants practiced keeping static posture (10 minutes) and dynamic weight shift. Each session had 50 minutes, with 12 sessions over 6 weeks.	The experimental and control groups were comparable in the pretest. After training, both groups performed better on the Berg Balance Scale, the Dynamic Gait Index, fixed-time Up-and-Go test, and the post-test and follow-up Parkinson's Disease Questionnaire than pre-test. However, no significant differences were found between these two groups at post-test and follow-up.	Ib

et al., 2017) suggest effectiveness in programs applied to the elderly. However, in people with Parkinson's disease, the comparison between groups was not significant, as both the experimental and control groups had improvements. Despite this last result (Yang et al., 2016), the analysis suggests improvement of frailty, in the physical and cognitive dimensions. Although the physiological process of aging contains in itself a decrease of functions and consequent loss of functionality, this result was expected, continued training, lasting from 1 month to 1.5 months, with sessions ranging from 30-50 minutes, performed 3 time per week, led to these improvements. The results are consistent with other studies. In fact, a meta-analysis on the use of Virtual reality therapy for rehabilitation of balance in the elderly showed positive results regarding improvements in dynamic and static balance (70% of studies), mobility (80%), flexibility (30%), gait (20%) and fall prevention (20%) (Amorim, Leite, Brizola, & Yonamine, 2018).

Regarding the use of balance training using Wii Fit, we found its presence in the following studies: i) in a study with a Wii Fit balance training program lasting one hour per session, three sessions per week for six weeks (Fu et al., 2015) ii) another supervised balance training program performed once a week for 6 weeks (Golla et al., 2018); iii) a 45-minute Wii fit program three days a week for 8 weeks (Padala et al., 2017) and iv) a program conducted during 14 training sessions, lasting 50 min each, twice a week (Gomes et al., 2018).

Intervention with Wii fit improved balance in the elderly and reduced risk and occurrence of falls (Fu et al., 2015), improved balance in seniors with stroke (Golla et al., 2018), improved balance in seniors (Padala et al., 2017) and improved progress in postural control and gait of frail seniors (Gomes et al., 2018). This is in line with a systematic review that included studies on the use of Wii fit by the elderly at risk of falling, and improved balance results between 16 and 42% over baseline (Thomas et al., 2019).

At the level of Interactive Video Game-Based Exercise on Balance, 4 studies emerged. The ProBalance 3D program applied for 12 weeks, with 90 min sessions, 2 days a week (Gouveia et al., 2018). A program applied for 6 weeks (E. S. Hung et al., 2019), another study in which 20 minutes of Tetrax biofeedback games controlled by change in pressure center were performed 3 times a week for 6 weeks(Hung et al., 2016) plus a study in which exergame training was done 3 sessions per week for 12 weeks (Santos et al., 2019).

Improved quality of life in community-dwelling elderly with balance disorders (Gouveia et al., 2018); showed a positive effect on functional balance in people with peripheral diabetic neuropathy (E. S.-W. Hung et al., 2019); improved balance, functional capacity and proprioception in people with chronic hemiplegia (Hung et al., 2016); improved muscle strength and functional capacity in pre-frail older women (Santos et al., 2019). In a previous systematic review, it was also found that health-related quality of life instruments, study settings, exercise duration and frequency also varied across studies with the use of exergaming platforms. However, health-related quality of life improved in 3 out of 9 studies (Cacciata et al., 2019).

Technology-based exercise interventions have been reported to have good adherence and may provide a sustainable means of promoting physical activity and preventing falls in the elderly. (Valenzuela, Okubo, Woodbury, Lord, & Delbaere, 2018) . The Multidisciplinary Home-Telehealth Program to Prevent Falls was applied for 6 months and was feasible and effective in preventing falls in the elderly with chronic diseases and high risk of falling. (Bernocchi et al., 2019) . Nurse home visits with or without alert buttons carried out for 9 months had a positive effect on seniors' perception of frailty (Favela et al., 2013).

The intervention on Home Telemonitoring has been reported in 3 studies. A study on using text messaging to monitor and encourage physical activity (Henry & Moore, 2016); another study on the use of tele-exercise, where supervised resistance exercises were performed at home for 20 to 40 minutes a day, three times a week for 12 weeks (Hong et al., 2017) and another study, the third on telemonitoring case management, for 12 months (Upatising et al., 2013).

The results of this type of intervention indicated that an SMS/MMS physical activity intervention could be administered to people with neuro-cognitive impairment. (Henry & Moore, 2016) . It allowed for the increase of skeletal muscle mass and lower limb physical functioning with a view to improving sarcopenia in community-dwelling elderly (Hong et al., 2017). Frailty and mortality decreased in fragile and at-risk patients (Upatising et al., 2013).

A systematic review and meta-analysis previously performed did not provide sufficient scientific evidence that interventions in frail seniors may be protective against the included adverse outcomes, although some findings have suggested a decrease in these adverse outcome events, such as death and hospitalization (Van der Elst et al., 2018).

Research with larger and more homogeneous samples is needed to investigate the feasibility, acceptability and effectiveness of technology-based exercise programs over longer periods for home-dwelling frail seniors. Challenges in this regard include the use of experimental designs, the development of standardized and sensitive outcome measurements and the need for interventions that can be implemented to reverse or delay disability in fragile seniors in resource-poor settings.

FINAL CONSIDERATIONS

As the population ages, the number of seniors with frailty is expected to increase worldwide, with the consequent rise in spending on health and long-term care.

Frailty is a common and important geriatric condition characterized by age-related declines in multiple physiological mechanisms, leading to increased vulnerability to stressors and increased risk of adverse health outcomes. Given its multidimensional nature, reversing frailty requires a comprehensive and multidisciplinary approach.

With this review, it was possible to identify the main contemporary ICT-based intervention programs, on prevention/reduction in community-dwelling elderly people with fragility, namely Virtual reality/Augmented reality, Multidisciplinary Home-Telehealth Program to Prevent Falls, Nurse home visits with or without alert buttons, balance training using Wii Fit, Interactive Game-Based Video Exercise on Balance and Home Telemonitoring.

Most studies have shown evidence of the effectiveness of ICT programs for reversing or delaying disability in frail older adults, with positive effects on balance improvement, postural control, gait, cognition, quality of life and reduced frailty, the risk of falling and the incidence of falling, hospitalizations as well as mortality.

The limitations of the current SR, regarding content, lie in the variability of interventions and the sample, making the comparability of results difficult. Regarding the methodology, the limitations are related to the reduced data sources consulted. In addition, the languages in which most studies are presented require greater efforts for interpretation. However, it is considered that SR supports the construction of a protocol for the Alentejo region. Thus, it was timely, as knowledge about ICT use increased and perhaps by highlighting the gains, contributed to reduce frailty in the elderly, who live in the community.

REFERENCES

Amorim, J. S., Leite, R. C., Brizola, R., & Yonamine, C. Y. (2018). Virtual reality therapy for rehabilitation of balance in the elderly: a systematic review and META-analysis. *Advances in Rheumatology, 58.*

Andrew, M. K., Dupuis-Blanchard, S., Maxwell, C., Giguere, A., Keefe, J., Rockwood, K., & St John, P. (2018). Social and societal implications of frailty, including impact on Canadian healthcare systems. *The Journal of Frailty & Aging*, *7*(4), 217–223. doi:10.14283/jfa.2018.30 PMID:30298169

Bernocchi, P., Giordano, A., Pintavalle, G., Galli, T., Ballini Spoglia, E., Baratti, D., & Scalvini, S. (2019). Feasibility and Clinical Efficacy of a Multidisciplinary Home-Telehealth Program to Prevent Falls in Older Adults: A Randomized Controlled Trial. *Journal of the American Medical Directors Association*, *20*(3), 340–346. doi:10.1016/j.jamda.2018.09.003 PMID:30366759

Cacciata, M., Stromberg, A., Lee, J. A., Sorkin, D., Lombardo, D., Clancy, S., ... Evangelista, L. S. (2019). Effect of exergaming on health-related quality of life in older adults: A systematic review. *International Journal of Nursing Studies*, *93*, 30–40. doi:10.1016/j.ijnurstu.2019.01.010 PMID:30861452

Chen, Y. R., & Schulz, P. J. (2016). The Effect of Information Communication Technology Interventions on Reducing Social Isolation in the Elderly: A Systematic Review. *Journal of Medical Internet Research*, *18*(1), e18. doi:10.2196/jmir.4596 PMID:26822073

Favela, J., Castro, L. A., Franco-Marina, F., Sánchez-García, S., Juárez-Cedillo, T., Espinel Bermudez, C., ... García-Peña, C. (2013). Nurse home visits with or without alert buttons versus usual care in the frail elderly: A randomized controlled trial. *Clinical Interventions in Aging*, *8*, 85–95. doi:10.2147/CIA.S38618 PMID:23378751

Fonseca, A. (2018). *Boas práticas de Aging in Place. Divulgar para valorizar. Guia de boas práticas*. Lisboa: Fundação Calouste Gulbenkian / Faculdade de Educação e Psicologia — Universidade Católica Portuguesa.

Fu, A. S., Gao, K. L., Tung, A. K., Tsang, W. W., & Kwan, M. M. (2015). Effectiveness of Exergaming Training in Reducing Risk and Incidence of Falls in Frail Older Adults With a History of Falls. *Archives of Physical Medicine and Rehabilitation, 96*(12), 2096–2102. doi:10.1016/j.apmr.2015.08.427 PMID:26360975

Gobbens, R. J., Luijkx, K. G., Wijnen-Sponselee, M. T., & Schols, J. M. (2010). Towards an integral conceptual model of frailty. *The Journal of Nutrition, Health & Aging, 14*(3), 175–181. doi:10.100712603-010-0045-6 PMID:20191249

Golla, A., Muller, T., Wohlfarth, K., Jahn, P., Mattukat, K., & Mau, W. (2018). Home-based balance training using Wii Fit: A pilot randomised controlled trial with mobile older stroke survivors. *Pilot and Feasibility Studies, 4*(1), 143. doi:10.118640814-018-0334-0 PMID:30155268

Gomes, G. C. V., Simoes, M. D. S., Lin, S. M., Bacha, J. M. R., Viveiro, L. A. P., Varise, E. M., ... Pompeu, J. E. (2018). Feasibility, safety, acceptability, and functional outcomes of playing Nintendo Wii Fit Plus(TM) for frail older adults: A randomized feasibility clinical trial. *Maturitas, 118*, 20–28. doi:10.1016/j.maturitas.2018.10.002 PMID:30415751

Gouveia, B. R., Gouveia, É. R., Ihle, A., Jardim, H. G., Martins, M. M., Freitas, D. L., & Kliegel, M. (2018). The effect of the ProBalance Programme on health-related quality of life of community-dwelling older adults: A randomised controlled trial. *Archives of Gerontology and Geriatrics, 74*, 26–31. doi:10.1016/j.archger.2017.08.012 PMID:28941936

Greenhalgh, T., Procter, R., Wherton, J., Sugarhood, P., Hinder, S., & Rouncefield, M. (2015). What is quality in assisted living technology? The ARCHIE framework for effective telehealth and telecare services. *BMC Medicine, 13*(1), 91. doi:10.118612916-015-0279-6 PMID:25902803

Henry, B. L., & Moore, D. J. (2016). Preliminary Findings Describing Participant Experience With iSTEP, an mHealth Intervention to Increase Physical Activity and Improve Neurocognitive Function in People Living With HIV. *J Assoc Nurses AIDS Care, 27*(4), 495–511. doi:10.1016/j.jana.2016.01.001 PMID:26847379

Higgins, J., & Green, S. (2008). *Cochrane handbook for systematic reviews of interventions*. West Sussex: John Wiley & Sons Ltd. doi:10.1002/9780470712184

Hong, J., Kim, J., Kim, S. W., & Kong, H. J. (2017). Effects of home-based tele-exercise on sarcopenia among community-dwelling elderly adults: Body composition and functional fitness. *Exp Gerontol, 87*(Pt A), 33-39. doi:10.1016/j.exger.2016.11.002

Hung, E. S., Chen, S. C., Chang, F. C., Shiao, Y., Peng, C. W., & Lai, C. H. (2019). Effects of Interactive Video Game-Based Exercise on Balance in Diabetic Patients with Peripheral Neuropathy: An Open-Level, Crossover Pilot Study. *Evidence-based complementary and alternative medicine: eCAM, 2019*, 4540709. doi:10.1155/2019/4540709

Hung, E. S.-W., Chen, S.-C., Chang, F.-C., Shiao, Y., Peng, C.-W., & Lai, C.-H. (2019). Effects of Interactive Video Game-Based Exercise on Balance in Diabetic Patients with Peripheral Neuropathy: An Open-Level, Crossover Pilot Study. *Evidence-based complementary and alternative medicine: eCAM, 2019*, 4540709. doi:10.1155/2019/4540709

Hung, J. W., Yu, M. Y., Chang, K. C., Lee, H. C., Hsieh, Y. W., & Chen, P. C. (2016). Feasibility of Using Tetrax Biofeedback Video Games for Balance Training in Patients With Chronic Hemiplegic Stroke. *PM & R, 8*(10), 962–970. doi:10.1016/j.pmrj.2016.02.009 PMID:26968609

JBI. (2011). *Joanna Briggs Institute Reviewers' Manual.* Adelaide: The Joanna Briggs Institute. University of Adelaide.

Kamińska, M. S., Miller, A., Rotter, I., Szylińska, A., & Grochans, E. (2018). The effectiveness of virtual reality training in reducing the risk of falls among elderly people. *Clinical Interventions in Aging, 13*, 2329–2338. doi:10.2147/CIA.S183502 PMID:30532523

Lee, C.-H., Kim, Y., & Lee, B.-H. (2014). Augmented reality-based postural control training improves gait function in patients with stroke: Randomized controlled trial. *Hong Kong Physiotherapy Journal, 32*(2), 51–57. doi:10.1016/j.hkpj.2014.04.002

Magalhaes, K. A., Giacomin, K. C., dos Santos, W. J., & Firmo, J. O. (2015). A visita domiciliária do agente comunitário de saúde a famílias com idosos frágeis. *Ciencia & Saude Coletiva, 20*(12), 3787–3796. doi:10.1590/1413-812320152012.07622014 PMID:26691803

Marek, K. D., Stetzer, F., Adams, S. J., Popejoy, L. L., & Rantz, M. (2012). Aging in place versus nursing home care: Comparison of costs to Medicare and Medicaid. *Research in Gerontological Nursing, 5*(2), 123–129. doi:10.3928/19404921-20110802-01 PMID:21846081

Matthew-Maich, N., Harris, L., Ploeg, J., Markle-Reid, M., Valaitis, R., Ibrahim, S., ... Isaacs, S. (2016). Designing, Implementing, and Evaluating Mobile Health Technologies for Managing Chronic Conditions in Older Adults: A Scoping Review. *JMIR mHealth and uHealth*, *4*(2), e29. doi:10.2196/mhealth.5127 PMID:27282195

Padala, K. P., Padala, P. R., Lensing, S. Y., Dennis, R. A., Bopp, M. M., Parkes, C. M., ... Sullivan, D. H. (2017). Efficacy of Wii-Fit on Static and Dynamic Balance in Community Dwelling Older Veterans: A Randomized Controlled Pilot Trial. *Journal of Aging Research*, *4653635*, 1–9. doi:10.1155/2017/4653635 PMID:28261500

Puts, M. T. E., Toubasi, S., Andrew, M. K., Ashe, M. C., Ploeg, J., Atkinson, E., ... McGilton, K. (2017). Interventions to prevent or reduce the level of frailty in community-dwelling older adults: A scoping review of the literature and international policies. *Age and Ageing*, *46*(3), 383–392. doi:10.1093/ageing/afw247 PMID:28064173

RNAO. (2007). *Falls Prevention. Building the Foundations for Patient Safety. Self-Learning Package*. Ontario: Nurses' Association of Ontario.

Rockwood, K., Fox, R. A., Stolee, P., Robertson, D., & Beattie, B. L. (1994). Frailty in elderly people: An evolving concept. *Canadian Medical Association Journal*, *150*(4), 489–495. PMID:8313261

Santos, G. O. R., Wolf, R., Silva, M. M., Rodacki, A. L. F., & Pereira, G. (2019). Does exercise intensity increment in exergame promote changes in strength, functional capacity and perceptual parameters in pre-frail older women? A randomized controlled trial. *Experimental Gerontology*, *116*, 25–30. doi:10.1016/j.exger.2018.12.009 PMID:30553026

Skjaeret, N., Nawaz, A., Morat, T., Schoene, D., Helbostad, J. L., & Vereijken, B. (2016). Exercise and rehabilitation delivered through exergames in older adults: An integrative review of technologies, safety and efficacy. *International Journal of Medical Informatics*, *85*(1), 1–16. doi:10.1016/j.ijmedinf.2015.10.008 PMID:26559887

Sousa, L. M., Firmino, C. F., Marques-Vieira, C. M., Severino, S., & Pestana, H. C. (2018). Revisões da literatura científica: Tipos, métodos e aplicações em enfermagem. *Revista Portuguesa de Enfermagem de Reabilitação*, *1*(1), 46–55.

Straudi, S., Severini, G., Sabbagh Charabati, A., Pavarelli, C., Gamberini, G., Scotti, A., & Basaglia, N. (2017). The effects of video game therapy on balance and attention in chronic ambulatory traumatic brain injury: An exploratory study. *BMC Neurology*, *17*(1), 86–86. doi:10.118612883-017-0871-9 PMID:28490322

Szturm, T., Betker, A. L., Moussavi, Z., Desai, A., & Goodman, V. (2011). Effects of an interactive computer game exercise regimen on balance impairment in frail community-dwelling older adults: A randomized controlled trial. *Physical Therapy*, *91*(10), 1449–1462. doi:10.2522/ptj.20090205 PMID:21799138

Thomas, E., Battaglia, G., Patti, A., Brusa, J., Leonardi, V., Palma, A., & Bellafiore, M. (2019). Physical activity programs for balance and fall prevention in elderly: A systematic review. *Medicine*, *98*(27), e16218. doi:10.1097/MD.0000000000016218 PMID:31277132

Upatising, B., Hanson, G. J., Kim, Y. L., Cha, S. S., Yih, Y., & Takahashi, P. Y. (2013). Effects of home telemonitoring on transitions between frailty states and death for older adults: A randomized controlled trial. *International Journal of General Medicine*, *6*, 145–151. doi:10.2147/IJGM.S40576 PMID:23525664

Valenzuela, T., Okubo, Y., Woodbury, A., Lord, S. R., & Delbaere, K. (2018). Adherence to Technology-Based Exercise Programs in Older Adults: A Systematic Review. *Journal of Geriatric Physical Therapy*, *41*(1), 49–61. doi:10.1519/JPT.0000000000000095 PMID:27362526

Van der Elst, M., Schoenmakers, B., Duppen, D., Lambotte, D., Fret, B., Vaes, B., & De Lepeleire, J. (2018). Interventions for frail community-dwelling older adults have no significant effect on adverse outcomes: A systematic review and meta-analysis. *BMC Geriatrics*, *18*(1), 249. doi:10.118612877-018-0936-7 PMID:30342479

Vilelas, J. (2017). *Investigação. O processo de construção do conhecimento*. Lisboa: Edições Sílabo.

WHO. (2015). *World report on ageing and health*. Geneve: World Health Organization.

Yang, W. C., Wang, H. K., Wu, R. M., Lo, C. S., & Lin, K. H. (2016). Home-based virtual reality balance training and conventional balance training in Parkinson's disease: A randomized controlled trial. *Journal of the Formosan Medical Association*, *115*(9), 734–743. doi:10.1016/j.jfma.2015.07.012 PMID:26279172

Chapter 8
Technology to Improve Elderly Nutrition:
An Approach From Social Science

Borja Rivero Jiménez
https://orcid.org/0000-0002-3691-0968
Universidad de Extremadura, Spain

David Conde Caballero
https://orcid.org/0000-0002-5967-4371
Universidad de Extremadura, Spain

Beatriz Muñoz González
Universidad de Extremadura, Spain

Lorenzo Mariano Juarez
Universidad de Extremadura, Spain

ABSTRACT

The ageing of the population is one of the main emerging problems for this century. Knowledge and understanding of the food ideologies and practices of this adult population is a vital issue in health policies and interventions. With the traditional tools and assumptions of ethnographic fieldwork, the research is oriented towards a series of objectives in order to complete the limited knowledge on these issues. Through some of the categories that emerge from the fieldwork, the authors analyze the ideology, practices, and representations on food in the adult population and try to propose some spaces from where technology can work on solutions.

DOI: 10.4018/978-1-7998-1937-0.ch008

INTRODUCTION

The ageing of the population emerges as a central theme in public policies at the end of the last century and is presented as a challenge to be faced effectively in the 21st century. Average life expectancy in Spain has risen to unprecedented levels, where we have doubled the figure in just four generations. The main causes pointed out in this change are related to the intense fall in mortality as a consequence of the improvement in the health conditions of the population, which are based above all on a better quality of nutrition and universal health care. It was unthinkable at the beginning of the last century to live well beyond the age of 40; today our life expectancy has increased to such an extent that people aged 65 and over already account for 18.7% (8,701,380 people) of the entire population (INE, 2014). By the year 2064, according to the National Statistics Institute (Abellán García, Rodríguez-Laso, Pujol Rodríguez, & Barrios, 2017), more than 33% of the population of developed countries will be over 65, 38.7%; in the case of Spain, reaching 222,000 centenarians compared to 12,000 today.

The implications of these population dynamics are the subject of discussion due to their evident impact on aspects such as labour relations, health and welfare systems and pension policy, but also on social aspects such as family models or the social construction of feelings. The challenges posed by this scenario are huge and are aggravated in some regions of Europe - such as Alentejo in Portugal or Extremadura in Spain - where movements of urban concentration converge in processes of depopulation of the rural milieu, inhabited mainly by elderly people who are getting older and alone. According to IMSERSO (Instituto de Mayores y Servicios Sociales, 2015), in 2014 older people represented 27.9% of the population of municipalities with less than 2,000 inhabitants, a figure that reached up to 40% in some localities of Extremadura (INE, 2018).

It is a question of vital relevance in health policies and interventions to reach knowledge and understanding of food ideologies and practices that underlie this type of adult population. There seems to be some consensus in the scientific literature in pointing out the relationship between food and quality of life (Arbonés et al., 2003; Schneider, 2006; World Health Organization, 2003). In the case of the elderly, in particular, the particular vulnerability of both nutrition and food is often underlined. Some authors agree that this is a major public health problem (Brownie, 2006; DiMaria-Ghalili & Amella, 2005; Seiler, 1999). Despite this, the available literature on ageing and nutrition has had a bias that has revolved around the analysis of specific health problems or has focused on institutionalized settings. We know very little about the practices and ideologies of older people living in rural areas. We cannot forget at this time that food and nutrition are truly complex and multidimensional domains. When defining the determinants in the construction of ideologies around food or the representations of what is or is not a healthy food, they can be defined on the basis of physical and psychological aspects, but we cannot forget those social and cultural (Chen, Schilling, & Lyder, 2001; Pirlich & Lochs, 2001). Therefore, these emerge as first-rate attitudinal determinants in defining how older people are fed.

OBJECTIVES AND METHOD

1. Our research sets a series of objectives that aim to broaden the knowledge on the above mentioned topics. From articulated approaches on the impact of culture, the objectives we set ourselves are the following:
   a. To know the nutritional situation of the elderly population in rural areas.
   b. Describe cultural food practices and their association with ideologies, representations, supply and availability systems, economic issues and other elements that build food security in the areas of study.
   c. To relate technological innovation with the findings of our empirical research, both at the level of production or analysis and in the evaluation of the proposed theoretical models.

The qualitative research presented here is linked to traditional ethnographic fieldwork tools and assumptions (Hammersley & Atkinson, 1994; Velasco & Díaz de Rada, 2006). The set of localities that compose the object of study is located in the southwest of Spain, specifically the municipalities of Campillo de Deleitosa, Garciaz and Casares de Hurdes, in the province of Cáceres, and Garlitos and Malcocinado, belonging to the province of Badajoz, all of them in Extremadura. The municipalities have been selected on the basis of indicators that indicate specific characteristics: they are small populations (less than 1000 inhabitants) with a high rate of ageing, in contexts with difficulties of access to health resources, social services and food supply. The research techniques we intend to apply are described below. We point out the research technique used and the types of materials we are producing.

- In-depth interviews: Narratives with interview responses according to the worked semi-structured interview model
- Mapping and observation: Map and register of supply spaces, practices on this process, storage, preparation (cooking techniques, instruments...) and food consumption. Description of the food process with emphasis on the difficulties and limitations.
- Informal Conversations: Informal conversations, not always recorded, to improve the interview script and provide other empirical material.

- Focus group: Opinions, beliefs, perceptions, interests and attitudes regarding "appropriate" and "healthy" ways of eating.
- 24h menú recall: Standardized questionnaire with adaptations to the particularities of field work.
- Observation of food practices: Participant observation of practices and field diary entries.
- Household food inventories: Description of standard diet, collection of shopping lists, photographs of refrigerators, kitchens, preparation mode.

MAIN FOCUS OF THE CHAPTER

Some Categories of Analysis

This project offers an optimal space for joint and collaborative research in different fields and disciplines of knowledge. By way of example, we can describe here some of the categories of analysis in which we are working.

First of all, one of the main problems we have encountered in the field work is access to food for the elderly. There is some consensus on the definition of food access and storage as a central pillar of community food security (Godfray et al., 2010; Schmidhuber & Tubiello, 2007). Many studies have sought to delimit this issue around economic variables, where access restrictions are based exclusively on household income calculations. This, being a correct and very valid approach in our research context, is not limited to being the only one on which we should focus our attention. In the villages of our research there is an important limitation in the supply, with localities that do not have stores or supermarkets and need to travel several kilometers to be able to make this food supply. The circulation of food - "the field of the edible" - is conditioned from a structural framework, limiting the supply to private initiatives of itinerant sale. We must therefore bear in mind that the social construction of taste is thus based on complex relations between the ideological and the material.

In the same category of analysis, it should be remembered that trips to collection centres are usually defined in universal terms: distance from the house to the shop. However, these data require a more particular analysis, given the specificity of the population in areas where levels of functionality or dependence are different from those of the majority of the population, mainly due to the high degree of ageing population. As these variables in these domains change, so does distance, increasing in many cases. We also need to look at the statistics more closely. There are data available that could tell us whether or not a family has a vehicle. In any case, at the micro level, we need to know the use that the person in charge of purchasing food can make of this vehicle. In the case of the elderly rural context of Extremadura, women have a much more limited capacity for use. In the fieldwork we have been able to see how the use of the vehicle for female activities - the purchase would still fall within the responsibility of women today - is subordinated to other male uses, such as going to the "bar". Statistics and figures must incorporate the concept of agency into the equation.

Food decisions, which have such a great impact on the health of populations, are not only limited by purely material aspects. On the contrary, it is crucial to know the ideologies and their construction processes, the second major category we face here. We need to answer the question of what, but above all how and why. It has been studied, for example, how the media play a crucial role in this regard through the dissemination of information and knowledge. This is so much so that the dissemination of information on medicine, public health and nutrition sciences through these media is an area of concern for many health and social scientists (Fineberg & Rowe, 1998; Hackman & Moe, 1999; Maheshwar, Narender, Balakrishna, & Rao, 2018), who point out how in many cases they contribute to the creation of myths or the propagation of misconceptions.

The current level of analysis allows us to affirm that the notion of "healthy" of this population group is far from medical and nutritional prescriptions. We need to provide data that not only show the gap, but also provide explanations to clarify these construction processes.

SOLUTIONS AND RECOMMENDATIONS

In our study, interdisciplinary work is also crucial in the diagnostic phase. We work on the mapping of study areas with a variable representation of distances and difficulties depending on factors such as functionality, but also social position or gender. Our intention is to offer tools that allow to visualize existing problems in a more precise way. This interdisciplinary relationship between social sciences and technology can also be seen in the collaborative work on technological research tools. Some of the ones we're working on would be:

- **Application to Improve Food Studies:** We are currently working on the design of an application to improve food studies, to speed up data collection, including descriptions of observation units. This app -called "Feedelio"- has been developed on the Android platform. It has been optimized to work in versions equal or superior to API 22, that is to say, Android 5.1. This translates into compatibility with 80.2% of Android devices. In it, we have looked for a useful application in the field work, for which we have minimized to the maximum the number of windows as well as clicks. The addition options fall only on a floating button that remains visible. The root element would always be the "Research", from which one would access the set of "observations" and that of "informants" that would form part of the ethnography. Each informant would be interviewed obtaining the information in different sets: 24 Recall Menu; anthropometric data or audio or video recording of the interview.

- **Structural constraints:** the consumption of fresh food, such as fish, for example - constitute a space where technological proposals can be developed to improve the diet of the elderly in these villages. During our conversations with some of the street food sellers, they admitted that they carried what they knew they could sell, underlining the capacity of the buyers to delimit their sale. This does not mean that this is a statement that is completely in line with reality. The sale of non-perishable products implies a lower risk for the entrepreneurs, who would assume with it lower losses. However, we could work on systems that allow us to define purchase lists of fresh products that do not imply a risk for business investment or to articulate actions from the administration to overcome these logistical problems. Technology has a lot of space to work here.

But there are also many more possibilities. From the analysis of food ideologies and practices we can take a first step for technologists to provide solutions that affect these construction processes. For example, if low liquid consumption is detected, technologists could provide solutions that allow, for example, reminders through messages on electronic devices. If we detect that health education in nutritional terms is not achieving its objective, the joint effort with technologists can define new tools or new languages to build these health education messages. Today it is not uncommon to talk about electronic prescriptions, just as there is already much scientific production on the reach of the mobile phone as a communication tool between health professionals and the population (Coiera, 2006; Perera, 2012; R. C. Wu et al., 2010; R. Wu et al., 2011). Some studies have shown its capacity to improve the quality of life of older people, to the extent that it has been used as a communication tool in health education or in the prevention of problems associated with pathologies such as diabetes or vascular problems (Melanson, 2010; Tucker et al., 2010).

CONCLUSION

The work on food and the ageing of the population in rural areas seems today inseparable from the contributions that can be made from technological innovation. We have referred here to aspects of the production of empirical materials, but social approaches and methodologies can also contribute to the analysis and evaluation of these technological solutions. In this sense, it is necessary to take into account the specificities of our study population, but it is also true that technological solutions must be adapted, not limiting themselves to the "known space", but to what is about to be developed. When we conclude our research, there may be new forms of food prescribing in which health professionals can control a family's diet by helping them choose the healthiest option.

Finally, the intersections between sociocultural approaches and technology come from the field of interventions. Technological proposals can be successful and attractive in laboratories, but they need to be functional in real life. Thus, the relationship between technology and society is crossed by factors such as age, rurality index or gender. Therefore, ethnographic research will allow the analysis of microsocial contexts that provide us with information and define possible problems derived from uses, or what is the same, and following Lowrie (Lowrie, 2018), we will try to understand how technology is articulated within social processes and the effect it has (or could have).

ACKNOWLEDGMENT

This work was supported by the 4IE project (0499_4IE_4_PLUS_4_E) funded by the Interreg V-A España-Portugal (POCTEP) 2014-2020 program.

REFERENCES

Abellán García, A., Rodríguez-Laso, A., Pujol Rodríguez, R., & Barrios, L. (2017). *12.000 centenarios en 2017 en España, ¿222.000 en 2066?* Retrieved October 15, 2018, from http://envejecimientoenred.es/centenarios_en_espana/

Arbonés, G., Carbajal, A., Gonzalvo, B., González-Gross, M., Joyanes, M., Marques-Lopes, I., ... Vaquero, M. P. (2003). Nutrición y recomendaciones dietéticas para personas mayores. *Nutrición Hospitalaria, 18*(3), 109–137. PMID:12875088

Brownie, S. (2006). Why are elderly individuals at risk of nutritional deficiency? *International Journal of Nursing Practice, 12*(2), 110–118. doi:10.1111/j.1440-172X.2006.00557.x PMID:16529597

Chen, C. C. H., Schilling, L. S., & Lyder, C. H. (2001). A concept analysis of malnutrition in the elderly. *Journal of Advanced Nursing, 36*(1), 131–142. doi:10.1046/j.1365-2648.2001.01950.x PMID:11555057

Coiera, E. (2006). Communication systems in healthcare. *The Clinical Biochemist., 27*(2), 89–98. Retrieved from https://www.ncbi.nlm.nih.gov/pubmed/17077879

DiMaria-Ghalili, R. A., & Amella, E. (2005). Nutrition in older adults. *The American Journal of Nursing, 105*(3), 40–50. doi:10.1097/00000446-200503000-00020 PMID:15729041

Fineberg, H. V., & Rowe, S. (1998). *Improving Public Understanding : Guidelines for Communicating Emerging Science on Nutririon, Food Safety, and Health.* Academic Press.

Godfray, H. C. J., Beddington, J. R., Crute, I. R., Haddad, L., Lawrence, D., Muir, J. F., ... Toulmin, C. (2010, February 12). Food security: The challenge of feeding 9 billion people. *Science, 327*(5967), 812–818. doi:10.1126cience.1185383 PMID:20110467

Hackman, E. M., & Moe, G. L. (1999). Evaluation of newspaper reports of nutrition-related research. *Journal of the American Dietetic Association, 99*(12), 1564–1566. doi:10.1016/S0002-8223(99)00384-3 PMID:10608952

Hammersley, M., & Atkinson, P. (1994). *Etnografía.* Barcelona: Métodos de Investigación. Paidós.

INE. (2014). Proyección de la Población de España 2014-2064: Notas de prensa. In Instituto Nacional de Estadística (INE). doi:10.1017/CBO9781107415324.004

INE. (2018). Encuesta continua de hogares. *Instituto Nacional de Estadística (INE).* https://www.ine.es/dyngs/INEbase/es/operacion.htm?c=Estadistica_C&cid=1254736176952&menu=ultiDatos&idp=1254735572981

Instituto de Mayores y Servicios Sociales (IMSERSO). (2015). *Informe 2014.* Las Personas Mayores en España.

Lowrie, I. (2018). Algorithms and Automation: An Introduction. *Cultural Anthropology, 33*(3), 349–359. doi:10.14506/ca33.3.01

Maheshwar, M., Narender, K., Balakrishna, N., & Rao, D. (2018). Teenagers Understanding and Influence of Media Content on their Diet and Health- Related Behaviour. *Journal of Clinical Nutrition & Dietetics*, *04*(02). doi:10.4172/2472-1921.100071

Melanson, D. (2010). *Sanofi-Aventis debuts iBGStar blood glucose meter for iPhone*. Retrieved October 15, 2018, from https://www.engadget.com/2010/09/21/sanofi-aventis-debuts-ibgstar-blood-glucose-meter-for-iphone/?guccounter=1

Perera, C. (2012). The Evolution of E-Health – Mobile Technology and mHealth. *Journal of Mobile Technology in Medicine*, *1*(1), 1–2. doi:10.7309/jmtm.1

Pirlich, M., & Lochs, H. (2001). Nutrition in the elderly. *Best Practice & Research. Clinical Gastroenterology*, *15*(6), 869–884. doi:10.1053/bega.2001.0246 PMID:11866482

Schmidhuber, J., & Tubiello, F. N. (2007). Global food security under climate change. *Proceedings of the National Academy of Sciences of the United States of America*, *104*(50), 19703–19708. doi:10.1073/pnas.0701976104 PMID:18077404

Schneider, M. (2006). Public health and the aging population. In *Introduction to public health* (2nd ed.). Academic Press.

Carneiro, I., De, D. C., & De Souza, R. (2013). *A Etnografia : Um Modo De Entender a Alimentação*. Academic Press.

Pettigrew, S., Worrall, C., Biagioni, N., Talati, Z., & Jongenelis, M. (2017). The role of food shopping in later life. *Appetite*, *111*, 71–78.

Seiler, W. O. (1999). Nutritional status of ill elderly patients. *Zeitschrift für Gerontologie und Geriatrie*, *32*(S1), I7–I11. doi:10.1007003910050174 PMID:10441797

Tucker, A. T., Maass, A., Bain, D. S., Chen, L. H., Azzam, M., Dawson, H., & Johnston, A. (2010). Augmentation of venous, arterial and microvascular blood supply in the leg by isometric neuromuscular stimulation via the peroneal nerve. *The International Journal of Angiology*, *19*(1), 31–37. doi:10.1055-0031-1278361 PMID:22477572

Velasco, H., & Díaz de Rada, A. (2006). *La Lógica de La Investigación Etnográfica*. Madrid: Trotta.

World Health Organization. (2003). *Diet, nutrition and the prevention of chronic diseases*. Geneva: WHO.

Wu, R., Rossos, P., Quan, S., Reeves, S., Lo, V., Wong, B., & Morra, D. (2011). An evaluation of the use of smartphones to communicate between clinicians: A mixed-methods study. *Journal of Medical Internet Research, 13*(3), e59. doi:10.2196/jmir.1655 PMID:21875849

Wu, R. C., Morra, D., Quan, S., Lai, S., Zanjani, S., Abrams, H., & Rossos, P. G. (2010). The use of smartphones for clinical communication on internal medicine wards. *Journal of Hospital Medicine, 5*(9), 553–559. doi:10.1002/jhm.775 PMID:20690190

Chapter 9
Interconnecting IoT Devices to Improve the QoL of Elderly People

Daniel Flores-Martin
Universidad de Extremadura, Spain

Alejandro Pérez-Vereda
University of Málaga, Spain

Javier Berrocal
https://orcid.org/0000-0002-1007-2134
University of Extremadura, Spain

Carlos Canal
University of Málaga, Spain

Juan M. Murillo
Universidad de Extremadura, Spain

ABSTRACT

The rate at which the internet is growing is unstoppable due to the large number of connected smart devices. Manufacturers often develop specific protocols for their own devices that do not usually follow any standards. This hinders the interconnection and coordination of devices from different manufacturers, limiting the number of daily activities that can be supported. Some works are proposing different techniques to reduce this barrier and avoid the vendor lock-in issue. Nevertheless, this interconnection should also depend on the context. In this chapter, the authors

DOI: 10.4018/978-1-7998-1937-0.ch009

propose a system to dynamically identify the interconnections required each specific situation depending on the context. This proposal has been tested in case studies focused on elderly people with the aim of automating their daily tasks and improving their quality of life. Further, in a world with an accelerated population aging, there is an increasing interest on developing solutions for the elderly living assistance through IoT systems.

INTRODUCTION

The Internet of Things (IoT) is becoming more and more important. This is due to the large amount of smart devices that are being developed. Recent studies estimate that by 2020 there will be 20-30 billion devices connected to the Internet (Nordrum, 2016; IronPaper, 2015). These devices can be applied for a multitude of fields such as smart cities, agriculture, automotive or healthcare (Haluza & Jungwirth, 2015). The purpose of these devices is to make people's lives easier by automating tasks or helping users to perform them. In healthcare, the IoT paradigm allows more personalized, collaborative and preventive care, where patients are able to monitor and manage their own health. Besides, the responsibility for healthcare is shared between patients and medical staff (Metcalf, Milliard, Gomez, & Schwartz, 2016). These solutions are particularly interesting, mainly due to limited resources or difficult access to them if we consider the ageing of the population and the depopulation of rural areas.

IoT devices can perform simple tasks such as monitoring blood pressure or glucose level, performing periodic reminders, enhancing drug management or notifying of certain events. These tasks are useful but the real potential of IoT devices lies in the interconnection between them to collaborate and to perform more complex tasks. Due to the great heterogeneity of devices on the market, where there are many different manufacturers and devices, this interconnection is not easy. In order to achieve this interconnection, each manufacturer usually develops its own communication protocols. This means that there is no defined communication standard and the risk of vendor lock-in increases. This phenomenon conditions users to acquire devices from the same manufacturers in order to achieve total compatibility, also complicating the possible migration to another in the future (Roman, Zhou, & Lopez, 2013), and even to set manually each device, something that can be tedious for people who do not have a certain technical knowledge.

Different works have promoted alternative methods to make IoT devices work with each other, such as specific frameworks, such as (Shrestha, Kubler, & Främling, 2014), where a framework is developed to integrate specific domain applications into IoT, or (Kim et al., 2016), which presents interfaces and interconnection procedures based on oneM2M (Swetina, Lu, Jacobs, Ennesser, & Song, 2014). The use of ontologies and the Semantic Web are also becoming very important to solve these interconnection problems (Szilagyi & Wira, 2016). The main objective of the Semantic Web is to improve the Internet by extending interoperability between computer systems using smart agents and applications that seek information without human intervention (Barnaghi, Wang, Henson, & Taylor, 2012). These works help to solve the problem of device interconnection, but it is not an easy task, because technological diversity of smart devices must be taken into account, as well as the correct handling of the context, which is not always considered.

Besides, the development of context-sensitive software has proved successful (Perera, Zaslavsky, Christen, & Georgakopoulos, 2014). IoT devices are becoming intelligent thanks to the information gathered about the context in which they are located, from near people or other devices. In order to reduce the interaction among people and devices, this interconnection must be adapted to the context. These drawbacks can be addressed by developing software capable of adapting its behaviour to people's needs (Perera et al., 2014; Taivalsaari & Mikkonen, 2017). In this way, several research areas can contribute to provide this adaptation, such us Context Oriented Programming (COP), Ambient Intelligent (AmI), Semantic Web, and Machine Learning (ML). Most of these paradigms allow us to define behaviours for different scenarios at design time, so the adaptation of the devices is limited to situations that developers have been able to identify, making it impossible to adapt them to other situations that may arise from the context.

The authors of this work have proposed the Situational-Context paradigm (Berrocal, Garcia-Alonso, Canal, & Murillo, 2016), where the context is treated as a way of analyzing the conditions that exist at a particular time and place identifying people's needs. In this work, the authors present an architecture that models the Situational-Context focused on healthcare for the elderly people domain, although it can be used for another domain. In addition, it allows to obtain data from users' profile, stored in their smartphones, to use them so that IoT devices can adapt their behaviour to people's needs. This process is carried out dynamically and at runtime, due to the different possibilities that can occur in a context are innumerable. Thanks to this, IoT devices can adapt their behaviour to situations not previously predefined.

MOTIVATIONS

Nowadays, the interconnection of IoT devices to achieve a coordinated work is still a problem that prevents to exploit the full potential of IoT paradigm.

To show the impact of this problem, we are going to use a scenario based on ageing and rurality. In the rest of this chapter the proposed scenario will be used to show the benefits of our work.

Juan is a 74 years old man who lives in La Calera in the southeast of Caceres, in the Las Villuercas Mountains. This morning, Juan went for a walk with his friend Emilio. They both have their mobile phones with them. Since the village is running out of inhabitants and they are getting older, their sons and daughters always ask them not to go out without their mobile phones in case something happens to them. Juan and Emilio are not aware of this, but their mobile phones can do much more than receive calls from their children. In addition, these devices are recording where they walk, where are them, with whom they are and are detecting each other so that their phones now know they are in company (Figure 1).

Figure 1. People tracking

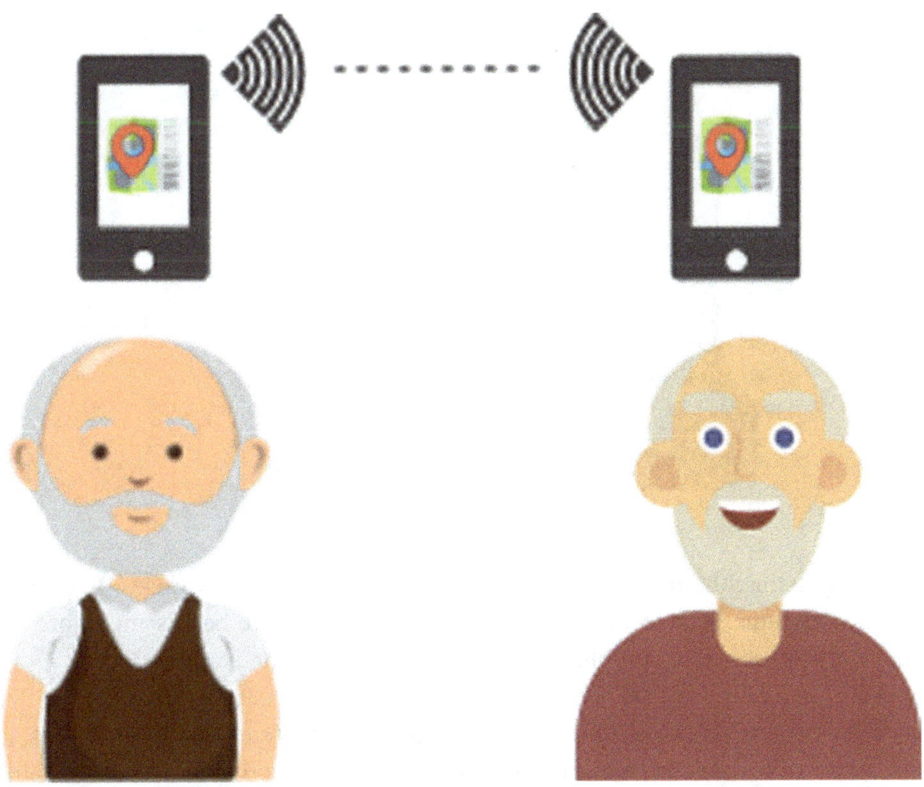

Juan has returned home and it's time to take his medicine. It is notified by the electronic pill dispenser that was given to him last month. This pill dispenser has also detected that there are no pills left for the next day (Figure 2). It is very important that Juan does not stop his heart treatment. Although his smartphone made the electronic prescription request, they were unable to bring his medication. There seems to have been a mistake at the pharmacy in Guadalupe. Fortunately, Emilio takes the same medication as Juan and received it last week. Juan and Emilio have received

Figure 2. Pill reminder

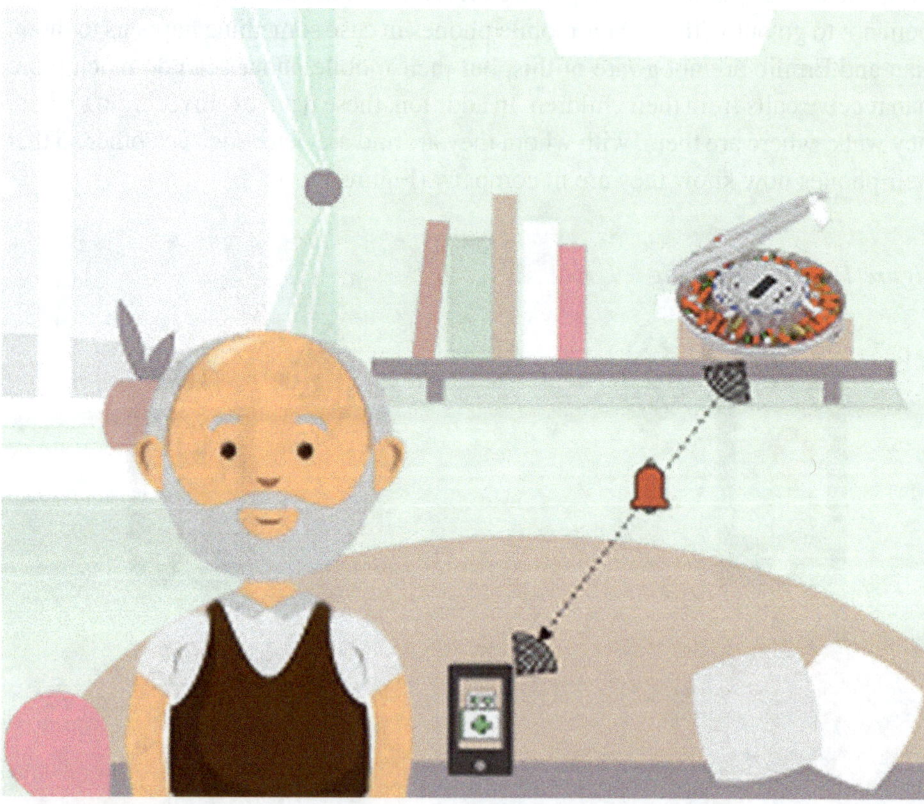

a message telling them that tomorrow Emilio must give Juan two doses (Figure 3).

The Semantic Web techniques and frameworks that have been seen before are not enough to solve this problem, since context information is needed.

This use case shows the need to interconnect different devices. In addition, this interconnection depends on the contextual information that surrounds the devices, so that all possible data can be had to carry out the interconnection in the best possible

Figure 3. Doses request flow

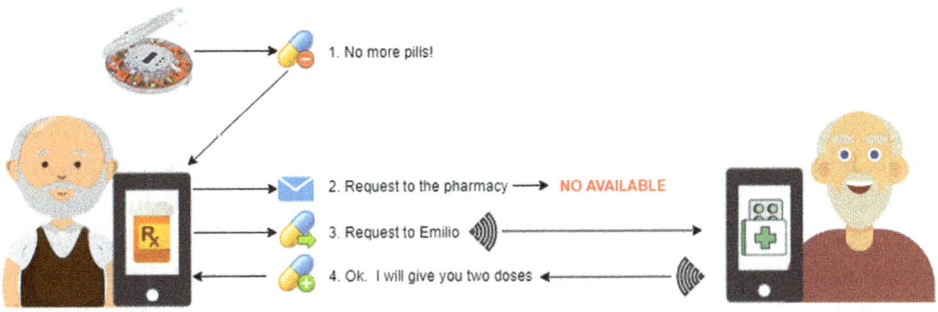

way. Therefore, we want to test the capacity of the Situational-Context to promote the generation of complex strategies that involve the orchestration of several devices.

SITUATIONAL-CONTEXT

Situational-Context is a way of analyzing the conditions that exist at a particular time and place in order to predict, at runtime, the expected IoT systems behaviour. It is composed of entities. These entities can be both IoT devices and people represented through their smartphones, indistinctly. In addition, they have two fundamental properties: *skills* and *goals*.

This model exploits the capabilities of smart devices to collect, store and calculate locally contextual information to build their virtual profile and the virtual profile of their owner. Therefore, the devices around it can reuse it to meet the user's preferences. Situational-Context defines that the virtual profile of an entity (IoT device or a person) must contain at least the following information:

- A Basic Profile that contains the raw contextual information dated with the status of the entity, the relationships with other devices and its history.
- A Social Profile. This profile contains the results of high-level inferences made on the Basic Profile.
- The Goals that details the state of the environment desired by the entity. These goals are deduced from the Basic and Social Profiles at runtime.
- The Skills that an entity has to make decisions and take actions capable of modifying the environment and aimed at achieving the goals.

Considering environments in which there are different entities and each of them has a virtual profile, Situational-Context can be defined as the composition of the virtual profiles of all entities involved in a particular situation.

Thanks to Situational-Context it is possible to analyze the context surrounding Juan and detect nearby entities, such as Emilio, or his smart pill dispenser, which can use its skill to make the electronic prescription when it detects that it is running out of doses of some type of pill, and thus be able to continue to provide Juan with his medication. In the same way, this could be applied to other entities such as Emilio (represented by his smartphone), Emilio's pill dispenser, or another IoT devices that they can have at home. Situational-Context aims, among others, to improve the QoL of people by avoiding having to invest so much time in configuring smart devices.

This paradigm has obtained previous results of interconnection of devices at the network level (Galán-Jiménez, Berrocal, Garcia-Alonso, Canal, & Murillo, 2017). We assume, therefore, that the connection through the network of IoT devices in a Situational-Context environment is feasible.

ENTITY REPRESENTATION ARCHITECTURE

Due to the detected need, we use the Situational-Context paradigm with which we intend to achieve a better interconnection of IoT devices and get the maximum benefit by adapting their behaviour to people's preferences at runtime. This favors the interaction of entities and allows them to be dependent on the context in which they are, at runtime. Its components are detailed in Figure 4.

Figure 4. Entity architecture

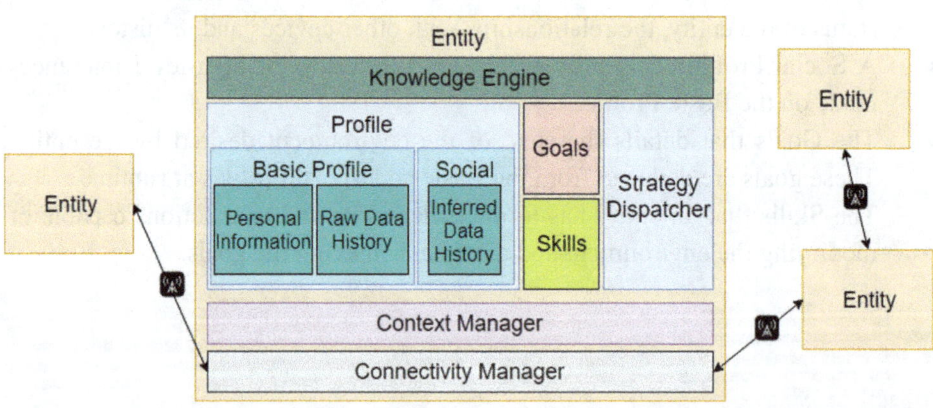

- **Connectivity Manager**: Establishes the physical connection between entities. It sends and receives information related to skills, goals, personal information, etc.
- **Context Manager**: Responsible for creating and updating contextual information. It contains the information of the entities belonging to the same situation in a given instant of time.
- **Profile**: Union of the Basic and the Social Profile of the entity.
    - **Basic Profile**: Basic information that identifies the entity, such as the identifier, manufacturer, model, date of manufacture, etc. (Personal Information). It also contains raw data about the history of interactions with other entities (Raw Data History).
    - **Social Profile**. Stores all inferred data from the basic profile (Inferred Data History). Thanks to this data, Juan's smartphone can know where Juan is moving or who he's accompanied by.
- **Skills**: Entity features. They produce a change in the context. For example, the pill dispenser can order pills from the pharmacy.
- **Goals**: They arise when one wants to obtain a state in a property of the environment that with the own capacities is not possible. For example, due to the situation that Juan's pill dispenser is empty, he must make the electronic prescription and also request some doses from his friend Emilio.
- **Strategy Dispatcher**: Devices can detect what goals there are in the environment, and which ones can be solved with their skills. A strategy is identified when it is detected how to coordinate the devices in the environment to solve the given goals. The complexity of strategies lies in the collaboration of entities to identify and solve needs. Returning to the example of Juan and Emilio, Emilio's pill dispenser must establish a strategy to give a few doses to Juan, but only if Emilio has plenty of pills.
- **Knowledge Engine**: It analyzes the history of the entity's activities to detect patterns and learn from them, with the goal of automating tasks in the future or detect routines.

This architecture achieves the interconnection of IoT devices at the features level. The interconnection is based on relating the skills of one entity with the goals of another. We know that the goals in an entity arise from the lack of skills when obtaining a desired state in the environment, so we must know how to perform this interconnection and that the goals can be resolved in the best way. Each entity has its own vision of the context, and knows the skills and goals of nearby entities, so that it can interact with them. This is achieved by integrating Situational-Context with Semantic Web and ontologies.

By looking that an ontology can represent the skills and goals of Juan's pill dispenser, we know what kind of goals could be covered by this entity. When Juan's pill dispenser detects that he has run out of pills, it interprets its social profile data and, as it knows that Emilio takes the same pills, and it can ask him for a couple of doses. In this way it will be able to automatically use its ability to cover the person need. The Semantic Web will be responsible for providing knowledge to this information, making the relationships between skills and goals are defined in a more human language, and also interpretable by machines.

To better explain the composition of the entities used in our scenario, some of the information stored in their virtual profiles is specified in Tables 1 and 2, where we can see Juan's pill dispenser and Juan, represented through his smartphone. Apart from the personal information, we observe that Juan's pill dispenser has a series of skills with which it can solve Juan's needs.

Based on the information coming from the virtual profile, each entity builds its own ontology. The purpose of this ontology is to relate the discovered entities through their skills and goals. The resolution of the goals of a given entity is to find a skill that is capable of solving it adequately. This mapping is done through simple queries with SPARQL. SPARQL is a RDF (Resource Description Framework) query

Table 1. Juan's pill dispenser

Personal info	Skills
Manufacturer - PDOne	**Pills management** - Reminder doses - Distribute - Recommendations
Model - One	
Family - HealthCare	**Pharmacy** - Request pills - Electronic receipt
Device - Pill dispenser	

Table 2. Juan

Personal info	Goals
Manufacturer - Huawei	**Pills management** - Reminder doses - Check dose amount - …
Model - P20 Lite	
Family - Smartphone - …	**Security** - Family notify - …

language and a W3C recommendation (Sirin & Parsia, 2007). RDF is a standard model for data exchange on the Web and is widely used as an organization scheme for ontologies (Lassila & Swick, 1999). Therefore, SPARQL contains capabilities to query the necessary and optional information from ontologies, and among other features, to identify which skill should be used to solve a given goal. This search is defined in a preliminary way through the name of the skill and goal. We are currently working on evolving the composition of these queries to make them more precise and complex. An example is shown below in Table 3.

Table 3. SPARQL query example

Query: context entities discovery	**Query: devices skills**	
#context devices discovery SELECT * WHERE { ? Entity a : Entity .}	# show devices skills SELECT * WHERE { ? Device a : Device . ? Device : hasSkill ?Skill .}	
Result	**Result**	
Entity	Entity	Skill
juanspilldispenser	juanpilldispenser	sk_reminderDoses
juan	Juanpilldispenser	sk_Distribution
Emilio	Juanpilldispenser	sk_requestPills
...	...	...

In our example, Juan needs to take his daily dose according to the medical prescription that his smartphone stores, but due to the lack of dose in the pill dispenser he cannot do it. In this case, thanks to the virtual profiles generated through Situational-Context, Juan knows that Emilio is taking the same medication and he can request him to send several doses. In addition, the interconnection of these entities, people and devices, is done in a totally dynamic way at runtime, so no previous configuration or manual action is necessary, which allows us to improve the people QoL by not having to be aware of the devices or having to invest our valuable time in configure them manually.

Virtual profiles are developed following the PeaaS (People as a Service) paradigm (Guillen et al., 2014) and using the novel tool developed by Tim Berners-Lee's team: Solid (Social Linked Data) (Mansour et al., 2016). Solid proposes a decentralized platform for social web applications, where user data is managed independently of the applications that consume this data, a proposal that is quite aligned with our work. Solid is a framework that can be used to implement the basic pillars of PeaaS, obtaining the following benefits (Berners-Lee, 2017): (1) True data ownership, where users should have the freedom to choose where their data resides and who is allowed to access it; (2) Modular design, because applications are decoupled from the data they produce, users will be able to avoid vendor lock-in, seamlessly switching between apps and personal data storage servers; and (3)Reusing existing data, developers will be able to easily innovate by creating new apps or improving current apps, all while reusing existing data that was created by other apps. This could be a good approach to build part of Situational-Context paradigm and could come in handful of benefits.

INTERCONNECTION FLOW

The devices interconnection in Situational-Context has a clear objective: the needs resolution. As we mentioned below, an entity has a need when its skills cannot achieve the desired state in the environment and it must draw on the skills of another one.

Through the Connectivity Manager, entities can connect to each other, and exchange information. For example, Juan's pill dispenser and Juan's smartphone can connect each other through Bluetooth.

This information is interpreted and updated by the Context Manager. At this point, the entity knows its own skills and goals, as well as those of the other entities in the context, and will know if it can solve any determined goal. Juan's pill dispenser knows that Juan does not have pills and that there are other elements in the environment with the skill to provide them, such as the pharmacy or Emilio's pill dispenser.

Then, Juan's smartphone will detect the information coming from the Profile, which contains the entity history and preferences that has a goal. Thanks to this information, Juan is reminded to have his doses by his pill dispenser every day.

Once the change to be made is detected, for example, to give a couple of doses to Juan, the Strategy Dispatcher will formulate a strategy and propose a change over the context. This strategy will consider the skills of the entity and also those of others that could contribute to solving the goal. Using an ontology, the strategy knows which skills and goals are related to each other. Once the strategy has been formulated it is carried out. Besides, it is stored in the profile in order to be able to infer on it and detect possible patterns, to facilitate the strategy development in the future. This whole process is carried out at runtime, without predefining the previous behaviour of the entities, as the solutions to be explored would be innumerable.

Figure 5 shows the interconnection diagram between the entities in the scenario.

For the specific case of the strategy of pills in the context of Juan, the pill dispenser takes into account the preferences of Juan and Emilio to distribute the pills so that Juan can receive his doses and Emilio has enough pills for the rest of

Figure 5. Interconnection between entities

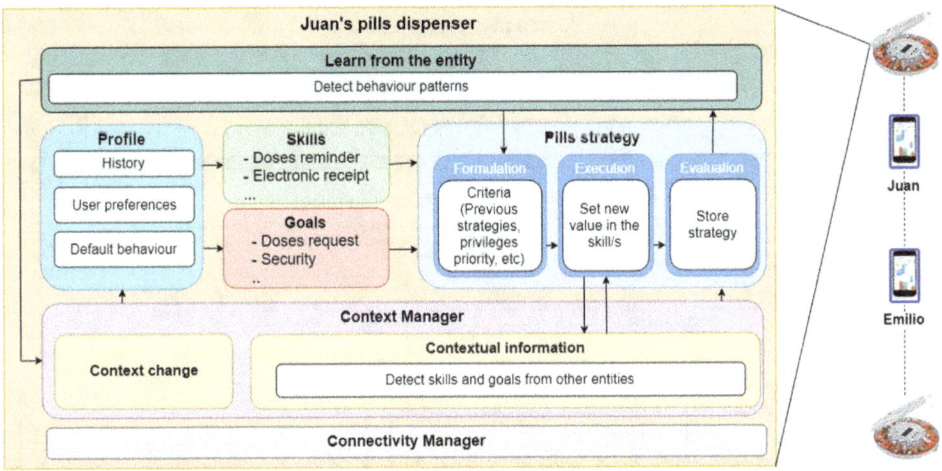

the days. Figure 6 shows the components of the architecture defined above from the point of view of the communication flow for this particular situation.

These strategies take into account other issues such as previous strategies, user privileges or their priority, when solving a need. Not all entities would have the same permissions within the context. We differentiate between the entity owning the context, and invited entities, and within these, we have several levels of privileges depending on parameters such as age within the context or level of importance. In this way, when it comes to covering a common need for several entities, those entities with more privileges are favoured, but also fulfilling the needs of the others. As the pillbox belongs to Juan, it must first satisfy his needs before those of the others. For example, if there were only a few doses left for him, none would be given to Emilio.

The execution of these strategies produces a change in the current context, modifying the behaviour of some entities and, in addition, learns which are the preferences of the entity or entities that are involved, so that, in future interactions, these strategies can be executed more precisely.

Similarly, the rest of entities such as Emilio's pill dispenser, or Juan and Emilio themselves, would have a representation similar to that of Juan's pill dispenser, and with identical behaviour.

RELATED WORK

As we discussed at the beginning of this research in (Flores-Martin, 2017), we can use different paradigms such as AmI, COP, SW and ML, to automate interactions

Figure 6. Communication flow for medication distribution

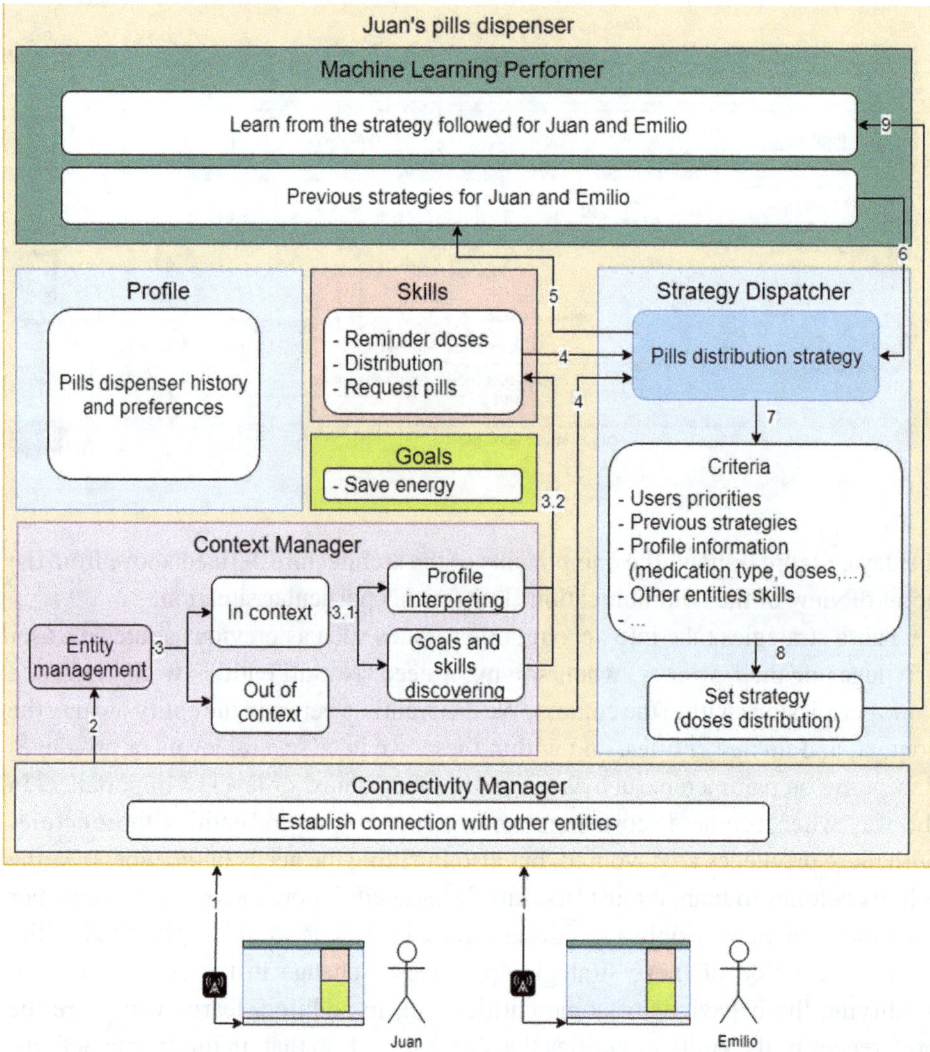

between users and IoT systems according to user preferences. In addition, solutions to improve integration between people and IoT systems through the use of smartphones such as People as a Service (PeasS) and Internet of People (IoP) were also discussed.

When we delve into Semantic Web aspects within the scope of IoT, we find several works that follow an objective similar to ours. SocioTal (Bernal Bernabé et al., 2017) is a project focused mainly on issues of security and data sharing, whose aim is to create a configurable and secure IoT environment that encourages people to contribute with their devices and information, providing appropriate tools and mechanisms that simplify complexity and encourage citizen participation. Gyrard et al. also address issues related to IoT and Semantic Web, and they even have developed their own framework to facilitate interaction between IoT devices from a template generator for different IoT domains (Gyrard, Datta, Bonnet, & Boudaoud, 2015), based on Semantic Web technologies to explicitly describe the meaning of sensor measurements. In (Datta, Bonnet, Gyrard, Da Costa, & Boudaoud, 2015), an architecture for personalized medical care in intelligent homes that allows continuous monitoring of physical parameters and processing of medical data is presented, where Semantic Web technologies are used to combine sensor data from different domains allowing interaction between heterogeneous devices.

As mentioned in Section 1, healthcare domain is gaining great importance within the IoT. We can find works focused on the care or treatment of the elderly. Yuehong et al. (Yuehong, Zeng, Chen, & Fan, 2016) provide an overview of IoT applications in the healthcare industry, based on a comprehensive literature review and discussion of researchers' achievements. This work is carried out from the perspectives of enabled technologies and methodologies, intelligent devices and systems based on IoT and the several applications of IoT in the healthcare industries. In (Pinto, Cabral, & Gomes, 2017), we find We-care, a system for the assistance of elderly people that is able to monitor and record the vital information of these people, as well as provide mechanisms to activate alarms in emergency situations. Along the same lines, Mainetti et al. (Mainetti, Patrono, Secco, & Sergi, 2016) have designed an Ambient System Living (AAL) system to create better living conditions for older people, capable of constantly monitoring their state of health through data from heterogeneous sources. Moreover, many IoT-based patient monitoring systems have a gateway between a sensor network and the Internet. In this sense, Rahmani et al. (Rahmani et al., 2015) propose a system called Smart e-Health Gateway, which assumes responsibility for managing the load of the sensor network and a remote health care center. This development addresses many challenges in ubiquitous health care systems, such as energy efficiency, scalability, and ubiquitous health monitoring and reliability issues.

In addition, if we combine Semantic Web with elderly care, we find an interesting project, SOPRANO (Wolf, Schmidt, & Klein, 2008), an extensible and open AAL platform for elderly people that aims to lead a more independent life in their family environment through a new generation of intelligent home with ambient intelligence.

We are aware that there are many proposals for the development of software whose behaviour adapts to the context, but that, to the best of our knowledge, do not cover in many cases the problems mentioned above, such as those related to the adaptation of devices to the conditions of the context at runtime. Therefore, the research challenges we address are several. First, the lack of a unified model of human-IoT interaction. IoT devices are produced by several manufacturers, each with its own interaction model. Secondly, the lack of an automatic negotiation model for the interaction between people and IoT devices according to people's preferences. Some of the works mentioned above pursue a similar goal to ours, in terms of achieving an adaptive context in IoT, but we want to make the interconnection of these IoT devices emerge from the situation itself. If these problems could be solved, there would be a better integration of people in IoT environments in terms of interoperability.

CONCLUSION

As the health care domain is becoming increasingly important, we are concerned about the idea of being able to connect as many smart devices as possible to make the lives of elderly people easier. However, the problem of interconnection in the IoT world is still present today due to the heterogeneity of devices on the market. The interaction between IoT devices is crucial for the resolution of strategies to support people daily tasks and must allow them to adapt their behaviours to people's needs, which often depends on the collaboration of several smart devices.

This work is another step towards achieving this interconnection in a dynamic way, thanks to technologies such as Situational-Context. Thus, we can adapt the behaviour of smart devices to the needs of people in real time, without the need to attend to previous configurations in design time.

ACKNOWLEDGMENT

This work was supported by the European Regional Development Fund (ERDF) and by 4IE project (0045-4IE-4-P) funded by the Interreg V-A España-Portugal (POCTEP) 2014-2020 program, by the Spanish Ministry of Science and Innovation through project RTI2018-094591-B-I00 (MINECO/FEDER, UE) and by the Department of Economy and Infrastructure of the Government of Extremadura (GR18112, IB18030).

REFERENCES

Barnaghi, P., Wang, W., Henson, C., & Taylor, K. (2012). Semantics for the Internet of Things: Early progress and back to the future. *International Journal on Semantic Web and Information Systems*, *8*(1), 1–21. doi:10.4018/jswis.2012010101

Bernabe, J. B., Elicegui, I., Gandrille, E., Gligoric, N., Gluhak, A., Hennebert, C., ... Nati, M. (2017, June). SocIoTal—The development and architecture of a social IoT framework. In *2017 Global Internet of Things Summit (GIoTS)* (pp. 1-6). IEEE.

Berners-Lee, T. (2017). *Solid vision.* https://solid.mit.edu/

Berrocal, J., Garcia-Alonso, J., Canal, C., & Murillo, J. M. (2016, June). Situational-Context: a unified view of everything involved at a particular situation. In *International Conference on Web Engineering* (pp. 476-483). Springer. 10.1007/978-3-319-38791-8_34

Datta, S. K., Bonnet, C., Gyrard, A., Da Costa, R. P. F., & Boudaoud, K. (2015, October). Applying Internet of Things for personalized healthcare in smart homes. In *2015 24th Wireless and Optical Communication Conference (WOCC)* (pp. 164-169). IEEE. 10.1109/WOCC.2015.7346198

Flores-Martin, D. (2017, November). Meeting IoT Users' Preferences by Emerging Behavior at Run-Time. In *International Conference on Service-Oriented Computing* (pp. 333-338). Springer.

Galán-Jiménez, J., Berrocal, J., Garcia-Alonso, J., Canal-Velasco, J. C., & Murillo, J. M. (2017). *Coordinating heterogeneous IoT devices by means of the centralized vision of the SDN controller.* Academic Press.

Guillen, J., Miranda, J., Berrocal, J., Garcia-Alonso, J., Murillo, J. M., & Canal, C. (2013). People as a service: A mobile-centric model for providing collective sociological profiles. *IEEE Software, 31*(2), 48–53. doi:10.1109/MS.2013.140

Gyrard, A., Datta, S. K., Bonnet, C., & Boudaoud, K. (2015, August). Cross-domain Internet of Things application development: M3 framework and evaluation. In *2015 3rd International Conference on Future Internet of Things and Cloud* (pp. 9-16). IEEE.

Haluza, D., & Jungwirth, D. (2015). ICT and the future of health care: Aspects of health promotion. *International Journal of Medical Informatics, 84*(1), 48–57. doi:10.1016/j.ijmedinf.2014.09.005 PMID:25293532

IronPaper. (2015). *Ironpaper.* https://www.ironpaper.com/webintel/articles/internet-things-market-statistics-2015/

Kim, J., Yun, J., Choi, S. C., Seed, D. N., Lu, G., Bauer, M., ... Song, J. (2016). Standard-based IoT platforms interworking: Implementation, experiences, and lessons learned. *IEEE Communications Magazine, 54*(7), 48–54. doi:10.1109/MCOM.2016.7514163

Lassila, O., & Swick, R. R. (1998). *Resource description framework (RDF) model and syntax specification*. Academic Press.

Mainetti, L., Patrono, L., Secco, A., & Sergi, I. (2016, July). An IoT-aware AAL system for elderly people. In *2016 International Multidisciplinary Conference on Computer and Energy Science (SpliTech)* (pp. 1-6). IEEE. 10.1109/SpliTech.2016.7555929

Mansour, E., Sambra, A. V., Hawke, S., Zereba, M., Capadisli, S., Ghanem, A., ... Berners-Lee, T. (2016, April). A demonstration of the solid platform for social web applications. In *Proceedings of the 25th International Conference Companion on World Wide Web* (pp. 223-226). International World Wide Web Conferences Steering Committee. 10.1145/2872518.2890529

Metcalf, D., Milliard, S. T., Gomez, M., & Schwartz, M. (2016). Wearables and the internet of things for health: Wearable, interconnected devices promise more efficient and comprehensive health care. *IEEE Pulse*, *7*(5), 35–39. doi:10.1109/MPUL.2016.2592260 PMID:28113167

Nordrum, A. (2016). The internet of fewer things. *IEEE Spectrum*, *53*(10), 12–13. doi:10.1109/MSPEC.2016.7572524

Perera, C., Zaslavsky, A., Christen, P., & Georgakopoulos, D. (2014). Context Aware Computing for the Internet of Things: A survey. *IEEE Communications Surveys and Tutorials*, *16*(1), 414–454. doi:10.1109/SURV.2013.042313.00197

Pinto, S., Cabral, J., & Gomes, T. (2017, March). We-care: An IoT-based health care system for elderly people. In *2017 IEEE International Conference on Industrial Technology (ICIT)* (pp. 1378-1383). IEEE. 10.1109/ICIT.2017.7915565

Rahmani, A. M., Thanigaivelan, N. K., Gia, T. N., Granados, J., Negash, B., Liljeberg, P., & Tenhunen, H. (2015, January). Smart e-health gateway: Bringing intelligence to internet-of-things based ubiquitous healthcare systems. In *2015 12th Annual IEEE Consumer Communications and Networking Conference (CCNC)* (pp. 826-834). IEEE.

Roman, R., Zhou, J., & Lopez, J. (2013). On the features and challenges of security and privacy in distributed internet of things. *Computer Networks*, *57*(10), 2266–2279. doi:10.1016/j.comnet.2012.12.018

Shrestha, N., Kubler, S., & Främling, K. (2014, August). Standardized framework for integrating domain-specific applications into the IoT. In *2014 International Conference on Future Internet of Things and Cloud* (pp. 124-131). IEEE. 10.1109/FiCloud.2014.29

Sirin, E., & Parsia, B. (2007, June). SPARQL-DL: SPARQL Query for OWL-DL. In OWLED (Vol. 258). Academic Press.

Swetina, J., Lu, G., Jacobs, P., Ennesser, F., & Song, J. (2014). Toward a standardized common M2M service layer platform: Introduction to oneM2M. *IEEE Wireless Communications*, *21*(3), 20–26.

Szilagyi, I., & Wira, P. (2016, October). Ontologies and Semantic Web for the Internet of Things-a survey. In *IECON 2016-42nd Annual Conference of the IEEE Industrial Electronics Society* (pp. 6949-6954). IEEE. 10.1109/IECON.2016.7793744

Taivalsaari, A., & Mikkonen, T. (2017). A roadmap to the programmable world: Software challenges in the IoT era. *IEEE Software*, *34*(1), 72–80. doi:10.1109/MS.2017.26

Wolf, P., Schmidt, A., & Klein, M. (2008, July). *SOPRANO-An extensible, open AAL platform for elderly people based on semantical contracts.* In 3rd Workshop on Artificial Intelligence Techniques for Ambient Intelligence (AITAmI'08), 18th European Conference on Artificial Intelligence (ECAI 08), Patras, Greece.

Yuehong, Y. I. N., Zeng, Y., Chen, X., & Fan, Y. (2016). The internet of things in healthcare: An overview. *Journal of Industrial Information Integration*, *1*, 3–13. doi:10.1016/j.jii.2016.03.004

Chapter 10
Evaluating Elders' Bio-Psycho-Social Health Dimensions Using Their Smartphones

Enrique Moguel
Universidad de Extremadura, Spain

José García-Alonso
https://orcid.org/0000-0002-6819-0299
Universidad de Extremadura, Spain

Javier Berrocal
https://orcid.org/0000-0002-1007-2134
Universidad de Extremadura, Spain

Juan M. Murillo
Universidad de Extremadura, Spain

ABSTRACT

The percentage of elder people in developed countries is increasing rapidly. A high percentage of them usually present multiple and chronic diseases. A patient with several diseases requires specific and coordinated care that is difficult to configure. Different frameworks can evaluate their functional status and identify the required care, together with the associated cost to the health system. Nevertheless, these frameworks are usually questionnaires that have to be periodically performed by the patients with the assistance of already overloaded professionals. In this chapter, the authors make use of mobile technologies to build a system capable of monitoring the activities of the elderly and analysing these data to assess their bio-psycho-social status. The experiments carried out show us that it correctly evaluates these patients and reduces the effort required by health professionals.

DOI: 10.4018/978-1-7998-1937-0.ch010

INTRODUCTION

Technology speeds up the communication between people. Technology provides convenience to use more than one method of communication. Now people can use email, social media, chat messengers, video conferencing, video calls, images, videos, symbols, diagrams, charts and emoticons etc. for the communication.

But technology has also impacted us positively and negatively in our daily life communication. And as it cannot be otherwise, in the lives of the elderly as well.

World's elderly have historically been late adopters to the world of technology compared to their younger compatriots, but their movement into digital life continues to deepen.

The aging of the population is a confirmed fact in most developed countries. Over 20% of people in developed countries are elderly (65 or more years old), and the growth of this age group means that it is likely to reach some 26% of the population of these countries in 2030 (Facts and Figures on Healthy Ageing and Long-term Care - EUROPEAN INNOVATION PARTNERSHIP - European Commission, 2013).

At present, the world is experiencing population aging, a trend that is both pronounced and historically unprecedented. Over the past six decades, countries had experienced only a slight increase in the share of people aged 65 years and older, from 8% to 10%. However, in the next four decades, this group is expected to rise to 22% of the total population, a jump from 800 million to 2 billion people (Bloom et al., 2015).

This trend is even more worrying in rural regions, for example, Extremadura in Spain or Alentejo in Portugal. This kind of regions has lower population density than the average, and they keep losing its young population to more socioeconomically developed regions. Therefore, they have a higher-than-average aged population while being economically disadvantaged with a fragile cultural and socioeconomic context. Additionally, due to low population density and youth migration to richer regions, elders frequently live alone (Berry & Kirschner, 2013).

Aging in these regions is not a problem by itself, at least not directly. However, as people become older, they are more prone to diseases such as cognitive impairment, diabetes, hypertension, and cardiovascular problems. Different studies indicate that a significant number of these diseases related to aging have their origin in deficient nutrition (Morley & Silver, 1995).

As these people get older, the likelihood of illnesses and chronic diseases increases. Different studies of the National Council on Aging show that more than 80% of older adults have at least one chronic disease, and it is estimated that at least 77% of them have two or more chronic diseases (Facts About Healthy Aging, 2015).

Patients with Multiple Chronic Diseases (MCD) require specific care totally created ad-hoc for their specific problems. These care are usually expensive (McPhail,

2016). Different studies, such as (Moguel et al., 2018) and (Escorpizo et al., 2011), have defined questionnaires to evaluate the bio-psycho-social dimensions of patients and configure the care required, minimizing the associated costs. Thus, healthcare professionals can identify the care that would allow patients to have a certain Quality of Life (QoL) at the minimal cost. Nevertheless, these tests have to be passed by already overburden healthcare professional. Consequently, they are not as frequently passed as it would be required to maintain the patients QoL.

Currently, different mobile technologies are being used to track different diseases to improve patients QoL. Specifically, Internet of Things (IoT) (Gubbi,Buyya, Marusic, & Palaniswami, 2013) and mobile devices (Arsand, Muzny, Bradway, Muzik, & Hartvigsen, 2015) are being used. First case, the paper presents a Cloud centric vision for worldwide implementation of Internet of Things. The key enabling technologies and application domains that are likely to drive IoT research in the near future are discussed. A Cloud implementation using Aneka, which is based on interaction of private and public Clouds is presented. And the second case, the work presents a design of a diabetes diary application for a smartwatch was completed using agile development methods. The system, including a two-way communication between the applications on the smartwatch and mobile phone. The designed smartwatch system displays the time, day, date, and remaining battery time. It also allows for the entry of carbohydrates, insulin, and blood glucose (BG), with the option to view previously recorded data. Users were able to record specific physical activities, program reminders, and automatically record and transfer data, including step counts, to the mobile phone version of the diabetes diary. The smartwatch system can also be used as a standalone tool. Users reported usefulness, responded positively toward its functionalities.

These technologies can also be used to monitor patient's context and automatically answer the questionnaires and track the evolution of the patient in the different bio-psycho-social dimensions.

In this book chapter, the authors detail a context-aware mobile application to perform this assessment. This application uses the mobile device built-in sensors, and other external sensors, to gather the patient's contextual information. In addition, it uses machine learning to identify his/her behaviors and how they evolve over time. This information is then used to evaluate her functional status and to identify the required care.

MOTIVATION

The aging of the population is increasing and, usually, these habitants have multiple, and possibly chronic, diseases, requiring specific cares. Some of the authors of

Figure 1. Architecture of the context-aware app

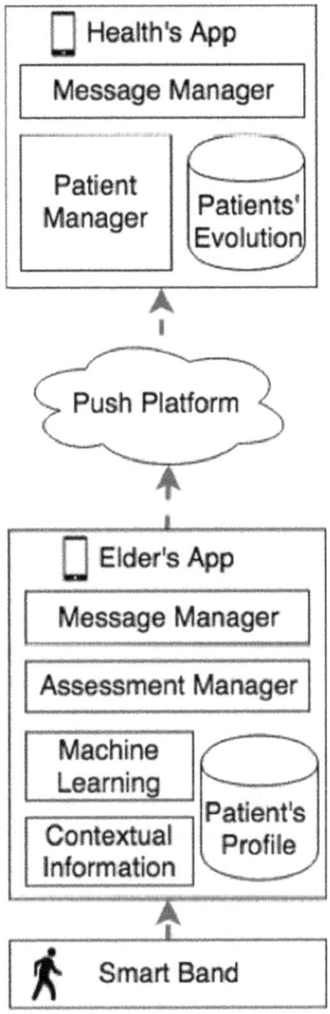

this book chapter have proposed a multidimensional assessment (Berrocal et al., 2018) to evaluate the elderly people' functionality. This framework measures four different areas: Body Functions, Body Structure, Activities and Participation, and Environmental Factors in order to identify the best possible treatment at the lower cost. Being as follows:

- **Body Functions:** In a similar way, this dimension evaluates matters such as consciousness functions, orientation functions, attention functions, sensation of pain, etc.

- **Body Structure:** This dimension is used to evaluate the condition of the skin, bones, etc.
- **Participation Activities:** This dimension is used to evaluate if the elderly can carry out a daily routine, have a conversation, can wash themselves o take care of areas of their body, etc.
- **Environmental Factors:** Finally, other aspects are evaluated in the platform such as family environment, friends, personal care providers, personal assistants and the elders health professionals.
- **General Functional Profile:** In this dimension matters such as self-management, learning and memory functions, communication or relationship with friends and caregivers are evaluated. In addition, all personal information such as age, marital status, weight, height, etc. is recorded in this dimension.

As the health professionals normally use a web platform to perform different assessment of an elder over time, all the information is stored. But this is a complex process that requires a huge effort of the health professional. In addition, this process should be repeated as the diseases evolve.

The scientific community has been devoting enormous effort to mitigate the problems. For instance, the success of IoT has led to the development of a large number of devices, which can obtain information about their users. Nevertheless, some characteristics essential for the success of these applications are: configuration effort, battery consumption and privacy.

IoT devices require users to configure them to gather information and act according to their preferences. Healthcare professional could configure these devices to elders, but eventual changes in their context would require their reconfiguration (Moguel et al., 2018). Increasing, again, their workload. During the last few years, some of the authors of this book chapter have been working on a new mobile computing model (Garcia-Alonso et al., 2019). This model allows mobile devices to gather the contextual information of his/her owner, store it to create a virtual profile and reuse it to reduce the reconfiguration efforts.

Another aspect of acquiring contextual information about the elderly person that should be taken into account is battery use. Most of the devices used in monitoring the elderly are mobile and, hence, small. They therefore have limited battery capacity. Many research studies have addressed this limitation proposing different techniques to reduce the resource consumption (Cho, Lee, Noh, Park, & Song, 2015). The authors of this book chapter have also proposed different techniques to reduce the battery and data traffic usage (Berrocal et al., 2017).

Finally, the privacy is a crucial aspect that is receiving much attention from the scientific community. An approach to preserve the privacy of the elderly is to keep their information in their own devices (Fiore, Caione, Zappatore, Mitri, &

Mainetti, 2017). This device then shares the necessary information with the required people, avoiding storing the elderly person's information in a centralized server and increasing its privacy.

In this chapter, the authors present a context-aware mobile application meeting the above detailed requirements. This application gathers the context of the patient to perform a multidimensional assessment of its health. In the next section, the researchers briefly detail the application architecture.

CONTEXT AWARE MOBILE APPLICATION

With the aim of easing the assessing of the functionality status of elderly people, the researchers designed and developed a system based on the previously detailed frameworks and technologies Fig. 1 shows the system's architecture.

The app for the elderly person gathers the patient's contextual information using different built-in sensors or external sensors. The data, and the frequency at which the information is gathered, is managed by the Contextual Information component depending on the user's activities (for instance, if he/she is running, the location is gathered more frequently). In addition, this component automatically reconfigures the different sensors and external devices used as the user's context evolve. All the gathered raw information is stored in the Patient's Profile database. That information is evaluated by the Machine Learning component to infer concrete data about the different dimensions evaluated. Concretely, it identifies the sleeping patterns of the patients, the activities done and their influence on the heart rhythm.

Obviously, the used sensors and the inferred information can only be used to evaluate some characteristics of the Body Functions and Activities and Participation dimensions (such as sleeping, some daily activities, etc.). For other characteristics (such as memory and hearing), the authors included specific activities, games and questionnaires in the mobile app to evaluate them. Therefore, they cannot be passively measured yet, but they are actively measured with the patient's participation.

Periodically, the Assessment Manager component analyses the inferred information in order to evaluate the patient's functional status. Currently, this task is weekly executed. Once the weekly assessment is completed, the results are sent to the Health app. To that end, the Elder's app uses the Message Manager component to send a push notification with that information. Hence, all the gathered and inferred information is stored only in the elders and professionals' mobile phone, increasing the data privacy and reducing the battery consumption since data do not have to be uploaded to a cloud environment.

The Health app receives the assessment result through the Message Manager component. That information is evaluated by the Patient Manager component to

Figure 2. Screenshot of the configuration view of the application

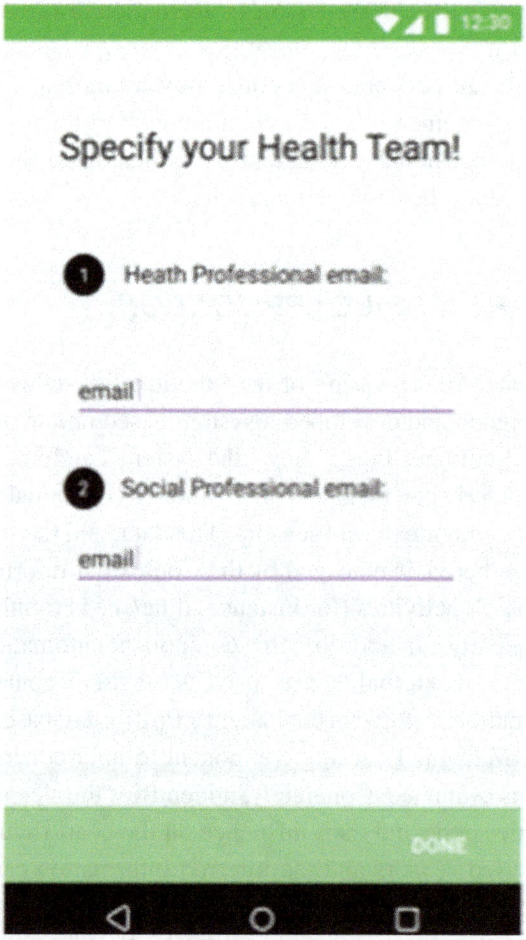

trigger any alarm if it has been an abrupt change in the elder's health, and to store it in the Patient Database. Fig. 2 and 3 shows some designs of the developed apps.

The applications detailed above were evaluated in a simulated environment in order to check their validity. To perform the experiment, 6 students were selected, 4 to undertake the role of the elderly and 2 that of the health professional. During the test, the students representing elderly persons performed their usual activities, and the student-professionals gathered the different assessments. Throughout the experiment, the student had to record all the actions they performed. Then, the recorded actions were used to manually perform the assessment framework and to compare the results. From that comparison the authors identified that both method provided similar results. In addition, the presented apps allowed professionals to save some time devoted to execute this assessment.

FUTURE WORKS

At the same time, the context aware mobile application is linked with the elders' smartphones. Therefore, each time a connected sensor or device performs an assessment of an elder, the updated information is stored in the virtual profile of the elder kept in the smartphone. The following example details how this information will be used to improve the interaction of the elder with other systems.

This potential solution provides two benefits. First and foremost, the enriched virtual profiles of the elderly simplify the interaction with other systems. And second, the integrations with the virtual profile allow us to use the rest of the profile information to notify health professional when the elder functionality or the activities suffers a change that is not represented in the assessment platform and even to automatically update the platform.

For example, the information will be provided from the smartphone so other systems can use it to adapt to the elders classification of functionality. For example, if the assessment of the participation activities of the elder determines that she has mobility problems, an adapted bed can detect this information and provide additional help when the user wants to stand up. Similarly, if the assessment detects hearing problems, the phones and other devices used by the elderly can dynamically adapt its volume to their user's needs, and even other people can be automatically notified when interacting with the elderly so they can make the appropriate adjustments.

Additionally, other example of how the information stored in the virtual profile of the elderly can be used to automatically update the assessment. One of the most relevant aspects of the virtual profile is the elderly daily routines. The virtual profile store the routines followed by an user and detects possible deviations from the routines to raise alarms and notify the appropriate caregivers. This information can be used to update the information in the assessment platform. For example, if the number of detected deviations from routines increases, it could cause an update in the assessment of the participation activities to reflect the new functionality levels of the elderly or an alert can be sent to a health professional indicating the need of an updated assessment.

Figure 3. Example of the chart shown to the health team

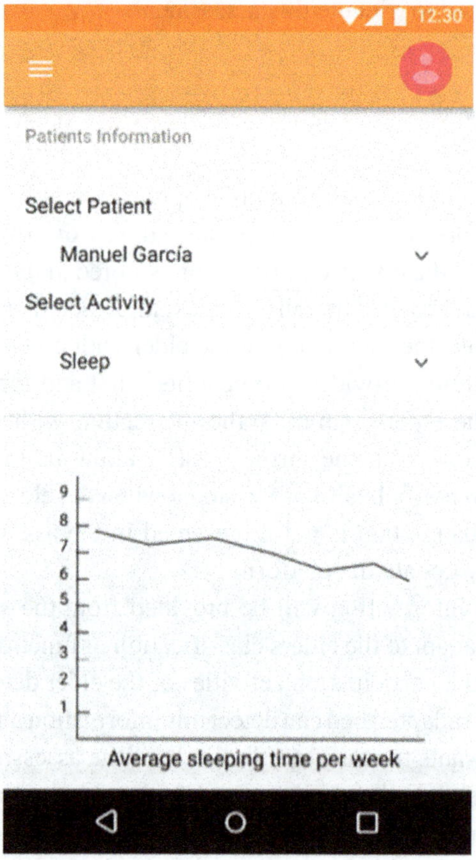

CONCLUSION

As mentioned above, the authors of this paper are working in the use of the Situational-Context to create an ecosystem of tools and systems to improve the quality of life of the elderly living in sparsely populated areas. As part of this effort, works like (Berrocal, Garcia-Alonso, Murillo, & Canal, 2017) or (Garcia-Alonso et al., 2018) present different techniques and proposals to this end.

Furthermore, eldercare is a very relevant topic and several researchers have proposed different alternatives to create virtual profiles of the elderly. For example, works like (Hervás, Bravo, & Fontecha, 2014) propose the use of a virtual profile of the elderly to assist them in their daily activities and to notify their relatives of potentially risky situations. Similarly, works like (Almeida et al., 2017) propose the use of IoT devices to increase the information gathered by the virtual profiles of the elderly. Finally, works like (Bouznad et al., 2017) propose the use of ontologies to improve the monitoring of the elders. All these works share several aspects with the one presented here. However, only this work is focused on the design of solutions for the healthcare systems of aged, sparsely populated regions.

Definitively, older adults experiencing MCD require complex to configure cares, and a constant evaluation of the evolution of their illnesses. In this book chapter, the authors have presented an application using new mobile technologies to semiautomate the monitoring and evaluation of this kind of patients. These applications allow health professional to remotely monitor different dimensions of the functional status of patients and with less effort. The researchers performed an experiment to validate the feasibility of the proposed system. Nevertheless, a more throughout experiment will be executed using real subjects

ACKNOWLEDGMENT

This work was supported by 4IE project (0045-4IE-4-P) and 4IE+ project (0499_4IE_PLUS_4_E) funded by the Interreg V-A España-Portugal (POCTEP) 2014-2020 program, by the Spanish Ministry of Science, Innovation and Universities (RTI2018-094591-B-I00), by the Department of Economy and Infrastructure of the Government of Extremadura (GR18112, IB18030), and by the European Regional Development Fund.

REFERENCES

Almeida, A., Fiore, A., Mainetti, L., Mulero, R., Patrono, L., & Rametta, P. (2017). An iot-aware architecture for collecting and managing data related to elderly behavior. *Wireless Communications and Mobile Computing*, *2017*, 2017. doi:10.1155/2017/5051915

Arsand, E., Muzny, M., Bradway, M., Muzik, J., & Hartvigsen, G. (2015, May). Performance of the First Combined Smartwatch and Smartphone Diabetes Diary Application Study. *Journal of Diabetes Science and Technology, 9*(3), 556–563. doi:10.1177/1932296814567708

Berrocal, J., Garcia-Alonso, J., Murillo, J. M., & Canal, C. (2017). Rich contex- tual information for monitoring the elderly in an early stage of cognitive impairment. *Pervasive and Mobile Computing*, *34*, 106–125. doi:10.1016/j.pmcj.2016.05.001

Berrocal, J., Garcia-Alonso, J., Murillo, J. M., Mendes, D., Fonseca, C., & Lopes, M. (2018, jun). Context-aware mobile app for the mul- tidimensional assessment of the elderly. In *2018 13th iberian confer- ence on information systems and technologies (cisti)* (pp. 1–6). IEEE. Retrieved from https://ieeexplore.ieee.org/document/8399239/

Berrocal, J., Garcia-Alonso, J., Vicente-Chicote, C., Hern'andez, J., Mikkonen, T., Canal, C., & Murillo, J. M. (2017, February). Early analysis of resource consumption patterns in mobile applications. *Pervasive and Mobile Computing, 35*, 32–50. doi:10.1016/j.pmcj.2016.06.011

Berry, E. H., & Kirschner, A. (2013). Demography of Rural Aging. In *Rural aging in 21st century America* (pp. 17–36). Dordrecht: Springer Netherlands; Retrieved from http://www.springerlink.com/index/10.1007/978

Bloom, D. E., Chatterji, S., Kowal, P., Lloyd-Sherlock, P., McKee, M., Rechel, B., ... Smith, J. P. (2015, February). Macroeconomic implications of population ageing and selected policy re- sponses. *Lancet, 385*(9968), 649–657. doi:10.1016/S0140-6736(14)61464-1 PMID:25468167

Bouznad, S., Chibani, A., Amirat, Y., Lyazid, S., Prestes, E., Sebbak, F., & Fiorini, S. (2017). Context-aware monitoring agents for ambient assisted living applications. In *European conference on ambient intelligence* (pp. 225–240). 10.1007/978-3-319-56997-0_18

Cho, D.-K., Lee, U., Noh, Y., Park, T., & Song, J. (2015, May). PlaceWalker: An energy-efficient place logging method that con- siders kinematics of normal human walking. *Pervasive and Mobile Computing, 19*, 24–36. Retrieved 2018-02-08, from https://www.sciencedirect.com/science/article/pii/S1574119214000583

Escorpizo, R., Finger, M. E., Glssel, A., Gradinger, F., Lckenkemper, M., & Cieza, A. (2011, June). A systematic review of functioning in vocational rehabilitation using the International Classification of Functioning, Dis- ability and Health. *Journal of Occupational Rehabilitation, 21*(2), 134–146. doi:10.100710926-011-9290-8 PMID:21328062

Facts About Healthy Aging. (2015, June). Retrieved 2018-02-08, from https://www.ncoa.org/news/resources-for-reporters/get-the- facts/healthy-aging-facts/

Facts and Figures on Healthy Ageing and Long-term Care - EUROPEAN INNOVATION PARTNERSHIP - European Commission. (2013, February). Retrieved 2018-02-08, from https://ec.europa.eu/eip/ageing/library/facts-and-figures-healthy-ageing-and-long-term-careen

Fiore, A., Caione, A., Zappatore, D., Mitri, G. D., & Mainetti, L. (2017). De- ploying Mobile Middleware for the Monitoring of Elderly People with the Internet of Things: A Case Study. In *Cloud Infrastructures, Services, and IoT Systems for Smart Cities* (pp. 29–36). Cham: Springer; doi:10.1007/978-3-319-67636-44

Garc'ıa-Alonso, J., Berrocal, J., Murillo, J. M., Mendes, D., Fonseca, C., & Lopes, M. (2018). Situational-context for virtually modeling the elderly. *9th international symposium on ambient intelligence.*

Garcia-Alonso, J., Berrocal, J., Murillo, J. M., Mendes, D., Fonseca, C., & Lopes, M. (2019, Jun.). Situational-Context for Virtually Modeling the Elderly. Springer. Retrieved from https://link.springer.com/10.1007/978-3-030-01746-0

Gubbi, J., Buyya, R., Marusic, S., & Palaniswami, M. (2013, September). Internet of Things (IoT): A vision, architectural elements, and future directions. *Future Generation Computer Systems, 29*(7), 1645–1660. Retrieved 2018-02-08, from https://www.sciencedirect.com/science/article/pii/S0167739X13000241

Herv'as, R., Bravo, J., & Fontecha, J. (2014). An assistive navigation system based on augmented reality and context awareness for people with mild cognitive impairments. *IEEE Journal of Biomedical and Health Informatics, 18*(1), 368–374. doi:10.1109/JBHI.2013.2266480 PMID:24403436

McPhail, S. M. (2016, July). Multimorbidity in chronic dis- ease: impact on health care resources and costs. *Risk Management and Healthcare Policy, 9*, 143–156. Retrieved 2018-02-08, from https://www.ncbi.nlm.nih.gov/pmc/articles/PMC4939994/

Moguel, E., Berrocal, J., Murillo, J. M., Garc'ıa-Alonso, J., Mendes, D., Fonseca, C., & Lopes, M. (2018, January). Enriched elderly virtual profiles by means of a multidimensional integrated assessment plat- form. *Procedia Computer Science, 138*, 56–63. doi:10.1016/j.procs.2018.10.009

Morley, J. E., & Silver, A. J. (1995, dec). Nutritional Issues in Nursing Home Care. *Annals of Internal Medicine, 123*(11), 850. Retrieved from http://annals.org/article.aspx?doi=10.7326/0003-4819-123-

Chapter 11
Emotion Identification With Smartphones to Improve the Elder Quality of Life Using Facial Recognition Techniques

Sheila Bonilla
Universidad de Extremadura, Spain

Enrique Moguel
Universidad de Extremadura, Spain

José Garcia-Alonso
https://orcid.org/0000-0002-6819-0299
Universidad de Extremadura, Spain

Javier Berrocal
https://orcid.org/0000-0002-1007-2134
Universidad de Extremadura, Spain

Juan M. Murillo
Universidad de Extremadura, Spain

ABSTRACT

The increase in the elderly population today is a fact. This group of people needs day-to-day care due to their age, and, in addition, they often have health problems. Technology can be used to mitigate these problems. However, it must be borne in mind that most of this population is currently unable to get the most out of electronic devices. To help elders benefit from these devices, systems adapted to their needs,

DOI: 10.4018/978-1-7998-1937-0.ch011

and preferences are needed. In particular, systems that use the elders' contextual information to integrate several aspects of eldercare and adapt them to each elder would provide significant benefits. In this case, the emotions will be used to recognize to what extent an elderly person needs care at certain times of the day and to adapt surrounding IoT systems to their needs and moods. For this purpose, this chapter proposes to use smartphones as the devices that centralize contextual information of the elders, focusing on emotion recognition.

INTRODUCTION

Today, thanks to advances in technology and communications, one of the fastest advancing electronic devices is the mobile phone. Nowadays, a large part of the population uses their mobile phones to communicate, search information, socialize, etc. Even in the context of elder population, there has been an increase in the uses of smartphones in recent years (Sánchez López, Fernández Alemán, Toval, & Carrillo de Gea, 2015).

A large part of the population in developed countries is formed by elder people (65 years of older). It is estimated that by 2030 this age group may reach 26% of the population (Rodrigues, Huber, Lamura, et al., 2012). On the other hand, in Spain, since 2012, 75.9% of people over the age of 65 use a mobile phone and, in addition, the use of this device has become a daily habit for them (Sánchez López et al., 2015).

In order to help this sector of the population, in addition to using mobile phones, more IoT (Internet of Things) devices are used everyday. These devices are connected to everyday objects through the Internet to add new or improved functionalities to them. Frequently, the elderly tend to use this type of device without being aware of it. For example, through medical care in intelligent homes, where the main objective of these systems is to have better control over the patient's health care, significantly reducing hospital visits and improving their quality of life. Another example in which IoT devices are used is the intelligent medication service, since the success in the treatment of any person depends to a great extent on taking the prescribed medicines at the right time. Due to this, smart pillbox or even smart pharmaceutical packaging were created (Núñez, Mendoza, Hernández, & Molinares, 2016) or (Morales Suárez-Varela, 2009). To use these devices need technical skills, since the must be initially con- figured so that they know how to satisfy their owners needs, for example the time at which the elderly should take their medicines. However, if these needs change, the devices must be reprogrammed.

Having this into account, the emotional state of the users is usually over- looked when gathering contextual information. However, the emotions displayed by user when performing certain action are of great interest to improve the systems behavior.

According to (Kulkarni, Shendge, Varma, & Kimmatkar, 2018) there are six basic types of emotions, which are: joy, sadness, surprise, fear, disgust and anger. Being able to identify these emotions will help improve the contextual information gathered in the system, and therefore, obtain systems better adapted to the needs and moods of their users. In the context of the elder population, this technique could be used to perform actions like detecting if the person has a problem at a certain moment of the day or even quite the opposite, due to the fact that this person has a positive emotional state.

For emotion recognition, numerous techniques are currently used, such as facial recognition through images or videos such as (Suk & Prabhakaran, 2014), (Claudino, de Lima, de Assis, & Torro, 2019) or (Gan, Chen, & Xu, 2019), but as far as the authors know it has not been studied how to include this in the everyday life of elderly people. In this book chapter, the authors present a technique to analyse the emotional state of the elderly, through facial recognition of emotions and the subsequent use of this information as part of the Situational Context, which allows for a better adaptation of IoT systems to the emotional state of elderly people.

In order to present our proposal, the rest of chapter is structured as follows: In Section 2, we will detail the background of this work focusing on emotion recognition and adaptation techniques based on contextual information; in Section 3, we will describe our proposal in which we will highlight the architecture and two case studies. Finally, in the last Section we will show the conclusions and future works.

BACKGROUND

Every year the number of IoT devices grows faster (Stergiou, Psannis, Kim, & Gupta, 2018), but the way to interconnect these devices does not change. For this reason, interconnection is a problem that exists today, so it is not possible to squeeze its full potential (Flores-Martin, Pérez-Vereda, Berrocal, Canal, & Murillo, 2018). This work aims to provide a response to these situations. With the help of facial recognition of emotions and the use of the Situational Context to gather information of the devices and adapt their behaviour to the users needs, we will be able to integrate different IoT devices with which to help improve the emotional state and quality of life of the elderly.

In the following sections we will show the possible techniques for facial recognition of emotions and then how we can adapt these techniques to other IoT devices through the virtual profile.

Techniques for Facial Recognition

Today, companies are deploying facial recognition technologies in a wide range of contexts with a increasing technological sophistication. At the simplest level, the technology can be used for facial detection, that is, simply to detect and locate a face in a photo or video (Mayron, 2015). Current uses of facial detection include refining search engine results to include only those results that contain a face, ensuring that the frame for a video chat feed actually includes a face, or developing virtual eyeglass fitting systems and virtual makeover tools that allow consumers to upload their photos online and "try on" a pair of glasses or a new hairstyle (Lv, Shao, Huang, Zhou, & Zhou, 2017). A more refined version of facial recognition technology allows companies to assess characteristics of facial images. For instance, companies can identify moods or emotions from facial expressions to determine a player's engagement with a video game or a viewer's excitement during a movie (Q. Wu, Zhao, & Jacopo, 2018). Companies can also place cameras into digital signs to determine the demographic characteristics of a face, such as age range and gender, and deliver targeted advertisements in real- time in retail spaces (C. C. Wu, Zeng, & Shih, 2015). This same technology could be used to identify the user who is going to use a certain mobile application.

Figure 1. Techniques for facial recognition

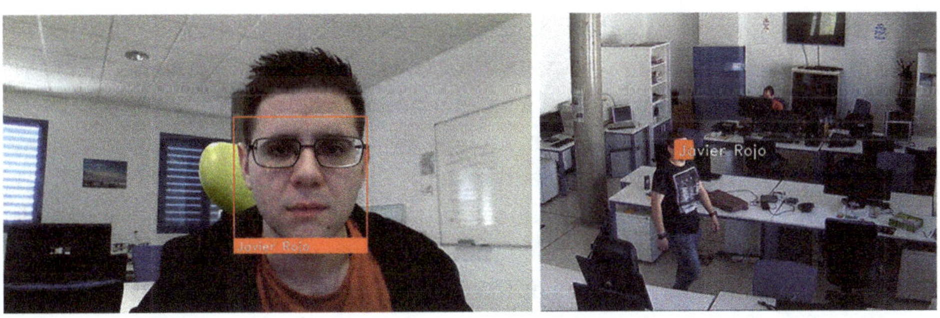

Techniques for the Recognition of Emotions

The field of research related to facial recognition of emotions, currently presents a large number of studies (Goyal, Upadhyay, Jadon, & Goyal, 2018) aimed at proving in some way, the detection of emotions. The mobile phone has a great influence on this part, as it helps to take videos or even photos that can help to detect them.

Most of the emotions recognition models follow a set of techniques, steps or even categorizations. Next, some of the most relevant will be detailed.

One of this studies use the detection of emotions through images (Li, Buenaposada, & Baumela, 2008). Its purpose is to present a system that detects the face of a person and classify it according to facial expression. In addition, it follows a set of very detailed techniques with which they can detect the face of the person, extract their discriminatory information and finally, be able to classify the expressions obtained.

On the other hand and Continuing with the recognition of images, the work (Kulkarni et al., 2018). Its objective is to analyze a possible facial image processing system based on people's emotions, following a specific structure and detailed step by step to reach the best possible solution.

In the field of detection of emotions through videos, there are works such as (Agarwal, Santra, & Mukherjee, 2018). Anubhad consists of a preliminary prototype designed to recognize facial expressions through videos in real time or even videos stored on the device itself (this includes a version for Windows and Android). The features used for facial expression recognition are based on two categories: geometric and appearance. Thanks to this categorization, as a result, a high percentage is obtained in the recognition of the six basic emotions mentioned above (joy, sadness, surprise, fear, disgust and anger) and the recognized emotions can be stored in the device themselves or they can be exported to be used by other systems or devices.

Adaptation Techniques/Virtual Profile

The virtual profile is used to adapt the needs of the elderly to IoT devices. This profile is based on the Situational Context (Berrocal, Garcia-Alonso, Canal, & Murillo, 2016) paradigm focused on analyzing the conditions that exist in places where there are Internet of Things systems. This model is used to gather all the information about the elder available in their devices and systems that interact in their normal lives. Using the Situational Context, the information gathering is transparent to people which implies that they do not need any technical knowledge or skill.

Before this study, the Situational Context did not have information related to emotions. Therefore, thanks to this work presented in this chapter, the information of the emotional state of a person at certain times of the day has been incorporated. This can help to enrich the context as well as being able to help it.

Through the information obtained, virtual profiles are generated that can be used to automatically adapt the behavior of IoT devices to the needs and preferences of each elder (Garcia-Alonso et al., 2018). For example, when a person is found to be sad, they are in their living room and it is also 5:00 pm. The system can put on the television program that this elder likes the most since his retransmission is currently being broadcasted.

Elderly people want to keep their autonomy, so that, whenever possible, they adapt their routines by adding new elements to their homes and/or using new technologies that facilitate the performance of their daily tasks and, at the same time, allow caregivers not to have to constantly accompany them (Berrocal, Garcia-Alonso, Murillo, & Canal, 2017). By adding more IoT devices, the sys- tem will capture more information in the virtual profile, which will make richer information so we can provide more efficient solutions to suit the elderly.

The authors of this book chapter previously presented a technological solution to make life easier for patients with dementia (Berrocal et al., 2017). Smartphones, smart clocks and other devices were used to control the location and vital symbols of a person with dementia. Caregivers could therefore be alerted when a parameter deviated from its normal values, for example, when the heart rate exceeded the values set by the caregiver, or when the affected person was in an area that the caregiver had not marked as safe.

From this, the researchers developed a mobile application to monitor elderly people with cognitive impairment with a certain degree of autonomy. The objective of this system is to detect the different daily routines of the user (schedules, movement patterns, etc.). Then, the smartphone monitors the user's daily activities and acts if any deviation is detected (for example, guiding the elderly to finish an activity or alerting their family members). The identification of routines is based on all available contextual information, such as time, location (indoors and/or outdoors), biometric data, family members or caregivers accompanying the elderly or the weather. The analysis of this information makes it possible to detect a wide variety of recurrent activities, along with all the contextual information associated with those activities. Identified routines are stored along with their contextual information and the transitions between them that the user follows. Finally, the authors defined an algorithm to identify deviations from routines, and to detect when, depending on the Situational Context it is necessary to activate an alert. All this allows us to identify a greater number of activities, better control the conditions in which each activity must be carried out and detect which deviations from the routines must trigger an alert.

The proposed virtual profile was initially composed of: a basic profile with the information of the elder, a social profile that stores high level information about the basic profile, goals which are deduced from the basic and social profile and finally, the skills to make decisions and changes in the environment (Moguel et al., 2018). But if, in addition to these components, the researchers add to this profile the daily routines of an elderly and, based on these routines, a facial emotion detector through which we store the emotional feeling of the elderly, and they will achieve the objective of making them richer in information, which will lead to IoT systems able to react to emotional changes in the elder.

Related Works on Emotion Recognition in Elderly Person

Facial recognition of emotions is a technique used in multiple investigations. Next, we will categorize the different uses of emotion recognition in elderly person:

- As we can see in paper (Lozano-Monasor, López, Vigo-Bustos, & Fernández-Caballero, 2017), they have developed an application for the recognition of emotions in elderly people from their facial expression, using a webcam. They are able to discriminate the six types of basic emotions (joy, sadness, surprise, fear, disgust and anger) and also the neutral expression. These six emotions are grouped into three categories: happiness, negative emotion and surprise. They have applied their technology in homes, placing a webcam in front of the elder and asking the person to simulate the facial expression associated with an emotion. The best results they obtained were in surprise and happiness. In this work, they aim to make the most of facial recognition of emotions by helping older people to detect anomalies in mood and be able to improve it through external stimulations. The main difference in the hardware used between this paper and ours is that they use a camera to detect emotions, while we have it integrated into the smartphone itself. On the other hand, their main objective is related to the elders being able to help them through external stimulations as we do, from their emotional state and with the virtual profile.
- On the other hand, there are studies such as (Dantcheva, Bilinski, Broutart, Robert, & Bremond, 2016), where the researchers have thought of a very important aspect: the need for a high level of care due to the loss of autonomy. Motivated by this, they propose a facial recognition of emotions through video in Alzheimer's patients. By testing these patients, their methods come to detect four different facial expressions which are: neutral, smile, sadness and speech. The researchers hope that their benefit will be in the face of positive emotions in which knowing their cause could be determined and replicated to increase the standard of living of the patients and that also leads to a delay in the development of Alzheimer's disease.
- On the other, there are works such as (Hossain & Muhammad, 2015), where the authors combine the facial recognition of emotions with other techniques, as we pretend with the Situational Context. This paper combines cloud computing with the development of cloud-based healthcare systems and services. Cloud computing has inspired healthcare professionals to remotely monitor patients' health while they are at home. To that end, this document proposes a cloud assisted voice and facial recognition framework for elderly health monitoring, where portable devices or video cameras collect voice

along with facial images and are delivered to the cloud server for possible analysis and classification. The patient status recognition system extracts speech characteristics and texture descriptors from facial images, and it then classifies them. The status that has been recognized is then sent to the remote care center, health professionals, and providers to provide the necessary services to provide uninterrupted health monitoring.

These three works pursue the same goal: to make life easier for the elderly through intelligent devices, whether IoT, smartphone or both. However, as far as the authors know, there is no work using the facial emotions of the elderly to adapt IoT systems to their needs and moods.

IMPROVING THE ELDERLY QUALITY OF LIFE BY USING EMOTION RECOGNITION

As mentioned above, an increasing percentage of the population uses electronic devices more easily. Thanks to the Situational Context paradigm, it is not necessary for elder to have a great deal of knowledge about electronic devices to take advantage of their capabilities.

The proposal presented in this chapter is an application capable of recognizing the emotional state of a person. This information is stored together with the existing virtual profiles proposed by the Situational Context. Using Anubhav's work (Agarwal et al., 2018) are recognized the six types of basic emotions using a video stored on the smartphone or capturing it in real time. In addition, the system has the possibility to export this information to other devices. This proposal includes the possibility of linking emotions with other contextual information.

The information obtained about emotions is later used to simplify or automate the interactions of the elder with different IOT devices. For example, for notifying family members or health team of a sudden change in the emotional state.

Additionally, the proposed system will store in a timeline the videos collected by the device alongside the emotional feeling and the time at which this recognition has been made. This will allow the system to monitor the usual emotional state of the elders and to detect a change in the elders daily routine and what may have caused this change according to the emotions detected combined with the rest of contextual information.

Architecture of the Proposal

For this proposal, an architecture has been developed with which intend to achieve the detection of emotions together with a better interconnection between different IoT devices and thus be able to get the maximum benefit. This architecture implies the interaction of different entities and the use of context information.

The components developed for the architecture detailed in Figure 2 are as follows:

- **Connectivity Manager**: establishes the physical connection between entities. Sends and receives information regarding skills, needs, personal information, etc.
- **Context Manager**: responsible for creating and updating contextual information. Contains the information of the entities belonging to the same situation in a given instant of time.
- **Profile**: union of the *Basic* and *Social Profile* of the entity.
    - **Basic Profile**: it is the basic information that identifies the entity (Personal Information). It contains raw data about the history of interaction with other entities (Raw Data History). It also contains the

Figure 2. Developed architecture to add change detection in a daily routine elderly

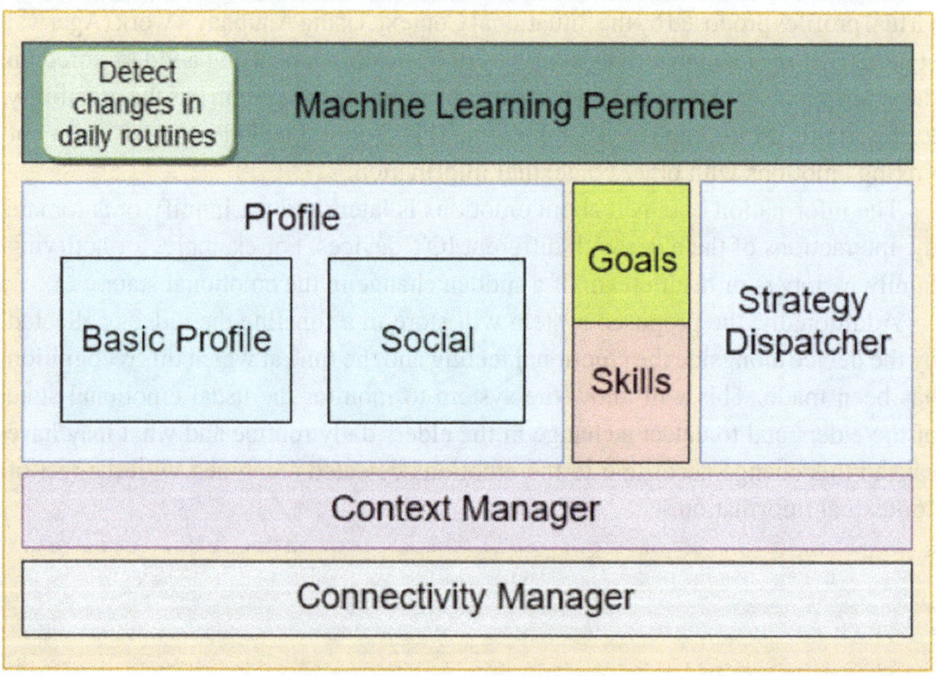

raw information about the entity's status, the relationships with other devices and its historic information.
    - **Social Profile**: it stores the set of all social data inferred by the basic profile (Inferred Data History).
- **Skills**: it produces a change in the context that is not possible with its own needs. It has the capabilities that an entity has to make decisions and perform actions capable of modifying the environment and aimed at achieving goals.
- **Strategy Dispatcher**: the devices can detect what needs there are in the context, and which ones can solve their skills, so a strategy is solved when there is a skill that can cover the need of an entity. The complexity of strategies lies in the collaboration of entities to identify and solve needs.
- **Machine Learning Performer**: this component analyzes the history of activities of the entity to detect patterns and learn from it, with the aim of automating tasks in the future.
    - **Detect changes in daily routines**: this component analyzes the daily routines that have been detected through the patterns of machine learning and, when a change occurs in these, proceeds to the detection of emotions.

For the study of the proposed system, the facial recognition through the smartphone will be made daily a minimum of three times. These three recognitions will always be done at the same time interval and are as follows:

- First recognition will be done early in the morning when it is detected that the elderly has woken up. The recognition will be made when the elderly takes the mobile for the first time in the day. In the case that the elderly does not use it, the mobile device will send him a notification with a warning.
- Second recognition, just after the midday meal. Through the daily routines the system will detect at the hour that the elder usually takes her lunch, for this reason it will have a stored hourly interval. After this interval, the first time the elderly person picks up the phone, the recognition will be made. Like in the previous case, if the user does not use its device the system sends a notification with a warning.
- Third recognition will take place after dinner. As in the second recognition, the elderly will have stored the time interval of his dinner. Therefore, after the interval, the first time the elderly picks up the mobile phone, the emotional recognition will be stored. As in the previous cases, if the user does not use its device, the system sends a notification with a warning.

The proposed architecture achieves an interconnection of IoT devices at the functional level. As the flow diagram in Figure 3 shows, the interconnection is based on relating an entity's daily routines to their owner emotions. In this case, when a change in a routine is detected the system will proceed to perform a facial recognition through a video of a total of ten seconds since the person takes his device. This video will be stored in the Raw Data History. Information about the emotion and date will be stored in Personal Information. When the emotion is detected and

Figure 3. Context manager flowchart

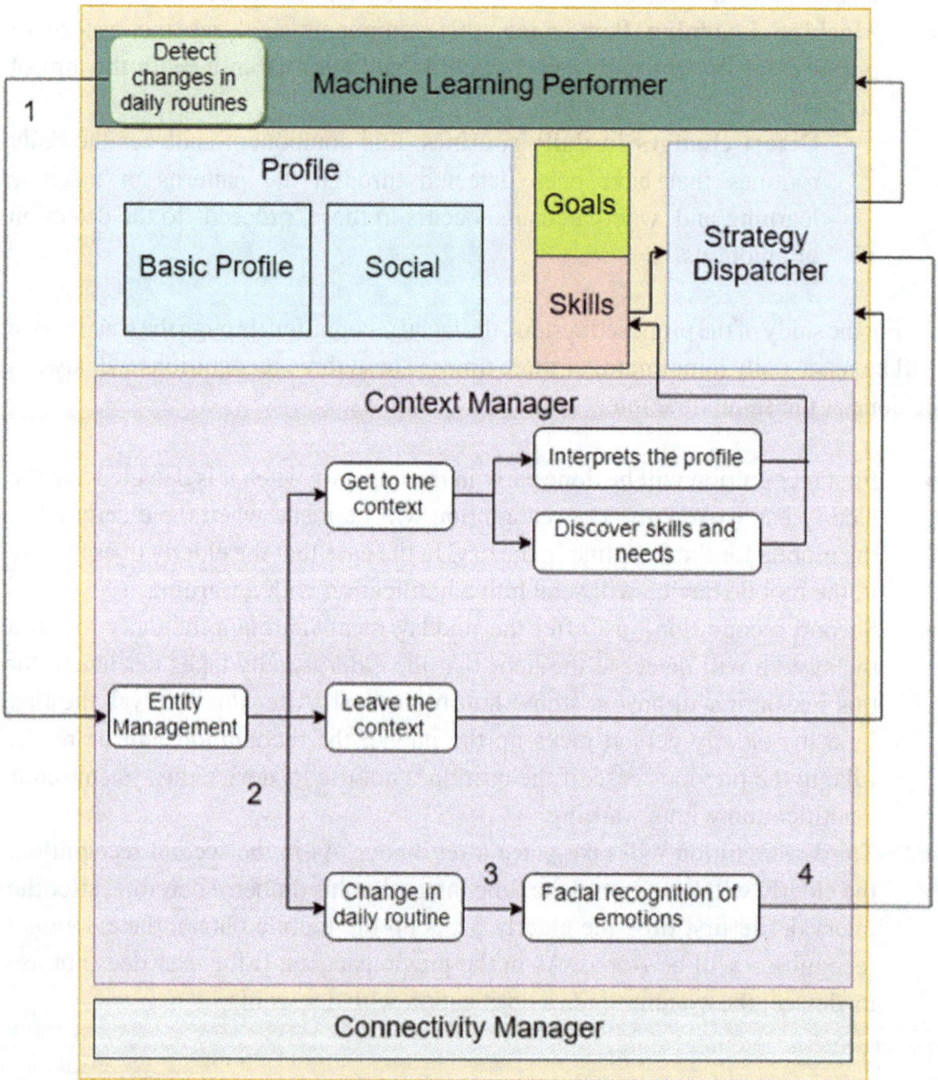

everything is stored in the device, the change of routine will be notified to a relative/ caregiver of the elderly, indicating through a text message/email that this person has not performed a daily routine and also indicating their emotional state.

If the elder at the time of recognition does not take the smartphone and the period of recognition ends. This information is not stored in the device so as not to cause an error.

Case Studies

As has been said before, facial recognition of emotions can be quite useful in helping the elderly. With the proposed architecture, everyday life can be made easier of the elderly. By detecting a change in their daily routine, their emotional state can be known and depending on the state in which the person is, act on it. In order to explain in more detail the situations of help for the elderly, two examples will be given below based on the following context:

The elderly mostly carry out daily routines such as going to buy bread, doing household chores, going out with friends to their usual park or even sitting in their village square to tell each other anecdotes. These routines are monitored, a change in these can indicate a change in your health or mood among others. In this specific case, two examples will be developed as follows:

- Juan has his daily routines monitored as discussed above. This person has his own mobile phone with which he makes calls and even communicates through social networks with his friends (for example, whatsapp), who also have smartphones. Through monitoring we can control when a routine is not performed in the usual range of hours.

Juan usually goes out with his friends to his village square around 12:00 a.m. But today Juan has not gone to his daily appointment. The system knows that Juan is not with his friends due to the interconnection of his smartphones, as they are far away. For this reason, the process of facial recognition of emotions begins. Once this recognition has been over, it knows that Juan emotion is happiness. Having this, the system can resort to the information that is stored in the device with the virtual profile. The last change stored on his smartphone is a video of his grandson playing football and for this, he has stayed home watching it. Later, when Juan goes to the square to chat with his friends, he wants to show them the video of his grandson playing football. This information is in the same situational context so he can share it with his friends so they can also see how well his grandson plays football.

- Irene, just as Juan, has her daily routines monitored. Irene receives her food every morning at 1:30 p.m. through a catering company that travels daily to these people's homes. She always eats at 2:00 p.m. In the meantime, she sets the table and prepares everything necessary. In this case, facial recognition is done after eating, so it is a fixed recognition that is done daily.

The food that the catering company has brought Irene today is the food that she has liked the least since she was little (grilled chicken), but these meals are standard for all the elderly and the company designs a common menu daily.

According to what her doctor has asked her, Irene must take pictures of her food every day in order to control the food that the caterer provides her. At 2:30 p.m. Irene picks up her phone, the time interval of her meal has already passed, thus activating the process of facial recognition of emotions. The recognition gets the feeling of anger because she didn't like the food. Joining the captured photo by the mobile device together with Irene's feeling of anger and the tastes the system has stored in virtual profile, the system can deduces that the food she has been brought to eat today is the food she likes the least.

Faced with this situation, Irene's mobile phone automatically sends a message to the catering company in which it shows that the food served to her today does not please her and with it she manages not to have this type of food sent to her in the future.

CONCLUSION AND FUTURE WORK

After different searches of the literature, nothing was found that was completely adapted to the objectives that were looking for. For this, in this chapter proposes a new paradigm. With the previously developed Situational Context, the authors have added a new functionality that helps to enrich it. This new function is the facial recognition of emotions, through which we can detect the emotional feeling of the elderly using a smartphone. With this recognition, the system obtains the emotional state of the person, which can be: joy, sadness, surprise, fear, disgust and anger. With this idea, the proposed system is able to improve the quality of life of the elderly through the recognition of emotions and it can act on this, sending notifications to family members or caregivers so they know how that person is at a certain time of day and because of what may be so.

Following this line, several validations are currently being carried out. Firstly, tests are being carried out on the smartphone's battery consumption to know the energy requirements of the system. On the other hand, the researchers of this chapter are looking at the level of data consumption. And finally, and most importantly, the authors seek the acceptance of the elderly to be able to record videos and thus reach the goal of recognizing emotions.

In future works the researchers will extend this proposal of facial recognition of emotions. The application will be developed for any Android device in which we can do tests on elderly people and that, correcting the flaws that may be in the categorization of emotions, the system can detect the emotion as accurately as possible. On the other hand, following with the Virtual Profile, the authors will continue enriching this profile adding new functionalities, besides integrating a greater number of IoT devices with which we can capture information and, to have in a more precise way the cause by which the old man changes his emotion in a certain moment of the day.

ACKNOWLEDGMENT

This work was supported by 4IE project (0045-4IE-4-P) and 4IE+ project (0499_4IE_PLUS_4_E) funded by the Interreg V-A España-Portugal (POCTEP) 2014-2020 program, by the Spanish Ministry of Science, Innovation and Universities (RTI2018-094591-B-I00), by the Department of Economy and Infrastructure of the Government of Extremadura (GR18112, IB18030), and by the European Regional Development Fund.

REFERENCES

Agarwal, S., Santra, B., & Mukherjee, D. P. (2018). Anubhav: Recognizing emotions through facial expression. *The Visual Computer*, *34*(2), 177–191. doi:10.100700371-016-1323-z

Berrocal, J., Garcia-Alonso, J., Canal, C., & Murillo, J. M. (2016). *Situational-Context: A Unified View of Everything Involved at a Particular Situation.* Springer. Retrieved from https://link.springer.com/10.1007/978-3-319-38791-8

Berrocal, J., Garcia-Alonso, J., Murillo, J. M., & Canal, C. (2017). Rich contextual information for monitoring the elderly in an early stage of cognitive impairment. *Pervasive and Mobile Computing*, *34*, 106–125. doi:10.1016/j.pmcj.2016.05.001

Claudino, R. G., de Lima, L. K. S., de Assis, E. D. B., & Torro, N. (2019, Dec). Facial expressions and eye tracking in individuals with social anxiety disorder: a systematic review. *Psicologia: Reflexão e Crítica*, *32*(1), 9. Retrieved from https://prc.springeropen.com/articles/10.1186/s41155-

Dantcheva, A., Bilinski, P., Broutart, J. C., Robert, P., & Bremond, F. (2016). *Emotion facial recognition by the means of automatic video analysis. Gerontechnology Journal.*

Flores-Martin, D., Pérez-Vereda, A., Berrocal, J., Canal, C., & Murillo, J. M. (2018). *Coordinación de Dispositivos IoT mediante Web Semántica y Ontologías en Situational-Context. JISBD.*

Gan, Y., Chen, J., & Xu, L. (2019, July). Facial expression recog-nition boosted by soft label with a diverse ensemble. *Pattern Recognition Letters, 125*, 105–112. doi:10.1016/j.patrec.2019.04.002

Garcia-Alonso, J., Berrocal, J., Murillo, J. M., Mendes, D., Fonseca, C., & Lopes, M. (2018). Situational-Context for Virtually Modeling the Elderly. *International symposium on ambient intelligence.*

Goyal, S. J., Upadhyay, A. K., Jadon, R., & Goyal, R. (2018). Real-life facial expression recognition systems: A review. In *Smart computing and informatics* (pp. 311–331). Springer. doi:10.1007/978-981-10-5544-7_31

Hossain, M. S., & Muhammad, G. (2015). Cloud-assisted speech and face recognition framework for health monitoring. *Mobile Networks and Applications, 20*(3), 391–399. doi:10.100711036-015-0586-3

Kulkarni, A., Shendge, A., Varma, V., & Kimmatkar, N. V. (2018). *Intelligent emotion detection system using facial images*. Academic Press.

Li, H., Buenaposada, J. M., & Baumela, L. (2008). Real-time facial expression recognition with illumination-corrected image sequences. In *Automatic face & gesture recognition, 2008. fg'08. 8th IEEE international conference on* (pp. 1–6). IEEE.

Lozano-Monasor, E., López, M. T., Vigo-Bustos, F., & Fernández-Caballero, A. (2017). Facial expression recognition in ageing adults: From lab to ambient assisted living. *Journal of Ambient Intelligence and Humanized Computing, 8*(4), 567–578. doi:10.100712652-017-0464-x

Lv, J.-J., Shao, X.-H., Huang, J.-S., Zhou, X.-D., & Zhou, X. (2017, March). Data augmentation for face recognition. *Neurocomputing, 230*, 184–196. doi:10.1016/j.neucom.2016.12.025

Mayron, L. M. (2015, May). Biometric Authentication on Mobile Devices. *IEEE Security and Privacy, 13*(3), 70–73. doi:10.1109/MSP.2015.67

Moguel, E., Berrocal, J., Murillo, J. M., Garcia-Alonso, J., Mendes, D., Fonseca, C., & Lopes, M. (2018). *Enriched elderly virtual profiles by means of a multidimensionalidad integrated assessment platform*. Academic Press.

Morales Suárez-Varela, M. T. (2009, April). la utilidad del pastillero para mejorar el terapéutico. *Atencion Primaria*, *41*(4), 185–191. doi:10.1016/j.aprim.2008.07.003 PMID:19328598

Núñez, C. A. V., Mendoza, P. S., Hernández, K. A., & Molinares, D. J. (2016). Internet de las cosas y la salud centrada en el hogar. *Salud Uninorte*, *32*(2).

Rodrigues, R., Huber, M., & Lamura, G. (2012). *Facts and figures on healthy ageing and long-term care*. Vienna: European Centre for Social Welfare Policy and Research.

Sánchez López, M. A., Fernández Alemán, J. L., Toval, A., & Carrillo de Gea, J. M. (2015). *Teléfonos inteligentes para la tercera edad: una revisión de aplicaciones móviles de salud*. Academic Press.

Stergiou, C., Psannis, K. E., Kim, B.-G., & Gupta, B. (2018). Secure integration of IoT and cloud computing. *Future Generation Computer Systems*, *78*, 964–975. doi:10.1016/j.future.2016.11.031

Suk, M., & Prabhakaran, B. (2014). Real-time mobile facial expression recognition system a case study. In *Proceedings of the IEEE conference on computer vision and pattern recognition workshops* (pp. 132–137). 10.1109/CVPRW.2014.25

Wu, C.-C., Zeng, Y.-C., & Shih, M.-J. (2015, Jun). Enhancing retailer marketing with an facial recognition integrated recommender system. In *2015 IEEE international conference on consumer electronics* (pp. 25–26). IEEE. Retrieved from https://ieeexplore.ieee.org/document/7216881/

Wu, Q., Zhao, W., & Jacopo, T. (2018, may). Towards Ob jective Assessment of Movie Trailer Quality Using Human Electroencephalogram and Facial Recognition. In *2018 IEEE international conference on electro/information technology* (pp. 0449–0452). IEEE. Retrieved from https://ieeexplore.ieee.org/document/8500283/

Chapter 12
Contribution of an Intelligent Virtual Assistant to Healthy Ageing in Adults With Type 2 Diabetes

Mara Pereira Guerreiro
UI&DE, Escola Superior de Enfermagem de Lisboa, CiiEM, Instituto Universitário Egas Moniz, Portugal

Isa Brito Félix
UI&DE, Escola Superior de Enfermagem de Lisboa, Portugal

João Balsa
https://orcid.org/0000-0001-8896-8152
Faculdade de Ciências, Universidade de Lisboa, Portugal

Maria Beatriz Carmo
https://orcid.org/0000-0002-4768-9517
BioISI, Faculdade de Ciências, Universidade de Lisboa, Portugal

Maria Adriana Henriques
https://orcid.org/0000-0003-0288-6653
UI&DE, Escola Superior de Enfermagem de Lisboa, ISAMB, Faculdade de Medicina da Universidade de Lisboa, Portugal

Afonso Cavaco
https://orcid.org/0000-0001-8466-0484
iMed.ULisboa, Faculdade de Farmácia, Universidade de Lisboa, Portugal

Ana Paula Cláudio
BioISI, Faculdade de Ciências, Universidade de Lisboa, Portugal

ABSTRACT

This chapter describes the development of a theory-driven and evidence-based digital intervention to facilitate self-care in older adults with Type 2 Diabetes (T2D) and, additionally, its contribution to healthy aging and the individual care plan. T2D is highly prevalent in older adults. Difficulties in adopting and maintaining desirable

DOI: 10.4018/978-1-7998-1937-0.ch012

self-care behaviors is associated with lack of glycemic control and subsequent complications, which significantly burden patients, their families, and the health system. The VASelfCare (Virtual Assistant Self-Care) intervention is a software application that provides an interface with a 3D anthropomorphic virtual assistant targeting three key self-care behaviors: medication-taking, physical activity, and a healthy diet. Other VASelfCare elements are intended for nurses providing diabetes consultations, including a web-based back-office with a patient data dashboard, which streamlines integration of care. The application prototype has been co-produced with older adults with T2D, primary care health professionals, and other stakeholders.

INTRODUCTION

The main objective of this chapter is to describe the development of a theory-driven and evidence-based digital intervention to facilitate self-care in older adults with T2D. Secondary objectives are presenting the contribution of the newly developed digital intervention to healthy aging and the individual care plan.

Our current lives are permeated by 'e-solutions'. Full digitalization is reaching all domains, including healthcare. Chronic conditions and their long-term treatments, such as the highly T2D, place a high burden, both individually and societally. Elderly T2D patients, due to the disease mild symptoms in the first years and its complex approach, tend to impinge on treatment adherence and lifestyle changes. Developing automatic and distant healthcare monitoring 'e-solution', tailored to incorporate useful information features as well as to increase motivation, is an excellent opportunity to have a positive impact on patients' behaviour, care plan outcomes and quality-adjusted life years.

The systematic and structured development of this digital self-care intervention is not only expected to maximize its likelihood of success and facilitate potential replication but may also inspire others researching the field.

Health care professionals may equally find the chapter valuable, as it illustrates how the use of a self-care application can enhance the care plan in face-to-face consultations, through shared clinical data. The fact that behaviour change techniques (BCTs) operationalization is exemplified within the application offers useful insights into its transferability to these consultations.

The chapter is composed of several sections. It starts with a background section, which provides information on healthy aging, as well as the epidemiology of diabetes and its clinical and economic impact, namely in older adults. Next, the evidence on the impact of mobile health in chronic disease management is discussed, focusing then on mobile applications to support diabetes self-management. The background section finishes with a brief description of applications based on relational agents.

The second section is about the VASelfCare project. It puts the project into perspective in the wider context of technology-based interventions, explains the methodological framework and describes the theoretical approach taken.

The third section presents the VASelfCare intervention design. It provides an account of the dialogues structure and creation and details how standardized behaviour change techniques were selected and operationalized.

The fourth section describes the VASelfCare prototype. Firstly, a general description of the prototype is provided, including its different views and the back-office dashboard. Then, the authors offer an overview of the technical aspects of the prototype architecture from an informatics standpoint.

The section that follows reports data on the involvement of target users in defining the application pre-requisites.

The sixth section deals with the potential value of VASelfCare to the individual care plan.

The conclusion section summarizes and discusses key points and elaborates on future research directions.

Throughout the chapter the authors resort to an extensive list of references, offering an overview on contemporary topics related to the development of self-care digital interventions, helpful for those seeking an update in the field. Moreover, the chapter provides visual presentations, including diagrams, VASelfCare print screens and graphs, to make information easily understandable to readers. Furthermore, suggestions on additional readings are offered for those interested in expanding their knowledge. Key terms are succinctly defined in a final section.

BACKGROUND

Healthy Aging

Longevity is one of the biggest achievements of modern societies. Life expectancy has increased across the World Health Organization (WHO) European Region, yet this does not necessarily mean more years in good health for all people (OECD/EU, 2018; World Health Organization, 2015). Aging is a dynamic and multifactorial process, associated with biological, physiological, environmental, psychological, behavioural, and social changes. These changes are linked with a rise in chronic conditions and reduced wellbeing (Suzman, Beard, Boerma, & Chatterji, 2015). In fact, aging is not only a major risk factor for a number of chronic diseases, but also for frailty and increased vulnerability. Most health problems in older age are the result of chronic diseases. Many of these can be prevented or delayed by engaging in healthy behaviours (World Health Organization, 2015). The management of long-term conditions in later life, such as diabetes, places a substantial burden on health care systems, representing a major global public health challenge.

The WHO Global Strategy and Action Plan on aging provides a policy framework to ensure a worldwide response to this phenomenon. One of the priorities is improving older people's access to clinical interventions able to maintain their capacities and enhance healthy aging trajectories (World Health Organization, 2017). "Ageing well" must be regarded as a global priority; longer lives can be a valuable resource, both for individuals and for society.

Healthy aging is defined as the process of developing and maintaining the functional ability that enables well-being in older age (World Health Organization, 2015), reflecting an ongoing interaction between individuals and their environments (Beard et al., 2016). It requires a multi-modal, societal approach that transcends health systems, as depicted in Figure 1. The health status of older adults is heterogeneous, ranging from the preserved functional ability to no independence in activities of daily living. Such heterogeneity demands services and care tailored to individual needs.

Figure 1. Requirements for healthy aging (based on WHO infographics)

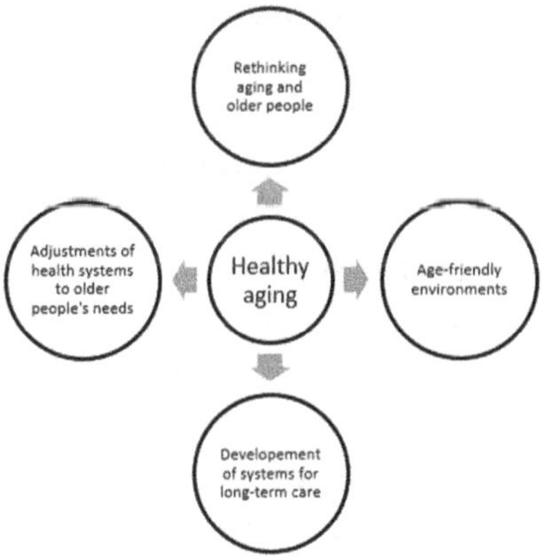

Diabetes in Older Adults

Around the world, 90% of diabetic adults suffer from type 2 diabetes mellitus (T2D) (Zheng, Ley, & Hu, 2018). Globally, T2D affects approximately 425 million adults (20-79 years) and is expected to rise to 629 million by 2045 (Cho et al., 2018).

Older adults are at high risk for developing T2D due to the effect of genetic, lifestyle and aging influences. Diabetes in older adults is a mounting public health burden, as they represent one of the fastest growing segments of the diabetes population. American data indicate that around one-quarter of people over 65 years have diabetes and one-half of older adults have pre-diabetes (Centers for Disease Control and Prevention, 2017). European data show that 19.3 million people aged 60-79 have diabetes, compared with 11.7 million people aged 40-59 and only 1.8 million aged 20-39. While more men than women have diabetes in middle-age (between 40 and 59 years old), a greater number of women have diabetes after age 70, mainly because they live longer (OECD/EU, 2018, p. 106). Portuguese data is essentially identical to global statistics: more than a quarter of the Portuguese population between 60 and 79 years old has diabetes and the aging of the Portuguese population has resulted in a 13.5% increase in diabetes prevalence between 2009 and 2015 (Sociedade Portuguesa de Diabetologia, 2016).

Managing hyperglycaemia in T2D requires a healthy diet, physical activity and, often, antidiabetic medication, which may include insulin injections, (Chrvala, Sherr, & Lipman, 2016; García-Pérez, Álvarez, Dilla, Gil-Guillén, & Orozco-Beltrán, 2013; Lavie et al., 2010; Munshi, 2019). Lifestyle interventions showed significant benefit in a number of risk factors associated with cardiovascular disease in persons with T2D (Chen et al., 2015); changing lifestyle is critical for the prevention and management of the disease (American Diabetes Association, 2019a, 2019b).

Difficulties in adhering to diabetes management, which requires behavioural changes maintained indefinitely, is associated with a lack of glycaemic control in more than half of the patients (García-Pérez et al., 2013). The management of older adults with diabetes is further complicated by the physiological changes associated with aging, as well as comorbidities and functional impairment (Kalyani, Golden, & Cefalu, 2017; P. G. Lee & Halter, 2017).

Poor control of T2D leads to a greater risk of heart attack and stroke, sight loss, foot and leg amputation, and renal failure (American Diabetes Association, 2019a, 2019b; OECD/EU, 2018). Complications in the kidneys, eyes, the vascular system, and peripheral nerves can be fatal and are associated with considerable direct and indirect costs for health systems. An estimated 1.6 million deaths were directly caused by diabetes, which was ranked by WHO as the seventh leading cause of death in 2016 (Zheng et al., 2018) The health expenditure allocated to treat diabetes and prevent complications are estimated at about EUR 150 billion in 2017 in the European Union, with the average expenditure per diabetic adult estimated at about EUR 4 600 per year (International Diabetes Federation, 2017).

Inevitably, people with chronic conditions such as T2D will spend most of their time self-managing. For instance, British data indicate that people with chronic conditions spend on average 4 hours per year with a health professional; the remaining 8756 hours are spent self-managing (Self Care Forum, 2016). Interventions focused on facilitating self-care, supplementing the care provided by health care professionals, are therefore a promising avenue to improve diabetes management and outcomes. Older people may require additional self-management education and support, due to co-existing chronic conditions, polymedication and functional impairment (American Diabetes Association, 2019a). Self-management education and support should be patient-centred, tailored to individual needs and may be delivered using technology (American Diabetes Association, 2019a).

Mobile Applications to Support Healthy Aging and Diabetes Self-Management

As previously pointed out, the challenges of responding to healthy ageing include the alignment of health systems to the needs of older people and developing systems for long-term care. WHO regards the use of digital technologies for health as an important mean to address healthcare needs; mobile health (m-Health) plays a pivotal role, mainly through continuous coverage (World Health Organization, 2019). M-health interventions recommended by WHO comprise digital tracking of patients' health status and services and targeted communication, via mobile devices.

Unsurprisingly m-health has received considerable attention from researchers, as it supports self-care and/or monitoring and communication by health care professionals in a convenient, affordable and scalable fashion, potentially contributing to ease the burden posed by an ageing society on health systems. Although systematic reviews are not always conclusive, m-health has shown beneficial effects in chronic disease management, including improvement of health outcomes for cardiovascular diseases, asthma, and diabetes (de Jong, Ros, & Schrijvers, 2014; Free et al., 2013; J.-A. Lee, Choi, Lee, & Jiang, 2018)

Several systematic reviews have looked at the impact of technology to support diabetes self- management. For example, (Pal et al., 2013) found a small beneficial effect of computer-based interventions on blood glucose control in adults with T2D; the pooled effect on glycosylated haemoglobin A1c (HbA1c) was -0.2% based on data from 11 randomized controlled trials (RCTs), comprising a total of 2637 participants. Included studies encompassed a wide array of interventions to support T2D self-care, resorting to communication or processing technology (Pal et al., 2013). Mobile phone-based interventions had a larger effect on HbA1c (subgroup analysis: -0.5%; three RCTs; 280 participants).

Other systematic reviews have specifically addressed the impact of mobile-phone applications in relevant endpoints in T2D (Cui, Wu, Mao, Wang, & Nie, 2016; Hou, Carter, Hewitt, Francisa, & Mayor, 2016). For example, Cui et al. estimated an effect of these applications in HbA1c of -0.40% (1022 participants, six RCTs). This effect can be important if achieved by patients on their own, without the additional cost of involving healthcare professionals. In concordance with (Pal et al., 2013), Cui et al. found no significant improvements on endpoints such as blood pressure and lipids, which together can tackle cardiovascular risk factors and reduce mortality.

Other reviews critically analysed existing features of mobile diabetes applications. While many applications address healthy eating, monitoring, taking medication and being active, one common limitation is the lack of patient behaviour and education e.g. problem solving, healthy coping and risk reduction (Chomutare, Fernandez-Luque, Årsand, & Hartvigsen, 2011; Ye, Khan, Boren, Simoes, & Kim, 2018).

Applications Based on Relational Agents

One concern is whether digital technology will reach older people. An important aspect, though, is that the age-based digital divide is expected to progressively fade in the near future. For instance, a decade ago a Portuguese survey on the use of communication and information technologies showed that only 4.4% and 3% of respondents in the 65-74 age bracket used computers and the internet (INE, 2006); current data indicate an increase in this proportion to 29% and 27%, respectively (INE, 2015). While aging barriers impact the use of m-health in older adults (Wildenbos, Peute, & Jaspers, 2018), this age group has a growing interest to integrate technology in the self-management of chronic conditions (Gilbert et al., 2015; Kim & Lee, 2017).

The use of relational agents has emerged as an encouraging approach to engage older people (Bickmore et al., 2013; Bickmore, Caruso, Clough-Gorr, & Heeren, 2005). Health literacy in older people is limited in countries such as Portugal (Mota-Pinto et al., 2010; Paiva et al., 2017). In these circumstances, software with communication capabilities, such as speech, intonation or gaze and gestures through an anthropomorphic character is advantageous, as it requires minimal text comprehension. This is exemplified by a pilot study ascertaining the performance of a virtual versus a human nurse in explaining discharge instructions to low literacy patients. The study found similar knowledge levels in both groups, but participants were significantly more satisfied with the virtual nurse, due to perceptions of less pressure, fewer biases, and more receptiveness to questions than the human (Timothy W. Bickmore, Pfeifer, & Paasche-Orlow, 2007). Further evidence of the acceptability of relational agents in older, low literacy patients, was provided by a randomized controlled trial investigating the effect on the exercise of a daily interaction with a relational agent during two months in 21 older adults (Timothy W. Bickmore, Caruso, Clough-Gorr, et al., 2005). Most participants had low reading literacy; about half of the sample had never used a computer before or had used it only a few times. The intervention led to a significant increase in steps count; participants found the system easy to use and were highly satisfied (Timothy W. Bickmore, Caruso, Clough-Gorr, et al., 2005). The fact that relational agents are able to establish a high degree of empathy with users and a feeling of being cared for in face-to-face interaction is also expected to overcome attrition in use over time, a common limitation in digital interventions across different age groups.

A good illustration of a multi-behavioural intervention based on a relational agent is a study aiming to promote medication-adherence and physical activity in adults with schizophrenia (Timothy W. Bickmore, Puskar, Schlenk, Pfeifer, & Sereika, 2010). The pilot evaluation during one month in a sample of 20 subjects showed that the intervention was well accepted; self-reported medication and physical activity adherence were also very high (Timothy W. Bickmore et al., 2010).

Relational agents have seldom been used in diabetes management. One exception is a virtual coach designed to work across devices and give tailored feedback to adults with T2D on physical activity and medication adherence (op den Akker et al., 2011). Another exception is an intelligent diabetes lifestyle coach (Monkaresi et al., 2013), capable of integration with other health related applications to, for instance, adapt exercise recommendations to weather conditions. However, both publications lack data on usability or the effect on endpoints of interest. Recently, a relational agent designed as a health coach proved to be a feasible and acceptable approach for enhancing family communication in adolescents with type 1 diabetes and their parents (Thompson et al., 2019).

THE VASelfCare PROJECT

The VASelfCare project, which started in January 2018, aims to develop a viable prototype of a virtual assistant application to support older patients with T2D in self-care and to test its use in this group. The virtual assistant has been designed as a relational agent, targeting three self-care behaviours (diet, physical activity) and medication adherence.

Figure 2 puts VASelfCare into perspective in the wider context of technology-based interventions; all concepts are explained in the "Key terms and definition section".

The project, funded by grant number LISBOA-01-0145-FEDER-024250, 02/SAICT/2016, has been structured into phases and sub-phases, depicted in Figure 3.

The project methodological approach draws on the Medical Research Council (MRC) framework for developing and evaluating complex interventions, which was first proposed about two decades ago, in recognition of the difficulties of evaluating complex interventions, i.e. interventions "build up from a number of components, which may act both independently and inter-dependently" (Medical Research Council, 2000). This framework has been extensively used (Bleijenberg et al., 2018); it is comprised of four phases, depicted in Figure 4 (Craig et al., 2008). Rather than

Figure 2. Relationship between self-management applications and higher-level concepts

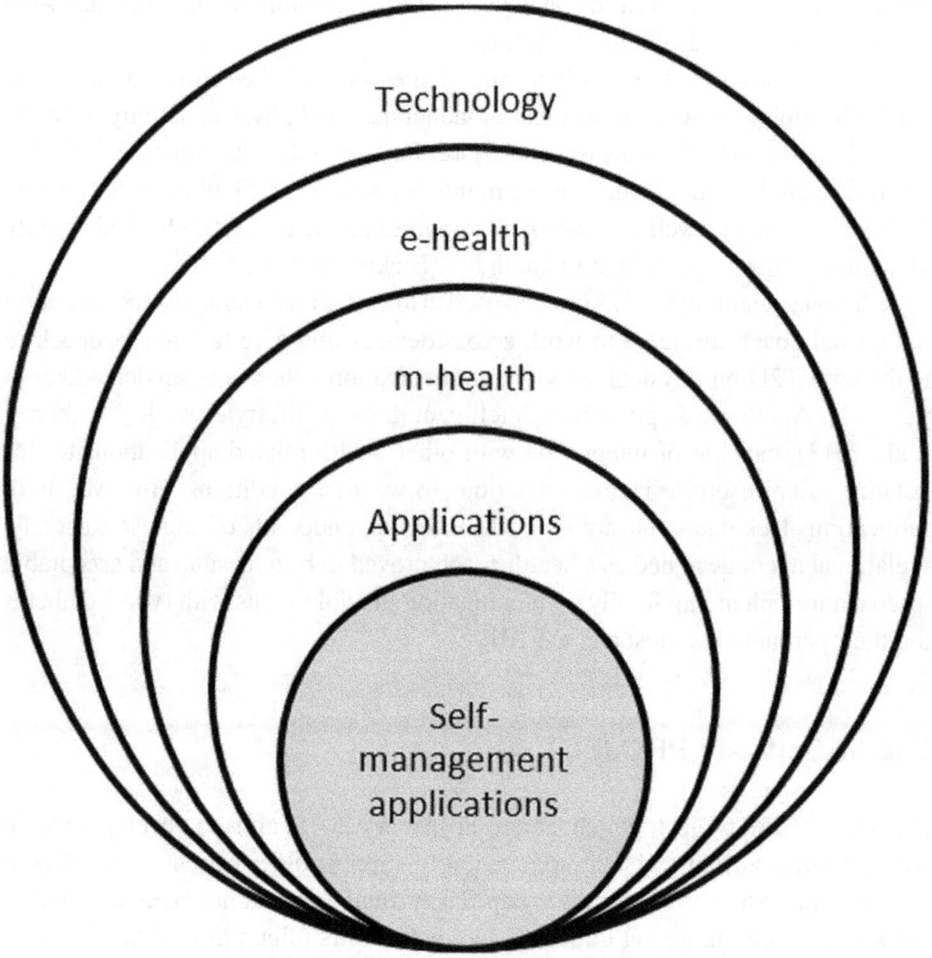

inflexible steps, these phases remind researchers of relevant issues pertaining to the development and evaluation of complex interventions.

Two phase 1 elements were incorporated in the methodological approach. Firstly, 'identifying or developing theory'. Best practice guidelines for developing interventions recommend using theory and suggest that theory-based interventions are more effective than counterparts without a theoretical underpinning (Craig et al., 2008). Behaviour change interventions are commonly designed without a target or successfully change theoretical constructs (Michie, van Stralen, & West, 2011). For example, in the field of medication adherence interventions, the absence of a

Figure 3. Overview of the VASelfCare project

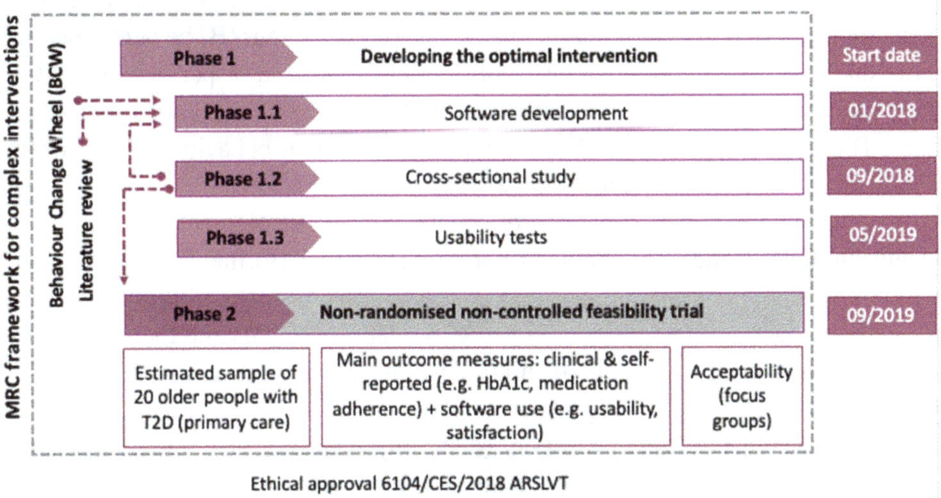

theoretical underpinning has been associated with limited effectiveness (Nieuwlaat et al., 2014; Patton, Hughes, Cadogan, & Ryan, 2017).

To improve the intervention design and its potential effectiveness, the Behaviour Change Wheel (BCW) framework was chosen (Michie, Atkins, & West, 2014). This framework enables a theoretical understanding of the change process, considering

Figure 4. Overview of the MRC framework phases

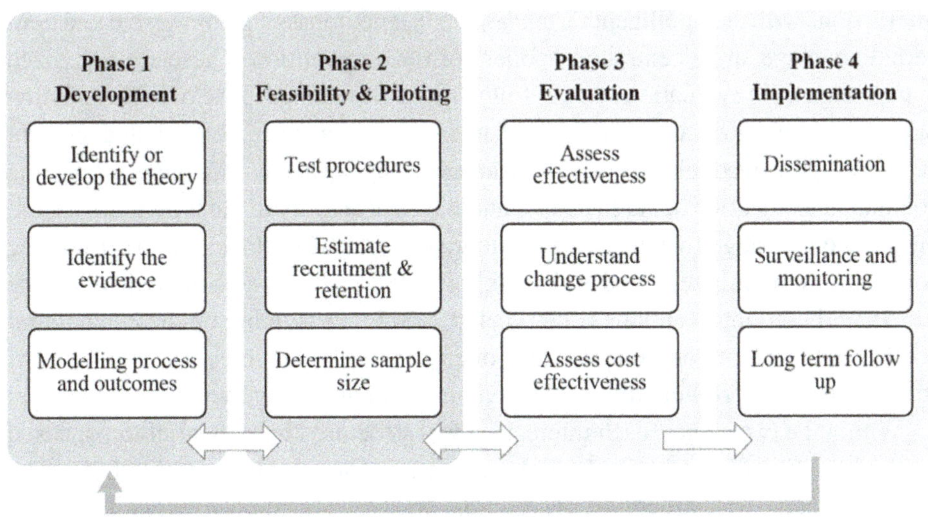

a wide range of influences on behaviour. It guides the intervention design in a systematic and structured fashion, grounded on the COM-B model of human behaviour. COM-B model proposes that for a given behaviour (B) be performed an individual must: be psychologically and physically capable of performing it (C); have social and physical opportunities to do so (O); and be motivated to carry it out (M) (Michie et al., 2014). The model recognizes that behaviour is part of an interacting system involving all these domains.

Another phase 1 element incorporated in the methodological approach was identifying the evidence. This included, but was not restricted to, literature searches on:

- The impact of interventions resorting to relational agents and their features;
- The impact of self-management applications for diabetes and its features;
- Guidelines for self-management of T2D;
- Features of beneficial lifestyle (diet, physical activity) and medication adherence interventions across a range of samples.

Phase 2 of the project (Figure 3) draws on phase 2 of the MRC framework (Figure 4). In phase 2 the prototype will be trialed for feasibility using patients enrolled in nursing consultations in participating primary care units. Such trial will be used to test sampling (namely inclusion and exclusion criteria), recruitment and data collection procedures. This information, together with data yielded, is expected to inform a possible future randomized controlled trial.

DESIGNING THE VASelfCare INTERVENTION

Interactions with the intelligent virtual assistant, encompassing both verbal and non-verbal language, are a central component of the intervention. These are organized in two stages: (1) evaluation and (2) follow-up. The main purpose of the evaluation phase is to collect data on variables of interest, such as user's knowledge, current behaviour, perceived self-efficacy or basic psychological needs. This enables tailoring content on medication adherence, diet and physical activity to the individual user in the subsequent stage (Migneault, Farzanfar, Wright, & Friedman, 2006). Tailoring content is commonly regarded as desirable and endorsed by meta-analytic evidence from web-based interventions (Lustria et al., 2013). Depending on the behavioural component, "evaluation" ranges from one to three interactions. The "follow-up" stage purports to promote desired behaviours or maintaining them.

Within the two stages, each interaction was structured in sequential steps, based on the literature (Timothy W. Bickmore, Caruso, Clough-Gorr, et al., 2005). The evaluation stage was structured in six steps: opening, social talk, assess, feedback, pre-closing and closing. The "opening" and "social talk" steps consist of greeting the user and inquiries about the general emotional and physical state, respectively. Questions on variables of interest are then posed ("assess"), such as on medication knowledge or healthy eating behaviours, followed by feedback on the answers collected. Finally, the content of the next interaction is described in the "pre-closing step" and a farewell is delivered ("closing"). The dialogues in the "follow-up" stage have three additional steps (Bickmore, Caruso, Clough-Gorr, et al., 2005); the first two ("opening" and "social talk") and the last two steps ("pre-closing" and "closing") correspond to those described in the previous stage. In the "review task" step, information is collected about previously agreed tasks or behaviours. Then, feedback is provided, and behaviour determinants are discussed when the user does not achieve the agreed goal ("assess"). The "counselling" step has a twofold purpose. Firstly, it offers strategies to overcome previously identified adherence barriers, if applicable. Secondly, it provides tailored educational content to users, based on the evaluation phase. In the "assign task" step, the user negotiates new goals with virtual assistant.

In addition to tailoring, other principles were employed to write comprehensive and optimal dialogues, including personalization, which broadly involves giving an indication that the software "knows who is talking to" (Migneault et al., 2006), and a helpful-cooperative communication style (Niess & Diefenbach, 2016). Examples of personalization are mentioning the user's name and referring to a relative or friend.

The BCW, the theoretical approach chosen, supported dialogue creation (Michie et al., 2014, 2013). Through the COM-B analyses, the BCW links COM-B domains to intervention functions (IFs) and subsequent policy categories most likely to achieve behavioural change (Michie et al., 2014, 2011). IFs represent how an intervention might change the target behaviour whilst policy categories are described as "types of decisions made by authorities that help to support and enact the intervention" (Michie et al., 2014), p. 235).

Additionally, IFs have been linked to a taxonomy of 93 replicable behaviour change techniques (BCTTv1) (Cane, Richardson, Johnston, Ladha, & Michie, 2015; Michie et al., 2013) which are considered the active ingredients of behaviour change. There is guidance on the BCTs better suited to certain IFs and their underlying theoretical domains (Cane et al., 2015; Michie, Johnston, Francis, Hardeman, & Eccles, 2008). This structured approach lends transparency to the process of intervention development and facilitates its subsequent implementation and evaluation (Michie et al., 2014).

From the list of 93 BCTs, the most appropriate for the VASelfCare intervention were selected based on:

- The most common BCTs under each IF (Michie et al., 2014) ;

- Effective medication adherence interventions from which BCTs could be derived (Nieuwlaat et al., 2014; Sapkota, Brien, Greenfield, & Aslani, 2015; Williams, Walker, Smalls, Campbell, & Egede, 2014);
- Effective BCTs reported on physical activity literature (Gillison, Rouse, Standage, Sebire, & Ryan, 2019) and diet (Cradock, ÓLaighin, Finucane, Gainforth, et al., 2017; Cradock, ÓLaighin, Finucane, Mckay, et al., 2017);
- Effective e-health interventions to improve glycaemic control in adults with T2D (Kebede, Liedtke, Möllers, & Pischke, 2017; Pal et al., 2013);
- A multidisciplinary discussion informed by the APEASE criteria (affordability, practicality, effectiveness and cost-effectiveness, acceptability, side-effects/safety, equity), in particular on the practicality of including BCTs in a digital technology intervention (Michie et al., 2014).

Suitable and potentially effective BCTs were incorporated in the interaction with the virtual assistant, particularly in the follow-up stage, in the "review tasks", "assess", "counselling" and "assign tasks" steps. Its implementation relied on tailoring, informed by the evaluation stage and previous interactions. Table 1 provides examples of BCTs operationalization. The process leading to the selection of BCTs and its operationalization has been described in detail elsewhere for the medication adherence component (Félix et al., 2019).

Dialogues were iteratively created by team members with a nursing, pharmacy, and sports sciences background. To ensure quality, guiding principles were agreed at the outset of the process, dialogue structure and content were discussed regularly, and independent double-checking of scripts was adopted. The latter included checking by an academic nutritionist, who was a member of the VASelfCare advisory board.

THE VASelfCare APPLICATION PROTOTYPE

General Description

The central element of the application is a virtual character called Vitória. This character has an anthropomorphic representation and is capable of speaking and expressing emotions through facial and body animations, depending on the context of the dialogue. Vitória communicates with the user via articulated speech (sound and subtitles), the users' input is collected via buttons or through recording values in the interface. Conveying emotions to users has been acknowledged as the cornerstone for engagement and long-term use (Timothy W. Bickmore et al., 2010).

A female 3D realistic model was chosen from Daz3D (https://www.daz3d.com/). This choice was supported by studies showing that realistic-looking virtual

Table 1. Examples of the operationalization of selected BCTs

BCT	Interactions with the virtual assistant: Medication	Interactions with the virtual assistant: Physical activity	Interactions with the virtual assistant: Diet	Other application features
Feedback on behaviour (2.2)	Verbal and visual information on antidiabetics – taking, via virtual assistant speech, using a helpful-cooperative communication style, and via a calendar.	Verbal and visual information on steps count, via virtual assistant speech, using a helpful-cooperative communication style, and via a chart.	Verbal information on fruit consumption, via virtual assistant speech, using a helpful-cooperative communication style.	Calendar depicting antidiabetics-taking (the same used by the virtual assistant).
Self-monitoring of behaviour (2.3)	Collecting data on antidiabetics-taking by the virtual assistant via a self-completed form.	Collecting data on daily steps count by the virtual assistant via a self-completed form.	Collecting data on vegetable consumption by the virtual assistant.	Record of daily steps count.
Problem solving (1.2)	The virtual assistant lists factors influencing antidiabetics adherence and generates strategies to overcome barriers or potentiate facilitators.	The virtual assistant lists factors influencing adherence to physical activity (walking) and generates strategies to overcome barriers or potentiate facilitators.	The virtual assistant lists factors influencing adherence to healthy eating and generates strategies to overcome barriers or increasing facilitators.	Not applicable.
Goal setting (behaviour) (1.1)	The virtual assistant asks whether the user intends to take oral antidiabetics as prescribed.	The virtual assistant and the user negotiate goals for steps count for the next day.	The virtual assistant asks whether the user intends to perform a specific healthy eating behaviour (e.g. read labels).	Not applicable

agents are more appropriate for medical tasks (Ring, Utami, & Bickmore, 2014; van Wissen, Vinkers, & van Halteren, 2016). Other applications have also employed female figures as relational agents, for example (Timothy W. Bickmore, Caruso, & Clough-Gorr, 2005; Timothy W. Bickmore, Caruso, Clough-Gorr, et al., 2005).

During the interaction, Vitória appears in a 3D scenario representing a living-room where details, such as the room luminosity and the landscape observed through the window, change according to the time of the day and season of the year. Figure 5 depicts the window with a winter scenario in the "Assess" step of medication adherence intervention. Exploring barriers to non-adherence involves a list of determinants that appear sequentially on the screen if the user selects "None of the options" (Figure 5). The inability of identifying non-adherence barriers triggers a referral to the nurse, particularly in case of repeated omission of doses.

The overall development of the application was guided by usability principles for older people (Arnhold, Quade, & Kirch, 2014). For example, redundancy of audio and subtitles may help reduce communication barriers, caused, for example, by lower eyesight accuracy and hearing deficits.

Figure 5. Interaction with Vitória in a medication adherence intervention

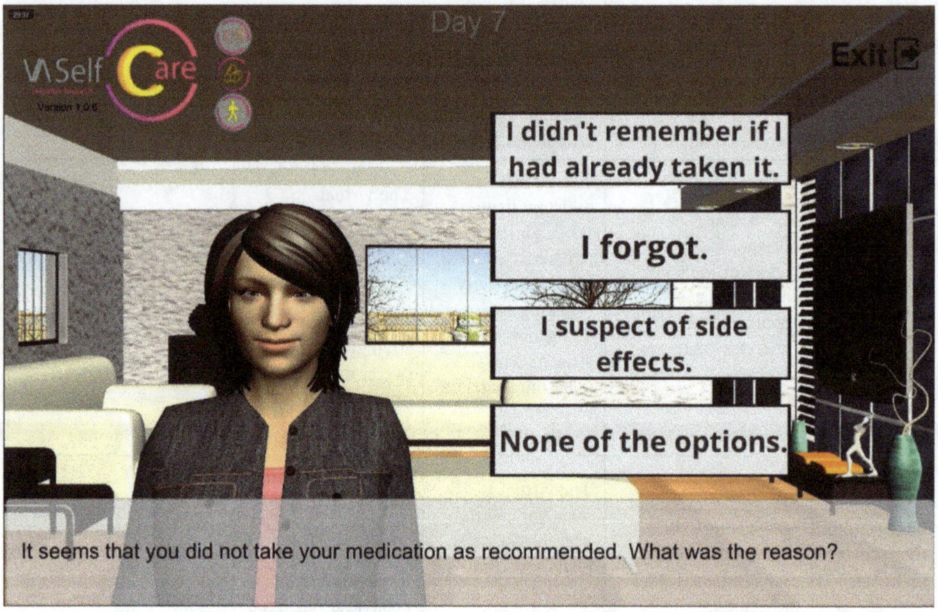
Day 7
VASelf Care
Exit
I didn't remember if I had already taken it.
I forgot.
I suspect of side effects.
None of the options.
It seems that you did not take your medication as recommended. What was the reason?

Figure 6. Application elements per target user

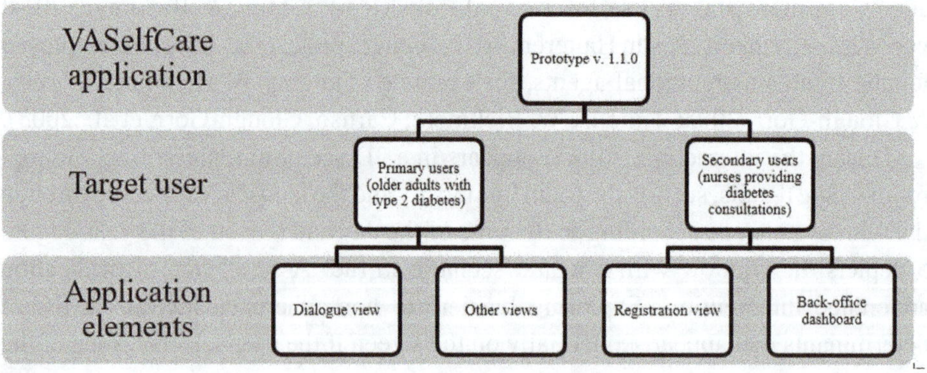

The application runs for a single user in tablets with Android operating system and does not require an Internet connection. This allows access for those without an Internet connection and, in turn, influenced software development options. Each tablet contains a local database that keeps all the interaction records of a particular user.

Figure 6 details the elements built-in the application per type of user. Primary care nurses and older adults with T2D have different initial views. The next sections present some of the functionalities provided by the VASelfCare interface. Both the registration view and the back-office dashboard contribute to the integration with current care pathways.

Registration View

To facilitate the integration of care, users' registration must be performed by the nurse delivering diabetes consultations. Nurses have responsibilities in educating and monitoring these patients; facilitating self-care is integral to the nurse-patient partnership (Henriques, Costa, & Cabrita, 2012).

User registration includes data such as height, weight, the prescribed antidiabetic medication, and the last HbA1c level. The application provides a specific password protected interface for this purpose.

Dialogue View and Other Views

When a person with diabetes logs in, the button "Enter" redirects to an initial menu with a number of options. Selecting the "Talk to Vitória" button starts the dialogue with the virtual assistant. The prototype is designed to allow only one full interaction with Vitória per day. A time-out of 30 minutes has been set up. After this predefined interval, the interaction is automatically cancelled and must be resumed from the outset next time the user selects this functionality.

The initial menu offers supplementary functionalities, organized in hierarchical menus:

- Knowing more (e.g., information about diabetes, diet information, including portion control and seasonal fruit and vegetables);
- Register data (e.g., input weight and blood glucose levels);
- My data (e.g., graphic or visual output of registered data over time, viewing assigned self-care plans);
- My diary (planning the weekly diary);
- My notes (inputting or consulting free text notes, e.g., such as questions to ask to in the next nursing diabetes consultation)
- About this application (e.g., quality assurance policy and data privacy).

"My data" view displays visual information based on data collected through the dialogue view (e.g. daily steps count, medication-taking, number of interactions with Vitória) or through inputted data in other views (e.g. blood glucose levels). Access to these other views is unrestricted.

Back-Office Application

A web browser application, the VASelfCare back-office, was developed to provide controlled access to the user's personal data and the interactions with the VASelfCare application. Data stored in the local database of each tablet is exported, via webservices, to a MySQL database hosted at an external server. This database keeps the data collected from all patients.

As the VASelfCare application can be used without an Internet connection, the content of the local database is exported to the project server whenever Internet access is available, including during nursing diabetes consultations.

Nurses and data administrator have access to contents according to their login credentials. While the nurses can only consult the information regarding their patients, subjected to patient consent, the administrator manages all data and can export anonymous database contents to CSV files, allowing examination of usage patterns and other pertinent analysis for improvement purposes.

Information for nurses is organized as a data dashboard, displaying data in a textual or graphical format, organized in several views through a menu. This information contributes to the integration of care, enabling monitoring and informing self-care support in nursing consultations.

Figure 7 and Figure 8 offer examples of the data dashboard for a fictitious patient. The dashboard tracks data from multiples sources:

Figure 7. VASelfCare back-office dashboard for nurses showing steps count and blood glucose levels charts

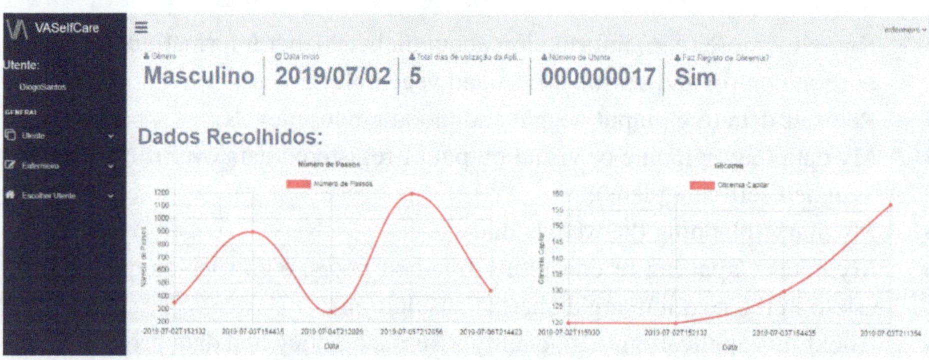

Figure 8. VASelfCare back-office dashboard for nurses showing the application usage

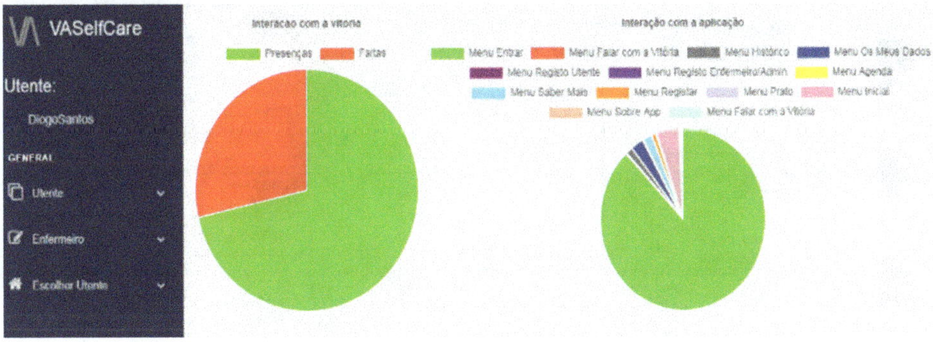

- Inputted by the nurses in the registration view;
- Recorded by the patient in the dialogue view (e.g. self-reported medication adherence and pedometer count) or other views (e.g. blood glucose levels);
- Stored by the application (e.g. number of interactions with Vitória).

Self-reported medication adherence data are converted into several indicators, including the number of missed doses and the level of adherence in percentage. While the commonly accepted 80% threshold for adherence is arguable (Baumgartner, Haynes, Hersberger, & Arnet, 2018), expressing the degree of treatment execution in an objective fashion may be valuable for nurses, namely to prioritize interventions targeting this component in relation to other components of self-care.

The Architecture of the Application

The application comprises three main components: VASelfCare Core, Dialogue Creator and Speech Generator (Figure 9), which are explained in the next sections.

VASelfCare Core

The VASelfCare Core is implemented in Unity3D (https://unity3d.com/pt) with C# scripts. Together they provide the user interface and the logic of the application, controlling the entire execution flow.

In particular, the execution flow is managed by the Application Controller, responsible for the logical sequence of the application plus for communicating with the other components of the VASelfCare Core and with the local database.

The other modules are the Dialogue Controller, the Speech Controller, and the Data Controller. The Dialogue Controller is in charge of the dialogue management.

Figure 9. VASelfCare application architecture

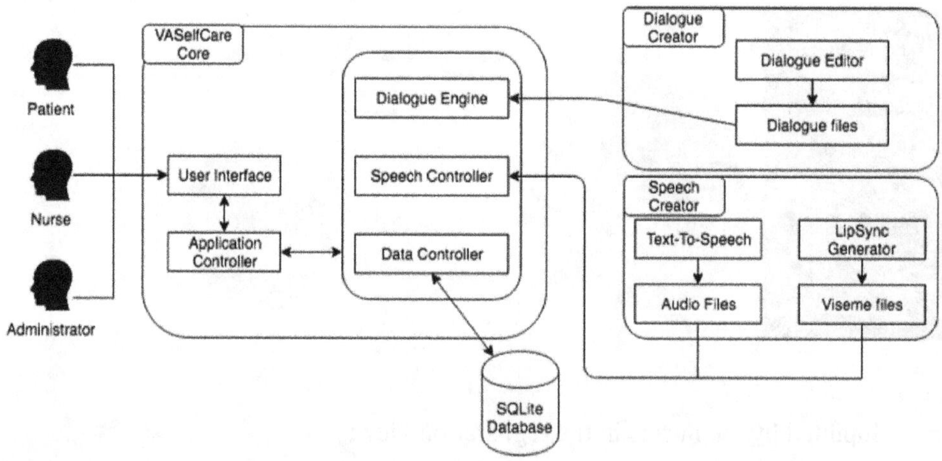

This component uses artificial intelligence techniques to define the dialogue flow. By incorporating context sensitive knowledge, and abstracting some dialogue components, the way the dialogue flow is managed gives the virtual assistant an intelligent dimension. The Speech Controller is the module that allows Vitória to speak, searching and activating the audio and viseme files that correspond to the on-going dialogue. Visemes are mouth animations that simulate phonemes articulation. Conversion of written dialogues to the viseme files is performed by a software previously developed (Cláudio, Carmo, Pinto, Cavaco, & Guerreiro, 2015). The Data Controller role is exchanging data with the local database. This embedded local database keeps track of clinical information inputted by the nurses and of all the user interactions. This information is relevant for the application to decide on the dialogue flow, providing a tailored and personalized interaction.

Dialogue Creator

The Dialogue Creator defines Vitória's speech and the choices presented to the user while the interaction takes place.

The graph system Yarn (https://github.com/InfiniteAmmoInc/Yarn) was chosen to build the dialogues, mainly due to its easy integration with Unity3D. Yarn provides an interface where the virtual assistant speech lines and the options presented to the user for answering are inserted in text boxes, designated by nodes. These are connected in a way that expresses the possible progressions of the dialogue during the interaction. Additionally, it allows the insertion of code lines that influence the dialogue flow.

Speech Generator

The Speech Generator combines audio and their corresponding viseme files to generated Vitória's speech.

The audio files are created using a commercial Text-To-Speech (TTS) software. The choice of Speech2Go (https://harposoftware.com/en/2-main/s-1/index/brand-speech2goivona/language-portuguese) was determined by the availability of voices in European Portuguese, the possibility of unlimited service and no expiration date. To facilitate users' experience the speech rate has been slowed down.

The viseme files are produced by the LipSync Generator, a software developed in-house (Cláudio et al., 2015), as previously mentioned.

Database

SQLite (https://www.sqlite.org/index.html) is employed in the local database. It is a software library that provides a database management system that encompasses a secure storage mechanism.

Co-Production of the Application Prototype

Software development was the first phase of the VASelfCare project, running in parallel with the cross-sectional study (Figure 3). The project embraces the principles of co production, in which digital technology is developed jointly with users, to understand their needs and preferences. Primary and secondary target users (older people with T2D and nurses, respectively) were iteratively involved in defining pre-requisites and testing usability.

Two additional layers of feedback were set up. Firstly, an Advisory Board, comprised of national and international experts in informatics, in research design and in clinical diabetology, as well as a patient representative. Secondly, a group of academic nurses with expertise in primary care.

This section reports the involvement of target users in defining pre-requisites. Evaluation of software requirements by academic primary care nurses has been reported elsewhere (Buinhas et al., 2019).

Participants and Procedure

Nurses, physicians and older people with T2D were purposively sampled within five primary care units (designated as USFs) of the Portuguese National Health Service. The involvement of family physicians was grounded on the potential for future integration of the application with the workflow of these professionals and also in recognition that self-care support may be provided in medical consultations.

A sample size of five to ten individuals in each group was envisaged. Participants were invited by the contact nurse in each primary care unit.

A previously piloted self-administered questionnaire was used as the instrument for data collection. The questionnaire consisted of three parts: social-demographic items, closed items on the prototype and open-ended questions about the prototype. Most items were common for both groups, but healthcare professionals had two additional open-questions and there were differences in three closed-questions. Participants responded to closed-questions on a 5-point Likert scale, with scores from *strongly disagree* (1) to *strongly agree* (5).

Data were collected in individual face-to-face sessions that lasted between 40 to 50 minutes, between July and October 2018. Firstly, the study was explained to participants by a member of the research team and written informed consent forms were signed. Then participants were asked to use a stable version of the prototype independently, guided by a script that covered a sample interaction with Vitória in the evaluation phase of the medication adherence component and other early prototype features. Members of the research team were available to clarify participants' doubts

Descriptive and bivariate statistics were conducted with the aid of *IBM SPSS statistics v.25* software. Missing data (item nonresponse) were excluded from the variable analysis. Textual data were analysed by deriving main themes related to the open-ended questions plus categories under these themes.

Results and Discussion

The sample described in Table 2 was comprised of 19 healthcare professionals (13 nurses and 6 physicians; 18 responses) plus nine adults with T2D.

Overall, the most frequent score was 4 (46,9%). Patients tended to have more positive opinions than healthcare professionals, but differences only reached statistical

Table 2. Socio-demographic profile of the pre-requisites sample

Healthcare professionals (n=19)	· 2 males 2 (10.5%), 17 females (89.5%) · Mean age 46 years (min 25; max 63) · Mean professional experience of 25 years (SD 11.17)
Adults with T2D (n=9)	· 5 males 5 (55.5%), 4 females (44.5%) · Mean age 71 years (min 66; max 89) · Education (n=8): ¼ basic schooling (n=2), ¼ secondary education (n=2), 50% higher education (n=4) · Roughly half (55.6%; n=5) reported using of tablets and/or smartphones daily; 1 participant with no experience

Figure 10. Opinion about Vitória's features (aggregated data – healthcare professionals and patients)

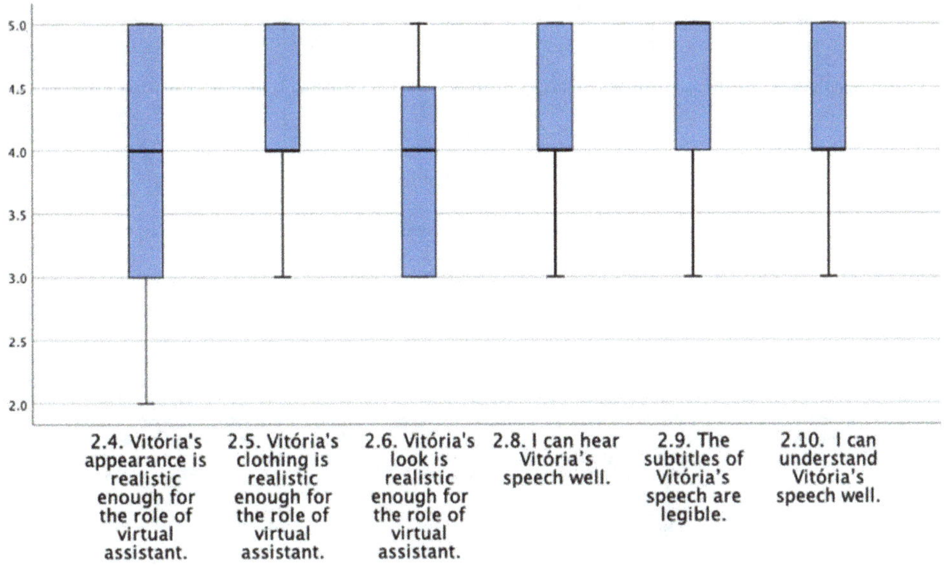

significance for item 2.7, concerning the virtual assistant's facial expression (mean value for professionals 3.37 vs older adults 4.33, t=3.00, p=0.006). Therefore, the remaining data were analysed together. Figure 10 presents the aggregated data on Vitória's features. Responses were, in general, very positive. As for Vitória's facial expressions, the realism of her appearance received the least encouraging opinions. This also emerged in textual data as a negative aspect under the theme technology; for example, one professional said that "Facial expressions are weird" (6_IDP1).

Respondents' opinions on other aspects of the interface were also generally positive (Figure 11). The statements that characters on the screen could be read well received only positive answers.

The application was found easy to use (mean 4.11, min 3, max 5; mean 4.56, min 4, max 5, for professionals and patients respectively). This was corroborated by findings under the category intuitiveness (theme technology): "Easy to handle and understand" (4_IDP1). The statement "I would like to try the application for a few weeks" received positive answers from patients (mean 4.56, min 4, max 5); healthcare professionals were more sceptical in this respect (mean 3.26, min 2, max 5). However, textual data indicates that both groups envisaged difficulties, as illustrated by the accounts of four patients under the technology theme "(People) are not used to use technology" (5_ID1).

Figure 11. Opinion about other interface characteristics (aggregated data – healthcare professionals and patients)

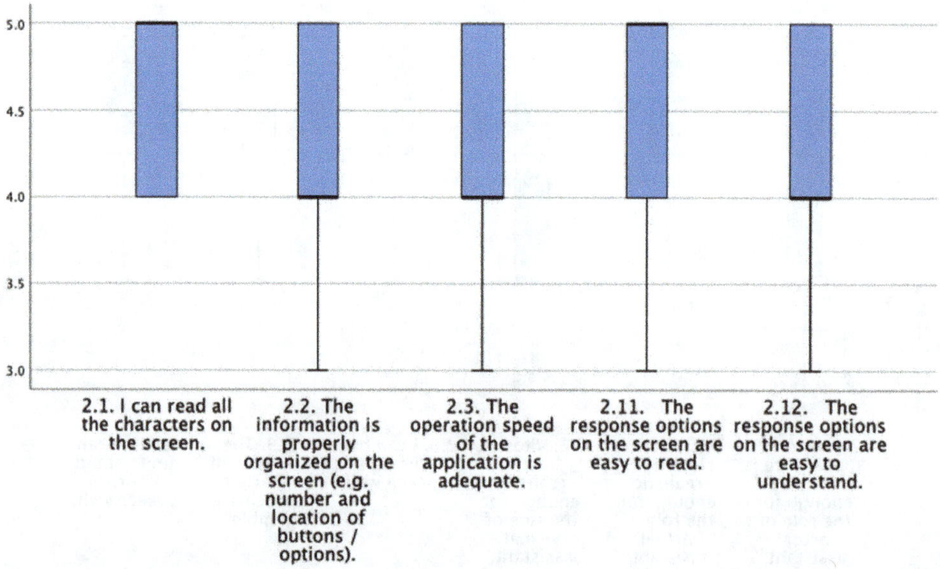

Results highlight the need for training older people with T2D in using a potentially new digital technology. This was already planned in the project protocol and mirrors the procedures adopted in similar studies, e.g. (King et al., 2017).

Patients and health professionals revealed somehow different views on Vitoria's feedback on their answers to questions posed in the evaluation phase. While patients were clearly satisfied (mean 4.56, min 4, max 5), health professionals mentioned that some aspects could be improved: "Address immediately the wrong answers in the evaluation phase" (2_IDP1). This issue merited discussion within the team; the overall positive opinion of patients and practical issues determined the maintenance of the initial approach.

In summary, answers to closed questions indicated, overall, a positive opinion about the prototype.

Textual data from both professionals and patients yielded numerous suggestions to inform pre-requisites, coded in four categories: "monitoring", "medication", "physical activity" and "diet". Data on negative aspects under several themes pointed out opportunities for improvement (e.g. background colours of the prototype were considered gloomy). These data have been addressed in the iterative software development process.

Interestingly, results from these tests with patients and health professionals are overall consistent with the ones obtained from academic nurses with expertise in primary care, which we have previously reported (Buinhas et al., 2019). Such consistency across distinct groups (academics, care providers and patients) is encouraging and endorses the approach we developed based on previous research and clinical literature for the Portuguese context. On-going usability tests, entailing a longer contact with the prototype, will provide additional data in this respect.

POTENTIAL CONTRIBUTION TO THE INDIVIDUAL CARE PLAN

Underlying both the VASelfCare prototype and the individual care plan (ICP) is the notion of patient empowerment, defined as the development of "self-confidence, self-esteem and coping skills to manage the physical, emotional and social impacts of illness in everyday life", equipping patients "to become "co-managers" of their condition in partnership with health professionals" (EMPATHiE Consortium, 2014).

The VASelfCare prototype contributes to the person-centeredness dimension of the ICP (Figure 12) by facilitating self-care through a mobile application for older adults with T2D. The ICP endorses the commonly accepted ethical principle that each person is primarily responsible for her own care; the role of the health system is to supplement the care process according to the person's needs, namely by considering the complexity of her health status and literacy level. Other ICP dimensions, depicted in Figure 12, are supported by the VASelfCare back-office dashboard. As previously explained, this dashboard summarizes pertinent data for T2D management originating from the mobile application use. Currently, these data are intended to be shared with nurses only but, subjected to end-user consent, the dashboard can be made available to other health professionals or, ideally, the entire

Figure 12. Relationship between the ICP dimensions and VASelfCare elements in diseased persons (T2D)

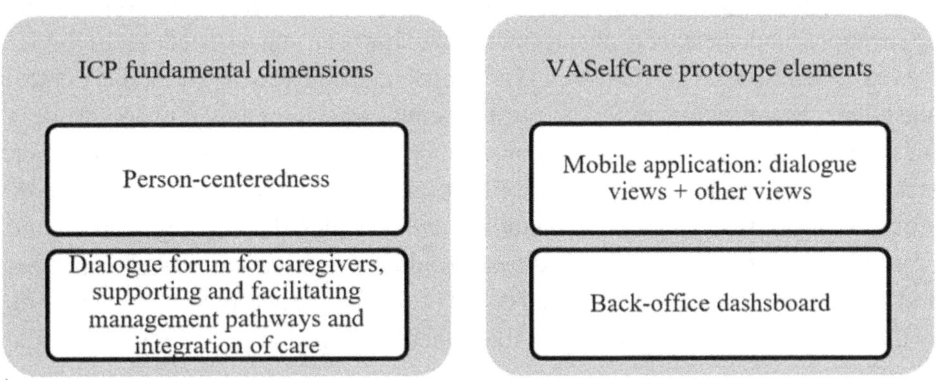

care team. Shared data among the care team is unusual in the Portuguese health system, where fragmented information within and across settings still prevails, with negative implications on efficiency and patient safety. Shared information can be valuable for decision-making about care and provides a common ground for communication between all caregivers, as posited by the ICP model.

ICP developers have conceptualized it in operational terms as an information front-office, shared by all care givers and fed by the electronic health record and additional relevant data, which could be inputted by any sector, level of care or care giver. In this integration paradigm, the VASelfCare back-office application could feed the ICP, should the channels to directly insert and read information be provided. This would also have the advantage of integrating self-care data with the ICP library, containing care guidelines for T2D, enabling easier personalization of treatment goals. An additional advantage would be making data available for automated analysis in processes aiding clinical decision support. An example would be the prediction of hypoglycaemic episodes or glycaemic control based on self-care data accompanied by suggestions for adjusting pharmacologic and non-pharmacologic treatment.

CONCLUSION

Key Points

The main objective of this chapter is to describe the development of a theory-driven and evidence-based digital intervention to facilitate self-care in older adults with Type 2 Diabetes (T2D). Secondary objectives are presenting the contribution of the newly developed digital intervention to healthy aging and the individual care plan.

T2D has an escalating prevalence globally and is associated with life-threatening complications, which are essentially preventable through effective diabetes control. Supporting diabetes self-management is regarded as paramount; as in most chronic diseases, people spend most of their time self-managing their condition. Mobile applications for diabetes self-management have shown an impact in reducing HbA1c. It is expected that VASelfCare can also contribute positively to glycaemic control and other relevant endpoints, by supporting behaviour change and/or maintenance in lifestyle (physical activity, diet) and medication-taking. This assumption, however, lacks empirical validation. The feasibility trial, which is the project's next phase, will determine the intervention viability and whether the investigation should proceed to a randomized controlled trial, to ultimately ascertain the effectiveness and economic endpoints. Such a trial could be a valuable addition to the literature, as the impact of mobile applications for diabetes self-management in older people has been researched infrequently. For example, the trials reviewed by (Cui et al., 2016) and (Hou et al., 2016) included mostly younger samples.

The assumption that the VASelfCare application prototype can contribute to healthy aging by maintaining functional ability (through the promotion of physical activity and healthy eating) warrants also empirical backing.

Developing a prototype specifically for older people is expected to overcome shortcomings of mobile application in this group, illustrated by Arnhold et al. (2014). Pre-requisites data and on-going usability tests support the appropriateness of the VASelfCare prototype for older adults. The feasibility trial, in which subjects will have longer contact with the prototype in a "real world" context, will further elucidate this aspect. Other distinctive features of the VASelfCare prototype, such as working without internet access, may render it more inclusive than commonly available mobile applications.

Co-production with stakeholders, and particularly primary users, is a strong point that may help technology succeeding (Dobson, 2019). While users' needs were not researched at the outset of the project, the iterative pragmatic approach for involving older adults with T2D, health professionals and experts throughout the development phase proved, so far, to be valuable. It has facilitated customization, it yielded opportunities to align the prototype with users' needs and it created a process for quality assurance, in the form of loop verifications. The decision of lifting requirements for the multi-behaviour intervention based on initial prototype features of a single component aided informed opinions by primary users often unaccustomed with self-management mobile applications.

Most m-Heath applications lack a theoretical ground for behaviour change. To maximize its clinical relevance the development of the VASelfCare prototype was guided by the BCW and imbedded in the MRC framework for complex interventions. Resorting to theory enables a better understanding of the behaviour change process (Patton et al., 2017) and tends to have a significant effect on outcomes (Webb, Joseph, Yardley, & Michie, 2010). Using the BCW allows, in turn, linkage with standardized behaviour-change techniques, enabling a clear description of the intervention active ingredients, which can facilitate replication.

FUTURE RESEARCH DIRECTIONS

Few studies have compared relational agents-based interventions with simpler digital technologies. Published evidence on relatively small and younger non-clinical populations presents contradictory results on the superiority of the relational agent approach (Mazzotta, Novielli, & De Carolis, 2009; op den Akker, Klaassen, & Nijholt, 2016). Another study with 178 patients (mean age 46.5 years ± 12.9) compared the acceptability of a relational agent versus a written form on a tablet screen for conducting a clinical structured interview to diagnose major depression disorder (Micoulaud-Franchi et al., 2016). Each subject completed the two digital tools in a randomized order. The relational agent had higher acceptability than the tablet and could avoid the decrease of satisfaction with repeated computerized clinical interviews (Micoulaud-Franchi et al., 2016).

Currently, it is not possible to claim the unarguable superiority of relational agents-based interventions. Further research is needed comparing this approach with the commonly available, text-only mobile applications, in terms of benefits and cost. As previously mentioned, once the intervention viability is established a larger, randomized controlled trial, could contribute to illuminate this issue.

Another research opportunity warranting exploration is adapting the prototype and its algorithms from a multi-behaviour intervention in a single disease to a multi-disease intervention. Digital products supporting self-care in more than a single chronic disease are largely under-researched, in spite of the prevalence of multimorbidity in older people.

Conversely, the prototype also has transferability potential into a simpler mobile application, addressing a healthy lifestyle (physical activity and diet) in non-diseased populations.

ACKNOWLEDGMENT

The authors are indebted to other VASelfCare team members for their contribution to software development (http://vaselfcare.rd.ciencias.ulisboa.pt/). This research was supported by Fundação para a Ciência e Tecnologia (FCT) and Compete 2020 [grant number LISBOA-01-0145-FEDER-024250]. It was also supported by FCT [Research Unit grant UID/MULTI /04046/2019 (to BioISI)].

REFERENCES

American Diabetes Association. (2019a). Older adults: Standards of medical care in diabetes. *Diabetes Care*, *42*(Supplement 1), S139–S147. doi:10.2337/dc19-S012 PMID:30559238

American Diabetes Association. (2019b). Lifestyle Management: Standards of Medical Care in Diabetes - 2019. *Diabetes Care*, *42*(Supplement 1), S46–S60. doi:10.2337/dc19-S005 PMID:30559231

Arnhold, M., Quade, M., & Kirch, W. (2014). Mobile applications for diabetics: A systematic review and expert-based usability evaluation considering the special requirements of diabetes patients age 50 years or older. *Journal of Medical Internet Research, 16*(4), 1–18. doi:10.2196/jmir.2968 PMID:24718852

Baumgartner, P. C., Haynes, R. B., Hersberger, K. E., & Arnet, I. (2018). A Systematic Review of Medication Adherence Thresholds Dependent of Clinical Outcomes. *Frontiers in Pharmacology, 9*, 1290. doi:10.3389/fphar.2018.01290 PMID:30524276

Beard, J. R., Officer, A., De Carvalho, I. A., Sadana, R., Pot, A. M., Michel, J. P., ... Chatterji, S. (2016, May 21). The World report on ageing and health: A policy framework for healthy ageing. *Lancet, 387*(10033), 2145–2154. doi:10.1016/S0140-6736(15)00516-4 PMID:26520231

Bickmore, T. W., Caruso, L., & Clough-Gorr, K. (2005). Acceptance and usability of a relational agent interface by urban older adults. *CHI '05 Extended Abstracts on Human Factors in Computing Systems - CHI '05*, 1212. doi:10.1145/1056808.1056879

Bickmore, T. W., Caruso, L., Clough-Gorr, K., & Heeren, T. (2005). 'It's just like you talk to a friend' relational agents for older adults. *Interacting with Computers, 17*(6), 711–735. doi:10.1016/j.intcom.2005.09.002

Bickmore, T. W., Puskar, K., Schlenk, E. A., Pfeifer, L. M., & Sereika, S. M. (2010). Maintaining reality: Relational agents for antipsychotic medication adherence. *Interacting with Computers, 22*(4), 276–288. doi:10.1016/j.intcom.2010.02.001

Bickmore, T. W., Silliman, R. A., Nelson, K., Cheng, D. M., Winter, M., Henault, L., & Paasche-Orlow, M. K. (2013). A randomized controlled trial of an automated exercise coach for older adults. *Journal of the American Geriatrics Society, 61*(10), 1676–1683. doi:10.1111/jgs.12449 PMID:24001030

Bickmore, T. W., Pfeifer, L. M., & Paasche-Orlow, M. K. (2007). *Health Document Explanation by Virtual Agents*. Intelligent Virtual Agents. doi:10.1007/978-3-540-74997-4_18

Bleijenberg, N., de Man-van Ginkel, J. M., Trappenburg, J. C. A., Ettema, R. G. A., Sino, C. G., Heim, N., ... Schuurmans, M. J. (2018). Increasing value and reducing waste by optimizing the development of complex interventions: Enriching the development phase of the Medical Research Council (MRC) Framework. *International Journal of Nursing Studies, 79*, 86–93. doi:10.1016/j.ijnurstu.2017.12.001 PMID:29220738

Buinhas, S., Cláudio, A. P., Carmo, M. B., Balsa, J., Cavaco, A., Mendes, A., ... Guerreiro, M. P. (2019). *Virtual Assistant to Improve Self-care of Older People with Type 2 Diabetes: First Prototype*. doi:10.1007/978-3-030-16028-9_21

Cane, J., Richardson, M., Johnston, M., Ladha, R., & Michie, S. (2015). From lists of behaviour change techniques (BCTs) to structured hierarchies: Comparison of two methods of developing a hierarchy of BCTs. *British Journal of Health Psychology*, *20*(1), 130–150. doi:10.1111/bjhp.12102 PMID:24815766

Centers for Disease Control and Prevention. (2017). National Diabetes Statistics Report: Estimates of Diabetes and Its Burden in the United States. Atlanta, GA: Centers for Disease Control and Prevention.

Chen, L., Pei, J.-H., Kuang, J., Chen, H.-M., Chen, Z., Li, Z.-W., & Yang, H.-Z. (2015). Effect of lifestyle intervention in patients with type 2 diabetes: A meta-analysis. *Metabolism: Clinical and Experimental*, *64*(2), 338–347. doi:10.1016/j.metabol.2014.10.018 PMID:25467842

Cho, N. H., Shaw, J. E., Karuranga, S., Huang, Y., da Rocha Fernandes, J. D., Ohlrogge, A. W., & Malanda, B. (2018). IDF Diabetes Atlas: Global estimates of diabetes prevalence for 2017 and projections for 2045. *Diabetes Research and Clinical Practice*, *138*, 271–281. doi:10.1016/j.diabres.2018.02.023 PMID:29496507

Chomutare, T., Fernandez-Luque, L., Årsand, E., & Hartvigsen, G. (2011). Features of Mobile Diabetes Applications: Review of the Literature and Analysis of Current Applications Compared Against Evidence-Based Guidelines. *Journal of Medical Internet Research*, *13*(3), e65. doi:10.2196/jmir.1874 PMID:21979293

Chrvala, C. A., Sherr, D., & Lipman, R. D. (2016). Diabetes self-management education for adults with type 2 diabetes mellitus: A systematic review of the effect on glycemic control. *Patient Education and Counseling*, *99*(6), 926–943. doi:10.1016/j.pec.2015.11.003 PMID:26658704

Cláudio, A. P., Carmo, M. B., Pinto, V., Cavaco, A., & Guerreiro, M. P. (2015). Virtual humans for training and assessment of self-medication consultation skills in pharmacy students. *10th International Conference on Computer Science & Education (ICCSE)*, 175–180. 10.1109/ICCSE.2015.7250238

Cradock, K. A., ÓLaighin, G., Finucane, F., Mckay, R., Quinlan, L. R., Ginis, K. A. M., & Gainforth, H. L. (2017). Diet Behavior Change Techniques in Type 2 Diabetes: A Systematic Review and Meta-analysis. *Diabetes Care*, *40*(12), 1800–1810. doi:10.2337/dc17-0462 PMID:29162585

Cradock, K. A., ÓLaighin, G., Finucane, F. M., Gainforth, H. L., Quinlan, L. R., & Ginis, K. A. M. (2017). Behaviour change techniques targeting both diet and physical activity in type 2 diabetes: A systematic review and meta-analysis. *The International Journal of Behavioral Nutrition and Physical Activity*, *14*(18), 1–17. doi:10.118612966-016-0436-0 PMID:28178985

Craig, P., Dieppe, P., Macintyre, S., Michie, S., Nazareth, I., & Petticrew, M. (2008). Developing and evaluating complex interventions: The new Medical Research Council guidance. *BMJ, 337*(a1655), 979–983. doi:10.1136/bmj.a1655

Cui, M., Wu, X., Mao, J., Wang, X., & Nie, M. (2016). T2DM self-management via smartphone applications: A systematic review and meta-analysis. *PLoS One, 11*(11), 1–15. doi:10.1371/journal.pone.0166718 PMID:27861583

de Jong, C. C., Ros, W. J., & Schrijvers, G. (2014). The Effects on Health Behavior and Health Outcomes of Internet-Based Asynchronous Communication Between Health Providers and Patients With a Chronic Condition: A Systematic Review. *Journal of Medical Internet Research, 16*(1), e19. doi:10.2196/jmir.3000 PMID:24434570

Dobson, J. (2019). Co-production helps ensure that new technology succeeds. *BMJ (Clinical Research Ed.), 366*, l4833. doi:10.1136/bmj.l4833

EMPATHiE Consortium. (2014). *EMPATHiE - Empowering patients in the management of chronic diseases - Final Summary Report.* Retrieved from https://ehff.eu/wp-content/uploads/2015/10/empathie_frep_en.pdf

Félix, I. B., Guerreiro, M. P., Cavaco, A., Cláudio, A. P., Mendes, A., Balsa, J., ... Henriques, A. (2019). Development of a Complex Intervention to Improve Adherence to Antidiabetic Medication in Older People Using an Anthropomorphic Virtual Assistant Software. *Frontiers in Pharmacology, 10*(June), 1–13. doi:10.3389/fphar.2019.00680 PMID:31281256

Free, C., Phillips, G., Watson, L., Galli, L., Felix, L., Edwards, P., ... Haines, A. (2013). The Effectiveness of Mobile-Health Technologies to Improve Health Care Service Delivery Processes: A Systematic Review and Meta-Analysis. *PLoS Medicine, 10*(1), e1001363. doi:10.1371/journal.pmed.1001363 PMID:23458994

García-Pérez, L. E., Álvarez, M., Dilla, T., Gil-Guillén, V., & Orozco-Beltrán, D. (2013). Adherence to therapies in patients with type 2 diabetes. *Diabetes Therapy : Research, Treatment and Education of Diabetes and Related Disorders, 4*(2), 175–194. doi:10.100713300-013-0034-y PMID:23990497

Gilbert, B. J., Goodman, E., Chadda, A., Hatfield, D., Forman, D. E., & Panch, T. (2015). The Role of Mobile Health in Elderly Populations. *Current Geriatrics Reports, 4*(4), 347–352. doi:10.100713670-015-0145-6

Gillison, F. B., Rouse, P., Standage, M., Sebire, S. J., & Ryan, R. M. (2019). A meta-analysis of techniques to promote motivation for health behaviour change from a self-determination theory perspective. *Health Psychology Review, 13*(1), 110–130. doi:10.1080/17437199.2018.1534071 PMID:30295176

Henriques, M. A., Costa, M. A., & Cabrita, J. (2012). Adherence and medication management by the elderly. *Journal of Clinical Nursing, 21*(21–22), 3096–3105. doi:10.1111/j.1365-2702.2012.04144.x PMID:22882751

Hou, C., Carter, B., Hewitt, J., Francisa, T., & Mayor, S. (2016). Do Mobile Phone Applications Improve Glycemic Control (HbA1c) in the Self-management of Diabetes? A Systematic Review, Meta-analysis, and GRADE of 14 Randomized Trials. *Diabetes Care, 39*(11), 2089–2095. doi:10.2337/dc16-0346 PMID:27926892

INE. (2006). *Sociedade da informação e do conhecimento - Inquérito à utilização de tecnologias da informação e da comunicação pelas famílias: 2006*. INE.

INE. (2015). *Sociedade da Informação e do Conhecimento - Inquérito à Utilização de Tecnologias da Informação e da Comunicação pelas Famílias*. INE.

International Diabetes Federation. (2017). *IDF Diabetes Atlas* (8th ed.). Retrieved from https://diabetesatlas.org/

Kalyani, R. R., Golden, S. H., & Cefalu, W. T. (2017). Diabetes and aging: Unique considerations and goals of care. *Diabetes Care, 40*(4), 440–443. doi:10.2337/dci17-0005 PMID:28325794

Kebede, M. M., Liedtke, T. P., Möllers, T., & Pischke, C. R. (2017). Characterizing Active Ingredients of eHealth Interventions Targeting Persons With Poorly Controlled Type 2 Diabetes Mellitus Using the Behavior Change Techniques Taxonomy: Scoping Review. *Journal of Medical Internet Research, 19*(10), e348. doi:10.2196/jmir.7135 PMID:29025693

Kim, B. Y., & Lee, J. (2017). Smart Devices for Older Adults Managing Chronic Disease: A Scoping Review. *JMIR mHealth and uHealth, 5*(5), e69. doi:10.2196/mhealth.7141 PMID:28536089

King, A. C., Campero, I., Sheats, J. L., Castro Sweet, C. M., Garcia, D., Chazaro, A., ... Bickmore, T. (2017). Testing the comparative effects of physical activity advice by humans vs. computers in underserved populations: The COMPASS trial design, methods, and baseline characteristics. *Contemporary Clinical Trials, 61*(April), 115–125. doi:10.1016/j.cct.2017.07.020 PMID:28739541

Lavie, C. J., Johannsen, N., Swift, D., Sénéchal, M., Earnest, C., Church, T., ... Blair, S. N. (2014). Exercise is Medicine—The Importance of Physical Activity, Exercise Training, Cardiorespiratory Fitness, and Obesity in the Prevention and Treatment of Type 2 Diabetes. *European Endocrinology, 10*(1), 18–22. doi:10.17925/EE.2014.10.01.18 PMID:29872459

Lee, J.-A., Choi, M., Lee, S. A., & Jiang, N. (2018). Effective behavioral intervention strategies using mobile health applications for chronic disease management: A systematic review. *BMC Medical Informatics and Decision Making*, *18*(1), 12. doi:10.118612911-018-0591-0 PMID:29458358

Lee, P. G., & Halter, J. B. (2017). The pathophysiology of hyperglycemia in older adults: Clinical considerations. *Diabetes Care*, *40*(4), 444–452. doi:10.2337/dc16-1732 PMID:28325795

Lustria, M. L. A., Noar, S. M., Cortese, J., Van Stee, S. K., Glueckauf, R. L., & Lee, J. (2013). A meta-analysis of web-delivered tailored health behavior change interventions. *Journal of Health Communication*, *18*(9), 1039–1069. doi:10.1080/10810730.2013.768727 PMID:23750972

Mazzotta, I., Novielli, N., & De Carolis, B. (2009). Are ECAs more persuasive than textual messages? In Lecture Notes in Computer Science (Vol. 5773, pp. 527–528). Springer. doi:10.1007/978-3-642-04380-2_75

Medical Research Council. (2000). *A Framework for Development and Evaluation of RCTs for Complex Interventions to Improve Health*. Author.

Michie, S., Atkins, L., & West, R. (2014). The Behavior Change Wheel: A Guide To Designing Interventions. London: Silverback Publishing.

Michie, S., Johnston, M., Francis, J., Hardeman, W., & Eccles, M. (2008). From Theory to Intervention: Mapping Theoretically Derived Behavioural Determinants to Behaviour Change Techniques. *Applied Psychology*, *57*(4), 660–680. doi:10.1111/j.1464-0597.2008.00341.x

Michie, S., Richardson, M., Johnston, M., Abraham, C., Francis, J., Hardeman, W., ... Wood, C. E. (2013). The behavior change technique taxonomy (v1) of 93 hierarchically clustered techniques: Building an international consensus for the reporting of behavior change interventions. *Annals of Behavioral Medicine*, *46*(1), 81–95. doi:10.100712160-013-9486-6 PMID:23512568

Michie, S., van Stralen, M. M., & West, R. (2011). The behaviour change wheel: A new method for characterising and designing behaviour change interventions. *Implementation Science; IS*, *6*(42), 1–11. doi:10.1186/1748-5908-6-42 PMID:21513547

Micoulaud-Franchi, J. A., Sagaspe, P., De Sevin, E., Bioulac, S., Sauteraud, A., & Philip, P. (2016). Acceptability of embodied conversational agent in a health care context. Lecture Notes in Computer Science, 10011, 416–419. doi:10.1007/978-3-319-47665-0_45

Migneault, J. P., Farzanfar, R., Wright, J. A., & Friedman, R. H. (2006). How to write health dialog for a talking computer. *Journal of Biomedical Informatics*, *39*(5), 468–481. doi:10.1016/j.jbi.2006.02.009 PMID:16564749

Monkaresi, H., Calvo, R. A., Pardo, A., Chow, K., Mullan, B., & Lam, M., … Cook, D. I. (2013). Intelligent Diabetes Lifestyle Coach. *Fifth International Workshop on Smart Healthcare and Wellness Applications (SmartHealth'13)*, 1–4.

Mota-Pinto, A., Rodrigues, V., Botelho, A., Veríssimo, M. T., Morais, A., Alves, C., ... de Oliveira, C. R. (2010). A socio-demographic study of aging in the Portuguese population: The EPEPP study. *Archives of Gerontology and Geriatrics*, *52*(3), 304–308. doi:10.1016/j.archger.2010.04.019 PMID:20510469

Munshi, M. (2019). *Treatment of type 2 diabetes mellitus in the older patient - UpToDate*. Retrieved September 16, 2019, from https://www.uptodate.com/contents/treatment-of-type-2-diabetes-mellitus-in-the-older-patient

Niess, J., & Diefenbach, S. (2016). Communication Styles of Interactive Tools for Self-Improvement. *Psychology of Well-Being*, *6*(1), 3. doi:10.118613612-016-0040-8 PMID:27335769

Nieuwlaat, R., Wilczynski, N., Navarro, T., Hobson, N., Jeffery, R., Keepanasseril, A., ... Haynes, R. (2014). Interventions for enhancing medication adherence [Review]. *Cochrane Database of Systematic Reviews*, (11), 1–730. doi:10.1002/14651858.CD000011.pub4 PMID:25412402

OECD/EU. (2018). *Health at a Glance: Europe 2018.* Summary in Spanish. doi:10.1787/fd41e65f-es

op den Akker, R., Klaassen, R., & Nijholt, A. (2016). Virtual Coaches for Healthy Lifestyle. In *Toward Robotic Socially Believable Behaving Systems - Volume II. Modeling Social Signals* (Vol. 106). doi:10.1016/j.neulet.2006.07.043

op den Akker, R., Klaassen, R., Lavrysen, T., Geleijnse, G., van Halteren, A., Schwietert, H., & van der Hout, M. (2011). A Personal Context-aware Multi-device Coaching Service That Supports a Healthy Lifestyle. *Proceedings of the 25th BCS Conference on Human-Computer Interaction*, 443–448. Retrieved from https://dl.acm.org/citation.cfm?id=2305316.2305397

Paiva, D., Silva, S., Severo, M., Moura-Ferreira, P., Lunet, N., & Azevedo, A. (2017). Limited Health Literacy in Portugal Assessed with the Newest Vital Sign Prevalência de Literacia em Saúde Inadequada em Portugal Medida com o Newest Vital Sign. *Acta Medica Portuguesa*, *30*(12), 861–869. doi:10.20344/amp.9135 PMID:29364799

Pal, K., Eastwood, S. V., Michie, S., Farmer, A. J., Barnard, M. L., Peacock, R., ... Murray, E. (2013). Computer-based diabetes self-management interventions for adults with type 2 diabetes mellitus. *Cochrane Database of Systematic Reviews*, (3). doi:10.1002/14651858.CD008776.pub2 PMID:23543567

Patton, D. E., Hughes, C. M., Cadogan, C. A., & Ryan, C. A. (2017). Theory-Based Interventions to Improve Medication Adherence in Older Adults Prescribed Polypharmacy: A Systematic Review. *Drugs & Aging*, *34*(2), 97–113. doi:10.100740266-016-0426-6 PMID:28025725

Ring, L., Utami, D., & Bickmore, T. (2014). The right agent for the job? The effects of agent visual appearance on task domain. Lecture Notes in Computer Science, 8637, 374–384. doi:10.1007/978-3-319-09767-1_49

Sapkota, S., Brien, J. A. E., Greenfield, J. R., & Aslani, P. (2015). A systematic review of interventions addressing adherence to anti-diabetic medications in patients with type 2 diabetes - Components of interventions. *PLoS One*, *10*(2), 1–17. doi:10.1371/journal.pone.0118296 PMID:26053004

Self Care Forum. (2016). *What do we mean by self care and why is it good for people?* Retrieved September 16, 2019, from http://www.selfcareforum.org/about-us/what-do-we-mean-by-self-care-and-why-is-good-for-people/

Sociedade Portuguesa de Diabetologia. (2016). Relatório Anual do Observatório Nacional da Diabetes 2016. In *Letra Soluvel - Publicidade e Marketing, Lda* (Vol. 1). Retrieved from https://www.clinicadadiabetes.pt/assets/docs/relatorio_anual_Diabetes_2016/

Suzman, R., Beard, J. R., Boerma, T., & Chatterji, S. (2015). Health in an ageing world - What do we know? *Lancet*, *385*(9967), 484–486. doi:10.1016/S0140-6736(14)61597-X PMID:25468156

Thompson, D., Callender, C., Gonynor, C., Cullen, K. W., Redondo, M. J., Butler, A., & Anderson, B. J. (2019). Using Relational Agents to Promote Family Communication Around Type 1 Diabetes Self-Management in the Diabetes Family Teamwork Online Intervention: Longitudinal Pilot Study. *Journal of Medical Internet Research*, *21*(9), e15318. doi:10.2196/15318 PMID:31538940

van Wissen, A., Vinkers, C., & van Halteren, A. (2016). Developing a Virtual Coach for Chronic Patients: A User Study on the Impact of Similarity, Familiarity and Realism. In A. Meschtscherjakov, B. De Ruyter, V. Fuchsberger, M. Murer, & M. Tscheligi (Eds.), *Persuasive Technology* (pp. 263–275). Cham: Springer International Publishing. doi:10.1007/978-3-319-31510-2_23

Webb, T. L., Joseph, J., Yardley, L., & Michie, S. (2010). Using the Internet to promote health behavior change: A systematic review and meta-analysis of the impact of theoretical basis, use of behavior change techniques, and mode of delivery on efficacy. *Journal of Medical Internet Research*, *12*(1), e4. doi:10.2196/jmir.1376 PMID:20164043

Wildenbos, G. A., Peute, L., & Jaspers, M. (2018). Aging barriers influencing mobile health usability for older adults: A literature based framework (MOLD-US). *International Journal of Medical Informatics*, *114*, 66–75. doi:10.1016/j.ijmedinf.2018.03.012 PMID:29673606

Williams, J. L. S., Walker, R. J., Smalls, B. L., Campbell, J. A., & Egede, L. E. (2014). Effective interventions to improve medication adherence in Type 2 diabetes: A systematic review. *Diabetes Management*, *4*(1), 29–48. doi:10.2217/dmt.13.62 PMID:25214893

World Health Organization. (2015). Chapter 3: Health in Older Age. In World Report on Ageing and Health (pp. 43–63). WHO.

World Health Organization. (2017). *Global strategy and action plan on ageing and health*. Retrieved from https://apps.who.int/bookorders

World Health Organization. (2019). *WHO guideline Recommendations on Digital Interventions for Health System Strengthening*. Retrieved from https://www.ncbi.nlm.nih.gov/pubmed/31162915

Ye, Q., Khan, U., Boren, S. A., Simoes, E. J., & Kim, M. S. (2018). An Analysis of Diabetes Mobile Applications Features Compared to AADE7™: Addressing Self-Management Behaviors in People With Diabetes. *Journal of Diabetes Science and Technology*, *12*(4), 808–816. doi:10.1177/1932296818754907 PMID:29390917

Zheng, Y., Ley, S. H., & Hu, F. B. (2018). Global aetiology and epidemiology of type 2 diabetes mellitus and its complications. *Nature Reviews. Endocrinology*, *14*(2), 88–98. doi:10.1038/nrendo.2017.151 PMID:29219149

ADDITIONAL READING

Balsa, J., Neves, P., Félix, I., Pereira Guerreiro, M., Alves, P., & Carmo, M. B. … Cláudio, A. P. (2019). Intelligent Virtual Assistant for Promoting Behaviour Change in Older People with T2D. In: P. Moura Oliveira., P. Novais & L. Reis (eds) Progress in Artificial Intelligence. EPIA 2019. Lecture Notes in Computer Science, vol. 11804, pp 372-83. Springer, Cham

Magyar, G., Balsa, J., Cláudio, A. P., Carmo, M. B., Neves, P., & Alves, P. … Guerreiro, M. P. (2019). Anthropomorphic virtual assistant to support self-care of type 2 diabetes in older people: A perspective on the role of artificial intelligence. *VISIGRAPP 2019 - Proceedings of the 14th International Joint Conference on Computer Vision, Imaging and Computer Graphics Theory and Applications*, 323–331.

Powers, M. A., Bardsley, J., Cypress, M., Duker, P., Funnell, M. M., Fischl, A. H., ... Vivian, E. (2015). Diabetes Self-management Education and Support in Type 2 Diabetes: A Joint Position Statement of the American Diabetes Association, the American Association of Diabetes Educators, and the Academy of Nutrition and Dietetics. *Journal of the Academy of Nutrition and Dietetics*, *115*(8), 1323–1334. doi:10.1016/j.jand.2015.05.012 PMID:26054423

KEY TERMS AND DEFINITIONS

Application (App): A computer program or group of programs designed for users, which rely on low level computer programs to work, such as operating systems.

Co-Production of a Digital Health Product: Involvement of primary users (and often other stakeholders) in product design or testing. The degree of involvement may vary from incorporating feedback to participation of users in research and development teams.

Digital Health Product: A product with an ultimate therapeutic purpose that works on computers or via the internet.

Electronic Health (E-Health): Provision of health care services or information exchange in the health context through computers devices and related technologies (e.g. the internet).

Mobile Health (M-Health): Provision of health care services or information exchange in the health context via wireless devices (e.g. smartphone, tablet, smart pill boxes) and related technologies (e.g. 3G and 4G systems mobile telecommunications, global positioning system, Bluetooth).

Older Person: Any individual aged 65 years or more.

Patient Empowerment: Actions aiming to educate an individual about one's disease, to promote shared decision making with professionals, in the extent desired by the individual, and to encourage self-management.

Relational Agent: Anthropomorphic virtual character designed to build rapport with users over time and establishing long-term relationships.

Self-Care: Tasks performed by an individual to maintain or restore one's health and to deal with disease, with or without the support of health professionals. It comprises, but it is not limited, to self-prevention, self-diagnosis, self-medication and self-management of disease and disability.

Self-Management: Tasks performed by an individual to minimize the impact of one's disease, with or without the support of health professionals. Tasks can holistically be categorized under medical management (e.g., taking medication, adhering to a diet, engaging in physical activity), role management (e.g., redefining life roles in light of a chronic disease) and emotional management (e.g., dealing with anger and frustration), and are related to a set of skills.

Technology: Application of technical processes or scientific knowledge for practical purposes.

Chapter 13
Integrated Continuous Healthcare Team Computer System Architecture

José Jasnau Caeiro
https://orcid.org/0000-0002-4760-726X
Instituto Politécnico de Beja, Portugal

Henrique Oliveira
https://orcid.org/0000-0001-8687-4291
Instituto de Telecomunicações, Instituto Superior Técnico, Portugal

Margarida Goes
https://orcid.org/0000-0001-6017-6874
Universidade Católica Portuguesa, Portugal

Manuel Lopes
https://orcid.org/0000-0002-7554-8041
Universidade de Évora, Portugal

César Fonseca
https://orcid.org/0000-0001-6975-612X
Universidade de Évora, Portugal

ABSTRACT

A computer-based pattern recognition system architecture destined to collect and process geographically referenced data about integrated continuous healthcare teams (ECCI) is presented and discussed in the chapter. These teams are part of Portugal's National Network of Integrated Continuous Care (RNCCI). The system is designed

DOI: 10.4018/978-1-7998-1937-0.ch013

to collect data about the displacement of each team during healthcare assistance. The pattern recognition system handles information about the costs related to the provided healthcare. The architecture is designed around open source software resources. Virtual machines and container-based technologies provide hardware independence. The Python programming language ecosystem is chosen for all the main components of the system.

INTRODUCTION

The no. 101/2006 Decree-law of Portugal (Government, 2006), creates the National Integrated Continued Healthcare Network, constituted by continued healthcare teams and units, and/or social support, and/or palliative care and actions. ECCI's (Integrated Continued Healthcare Teams) are defined as multidisciplinary teams that provide domiciled primary healthcare and social services to people with functional dependencies, terminal illness or are undergoing a convalescence process. These people are in situation that doesn't require them to be admitted but are unable to move autonomously. The ECCI teams may be constituted by a set of medical doctors, nurses, social workers and psychologists. All over the country there in was in the year 2016 a set of 279 teams (Administração Central do Sistema de Saúde, 2017) þ, see Table 1. There are a number of factors that contribute to the heterogeneity in terms of these teams such as:

- **The Area Covered by Each Team:** There are regions that are very large and rural thus making the ECCI team displacement an important cost issue. This is the case with the Alentejo and Center regions.
- **The Population Density:** There are densely populated areas such as the North and Lisboa and Tejo Valley whereas other areas in the country are sparsely populated such as Alentejo and the Center.
- **The Constitution of Each Team:** Each team has a varying number of doctors, nurses and other staff.

The elderly population in Portugal (PopulationPyramid.net, 2019) is already large and is growing and thus originates a strong and steady increase in the associated health care costs.

Machine learning systems have met during the last few years a rise in application fields. Some of these systems provide information that allow decision makers to take more informed policy decisions about a subject.

Table 1. Distribution of ECCI teams for each region of continental Portugal

Region	Area (Km2)	Inhabitants	Number of ECCI teams
North	21 278	3 689 173	84
Center	28 462	2 327 026	66
Lisboa and Tejo Valley	11 930	3 447 173	60
Alentejo	31 551	758 739	37
Algarve	4 997	451 006	32
Total	92 218	10 673 117	279

The system presented and discussed in the chapter will be designated throughout the document by ECCI-PR (ECCI- Pattern Recognition). This system's purpose is to present to decision makers managing integrated health resources, high level data analysis, using modern machine learning software tools applied to geographical located data, collected from ECCI team displacements. The system will provide information about the possibilities of cost optimization and improvement in service quality to the decision makers.

The system is built with open source components and is described in the next sections.

INTEGRATED CONTINUED HEALTHCARE PATTERN RECOGNITION SYSTEM

Machine learning is being introduced at all levels of decision-making systems. Healthcare is one area were the introduction of modern artificial intelligence technologies, such as pattern recognition machine learning based systems, may bring the most benefits. Healthcare is costly and complex and computer based systems may help decision makers to better use the available resources.

The ECCI-PR system is described in the following sections and the main architectural design decisions are presented, namely in terms of development and deployment.

THE SOFTWARE ECOSYSTEM

Each computer system starts by the choice of the operating system's, the systems architecture and the programming language used to glue the components of the system. This section presents the main decisions about the ECCI-PR system and the corresponding engineering design options. Every system design tries to be adopt the best practices available at the time of it's conception. This is the case for the ECCI-PR system. It embraces a reliable design by embracing a modern virtual machines approach and container technologies. The choice of programming language with a vibrant and very active community widely used and growing in popularity is also present in the ECCI-PR system design.

The Programming Languages Used for the System

The system is mainly developed with the adoption of a Python based ecosystem because of its rich set of APIs (Application Programming Interfaces). The most common way to install Python packages is through the PyPi software repository (https://pypi.org/) where there are more than 187 000 software projects available.

The Python programming language is relatively old in terms of the computer programming languages set. It's first stable version, 1.0, was presented in December 3, 1980, and nowadays the last stable version is 3.74. It is one of the most popular programming languages and gaining an increasing set of followers. The TIOBE Programming Community Index ranks Python as the 3rd most popular language (TIOBE Software BV (2019, July) with a 9.260% rating.

The main characteristics of this programming language are (Browning & Alchin, 2019):

- **Dynamic Programming:** The language is interpreted, dynamically typed and garbage-collected.
- **Multiparadigm:** Supports several programming paradigms such as: procedural; object-oriented and most of functional programming constructs.
- **Easy to Code and to Read:** Code readability is emphasized and many of the syntactic sugar present in other programming languages is not there.

The ECCI-PR systems uses the Python programming language packages to access geographical data (QGIS API and Postgis), to retrieve data from the PostgreSQL database server, to present the web user interface with GeoDjango and to submit the collected data to a machine learning analysis process with scikit-learn. In this chapter each software component will be further examined.

The Raspberry Pi GPS collection system uses the PAHO-MQTT Python package in conjunction with the gps package to send the geographic located data to ECCI-PR system.

There are some parts were other programming languages are used. Some minor Javascript pieces of code are used in the Node-RED flow since this is a Node.js based tool .

The Android based data collection system is programmed using a combination of Java and Kotlin code.

The Geographical Positioning Data Generating Systems

The collection of the ECCI teams displacement data is performed by two types of hardware systems:

Problems that often arise in complex software systems are the following:

- **IoT Based Hardware:** In this approach a Raspberry Pi 3 system is used as the main data generation system.
- **Smartphone Based Hardware:** In this approach a smartphone is used to generate the data.

Each ECCI team is accompanied by one of these systems. The ECCI data collection system will not reveal any personal details about the people that are visited by the medical teams. It will only register with a previously determined rate, the time and geographical position of the team. This will be stored in the ECCI-PR system.

The Raspberry Pi 3 IoT system is a small low cost, energy efficient, single-board computer, running a dedicated version of the Linux operating system (Donat, 2018). The Raspberry Pi computer is connected to a GSM/GPRS/GNSS hat (Raspberry Pi hardware module), that simultaneously receives GPS satellite data and connects to the Internet (Waveshare, 2019). The data produced by the system is sent via MQTT protocol to the ECCI-PR MQTT broker to be subsequently stored in the ECCI-PR PostGIS database. A data backup is locally performed. This data is also sent to the ECCI-PR at scheduled intervals using rsync. The IoT approach to geographical data collection is robust and inexpensive but more obtrusive than a smartphone.

Every smartphone has Internet connection as well as a GPS receiver. This provides an alternative to ECCI teams data collection. Modern Android programming is performed with the Kotlin language, nowadays Google's first choice (Google, 2019). The Kotlin programming language is compatible with Java but presents a major update in terms of software development since it introduces a Python alike approach to the syntax and a strong object-functional support (Hagos, 2018). The smartphone system sends data to the ECCI-PR PostGIS database using the same MQTT based approach. Also it keeps a copy of the data in the internal ROM memory to be later downloaded and sent to the database server.

Machine Learning Software

The ECCI-PR system processes the data using the scikit-learn Python based machine learning package (Pedregosa et al., 2011). The machine learning software classifies the displacement patterns of the ECCI's teams using a standard nearest-neighbors algorithm (Hauck, 2014). The data is classified into three cost vs efficiency classes. A matrix of costs associates each procedure, to a certain team. Each ECCI team reports which and how many procedures it performed during the day. This is introduced in the ECCI-PR database. The machine learning systems uses this information to classify the data into several categories.

The scikit-learn package is installed in the host machine. The host runs the Clear Linux operating system developed by Intel. This Linux distribution is fine tuned to run on Intel hardware and the machine learning software may run up to ten times faster than in other distributions .

The processed data is presented by the GeoDjango based web interface.

The User Interface

Two services are used to present a user interface: a Node-RED based server, that also collects MQTT data and sends it to the database server and a GeoDjango based server.

The Django Python based web framework is very popular and implements ver modern web development concepts. The GeoDjango extension allows an easy presentation of geographical data .

A Node-RED service is used to collect the MQTT data received from the clients and to introduce this data into the ECCI-PR database server. The Node-RED system also presents a simple view of the data sent by each ECCI team IoT or Android based data collection system.

VIRTUALIZATION AND CONTAINER TECHNOLOGIES

Problems that often arise in complex software systems are the following:

- **The Software is Complex:** The software system is composed of many components and the task of maintenance of each individual sub-system must be sub-delegated.
- **The Software System Must be Easily Redistributed and Redeployed:** Complex software must in many cases be put to work in different locations and with different physical hardware.

- **The Software Must be Maintained in an Easy and Controlled Way:** In systems that have to be available almost always and where disruption should be avoided all cost, the interruption periods must be very short but at the same time the maintenance of these systems must be possible.

In many ways virtualization and container technologies try to solve these problems increasing the reliability and availability of complex systems.

Virtualization

Virtualization in computing is defined as the abstraction of some physical component into a logical object (Portnoy, 2016). Software is executed on the virtual machines providing a separation from the underlying hardware. The first mainstream virtualization system appeared in the 1960's for IBM mainframes. A seminal paper on virtualization was published by (Popek & Goldberg, 1974). The roles and properties of virtual machines and corresponding monitors that are still used nowadays are presented. A virtual machine (VM) is defined as system that can virtualize all of the hardware resources: processors; storage; memory and networking. A Virtual Machinc Monitor (VMM), also callcd a hypcrvisor, is thc application/ software, that creates and manages the environment in which the virtual machines run. A layer diagram of a virtual machine based system is presented in Figure 1. In the lower layer of system is the physical hardware. In some systems the VMM may run directly on top of the hardware but in many cases the hypervisor runs on top of the host operating system. The hardware may supply more or less support to virtualization. When there is no support all the hardware is emulated. When there is hardware support for virtualization the VMs guest operating systems may run at speeds similar to the underlying host operating systems. Virtual machines provide greater flexibility in the operation of complex software systems. Whenever there are changes, malfunctions, maintenance periods or upgrades of the underlying host hardware or operating system/hypervisor, the virtual machines may migrate or be copied to another host. Also in terms of backup it is a benefit to use virtual machine monitors since they can easily handle snapshots of the VMs.

Container Technology

Although hardware virtualization brings many benefits in terms of system deployment during the last years a new paradigm emerged designated by container technologies (Mouat, 2015). Containers are an encapsulation of an application with its dependencies. They may look as a light form of virtual machines, since they

Figure 1. Layer diagram of the components of a virtual machine based system

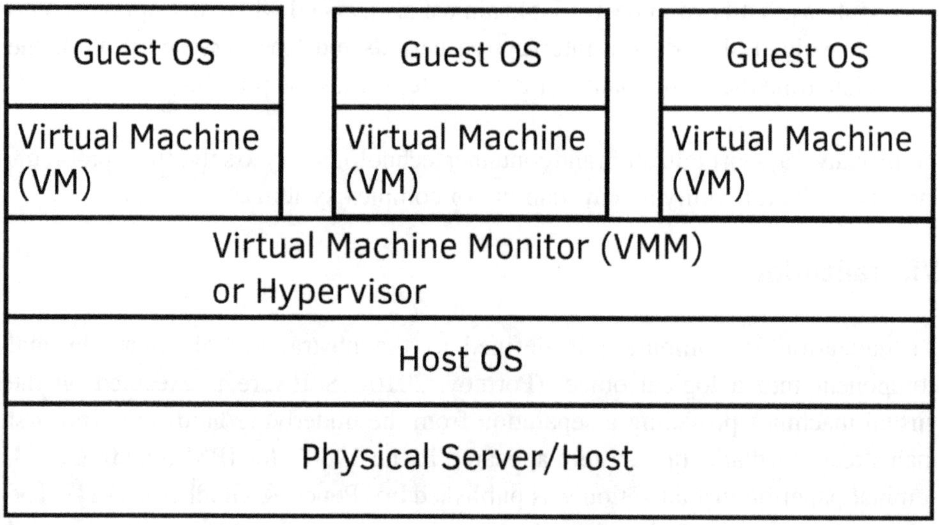

hold an isolated instance of an operating system, like a VM. Several advantages are present when using containers:

- Resources are shared with the host OS, which makes them more efficient. Containers can start and stop very rapidly and applications incur little or no overhead compared to applications running directly on the host OS.
- Containers are portable thus reducing the amount of bugs caused by subtle changes in the running environment.
- Containers are lightweight in their nature thus meaning that many containers may be run at the same time. Complex systems may be built using a combination of containers.
- Many hours of installation, test and deployment are saved when developing or when the host OS is changed.

A large publicly available set of container images are available at the Docker Hub site (Docker Inc., 2019b). Most of the images are available for download at no cost and present the Dockerfile from which they were build. A rating system by users shows the popularity of each container image. Most of the images present the corresponding installation and usage documentation.

A layer diagram of a container based system is presented in Figure 2. At the lower level we have the hardware and its corresponding physical server/host. On top of the hardware an operating system is running. The container engine is managed by the host OS and presents itself as a set of applications, libraries and a daemon process. Each containerized application uses its own set of libraries that may or not be common to another container. In Figure 2. the containerized application App 1 uses a set of Libraries A that are not used by the rest of the containers. The containers App 2 and App 3 share a set of libraries (Libraries B). Shared copies of the libraries and an incremental management of these libraries render the container deployed systems very slim in terms of storage requirements.

The goal of container technologies is to make applications portable and self-contained whereas virtualization fundamentally isolates from the underlying hardware.

Figure 2. Layer diagram of the components of a container based system

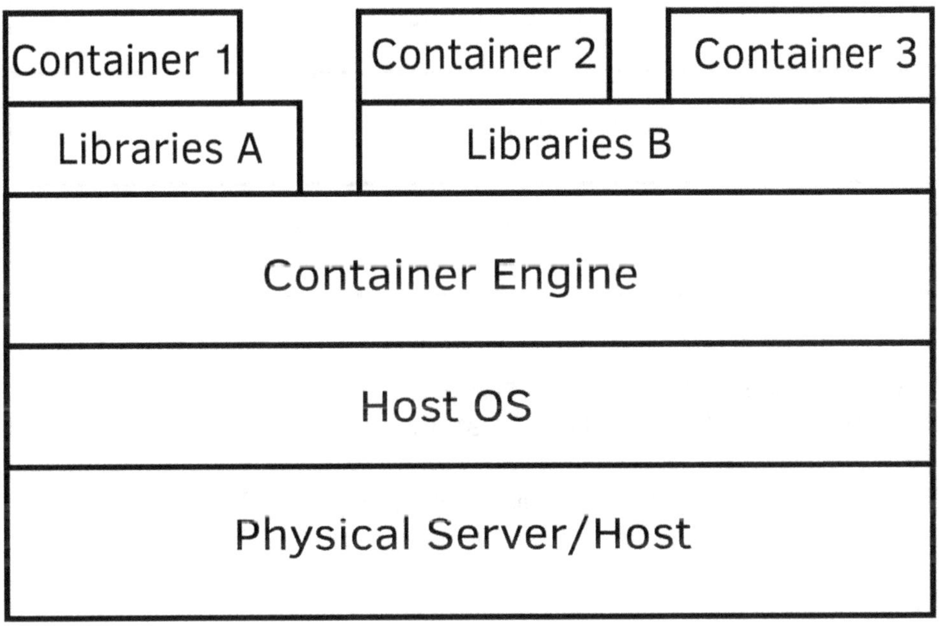

An advance in terms of container technologies are Kata Containers (Kata Containers, 2019). These provide an additional layer of isolation to applications by allowing a mix of virtualization and containerization. Each container process runs in a lightweight virtual machine with individualized kernels. Without sacrificing the advantages of traditional containerization an increased level of robustness and flexibility is presented by this approach. The architecture is presented in Figure 3. Containers A, B and C each has its own lightweight kernel.

Figure 3. Layer diagram of the components of a Kata container based system

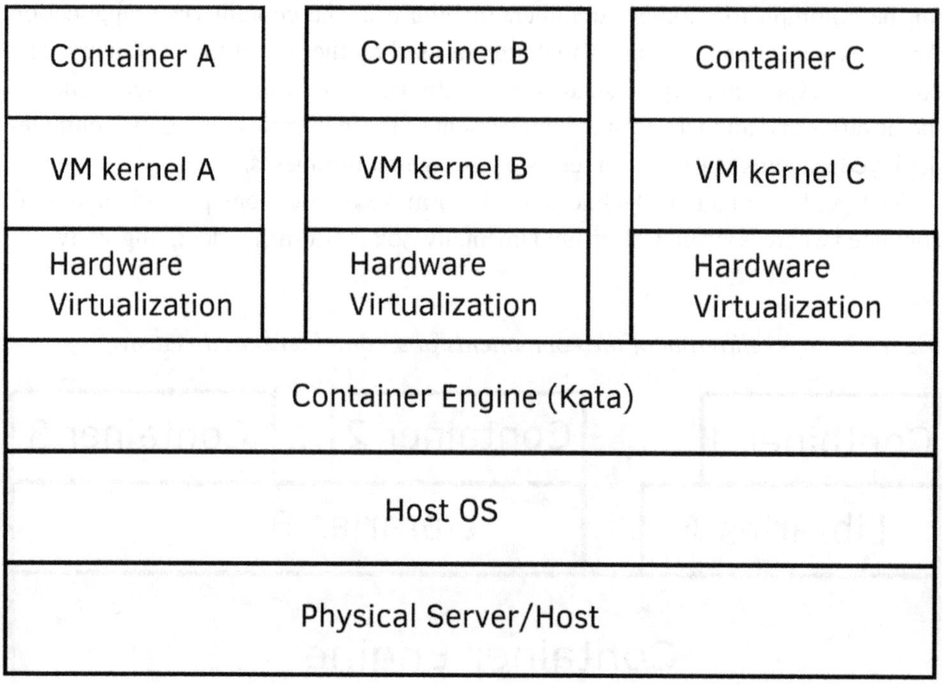

The Virtualized and Containerized Architecture of the ECCI-PR System

The ECCI-PR system adopts a combination of hardware virtualization and container technologies. The architecture of the system is presented in Figure 4.

Figure 4. Layer diagram of the ECCI-PR system

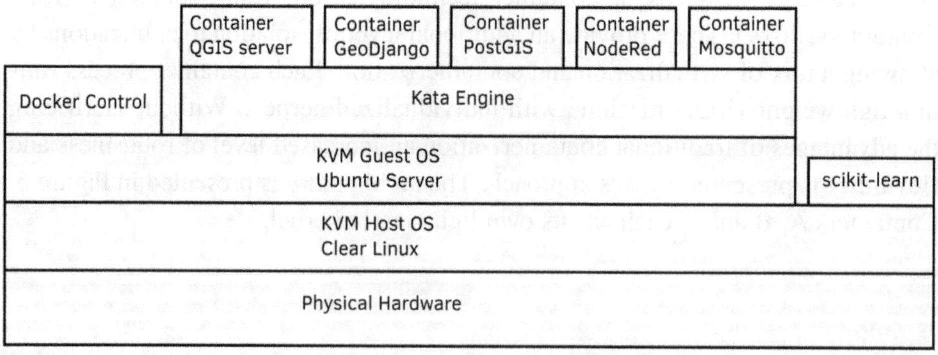

On top of the physical hardware runs the Clear Linux operating system. The host operating system provides support to running a KVM (Kernel Virtual Machine) VM, running an Ubuntu Server 18.04.2 (LTS) operating system. Ubuntu Server is a well documented and reliable Linux operating system with a 10 year support by Canonical, the company behind it.

The machine learning application is built with an ensemble of Python software, built around the scikit-learn package, running on the Clear Linux host. The container software solution is built with the Docker container version 18.09.7 integrated with Kata Containers (version 1.8.0-alpha2). In the guest VM run five Kata based containers:

- **QGIS Server:** This server provides geolocation data and maps to requests made from the central application built and server by the GeoDjango server.
- **GeoDjango Server:** The main application is built with Django with some geographical system extensions, namely support for a PostGIS server queries. This application provides the main user interface. It shows graphs and analysis results for the ECCI teams. The application calls the machine learning software on host server.
- **PostGIS Server:** The PostGIS server keeps the data collected from the ECCI teams and provides this data to the main application. This data can be requested by the host server when it runs the machine learning software.
- **Mosquitto MQTT Server:** This server is an MQTT broker system providing the means to communicate data coming from the ECCI teams and sending this data the NodeRed server.
- **Node-RED Server:** The Node-RED application provides a way to communicate with the MQTT server and store the ECCI data in the PostGIS server. It also provides a rude graphical interface that allows the user to check for the working of the ECCI data collection systems.

DATA COLLECTION, COMMUNICATION AND STORAGE

The data is collected with two different types of systems: an IoT based system and a smartphone system. In the system it is adopted a typical IoT data communication model. High latency is expected and the MQTT (Message Queuing Telemetry Transport) ISO standard (ISO/IEC PRF 20922) protocol is chosen for the data transmission (Hillar, 2017). It is based on a publish-subscribe model for messaging. It is designed to work on top of the TCP/IP protocol. A very limited network bandwidth is required. The MQTT server is designated as the “broker”. A client application may either publish or receive data using a subscription to a topic. Each client can connect to the broker. The data is hierarchically organized by topics and a tree of subtopics. Whenever a publisher client has a novel item of data to send, a control message with the information is sent to the broker system. Afterwards the broker server distributes the data to any receiver clients that have subscribed to the topic. The communication between clients and server may be encrypted using TLS.

The ECCI-PR system includes a MQTT broker server using a Docker container that implements an instance of the Mosquitto MQTT server software (Docker Inc., 2019a). The provider of the Mosquitto message broker open source software is the ECLIPSE Foundation (Eclipse Foundation., 2019a). The Eclipse Paho project, (Eclipse Foundation, 2019b), provides an open source client implementation of MQTT that is used in the ECCI-PR system for communication data generated at each ECCI team displacement device monitoring system, namely with the Raspbian OS. The Python implementation of this software is installed using the instructions available at (PyPi, 2019)

The Collected Data Storage

The data is collected from each ECCI monitoring system, using a Node-RED MQTT receiver. The data is published by a control message to the MQTT broker and then distributed to the NodeRed receiver using an appropriate topic subscription. The Node-RED application runs in a Docker container (https://hub.docker.com/r/nodered/node-red-docker/) on the guest VM. Node-RED is a flow-based programming tool. It allows an easy visual representation of the flow of data and the corresponding processing modules. The Node-RED application/server is open source and programmed in Node.js. The Node-RED based application sends request to store the data into the PostGIS database server after receiving and processing the MQTT subscribed information.

The PostGIS database server runs in a Docker container (https://github.com/appropriate/docker-postgis) using a PostgresSQL database server (https://www.postgresql.org/) with the PostGIS extensions (https://postgis.net/). This is an open source object-relational database server that is known for its speed and reliability (Juba, Vannahme, Volkov, 2015).

FUTURE RESEARCH DIRECTIONS

The collection of data from the ECCI team displacements may be supplemented with from other healthcare components. Namely it may be useful to find patterns between some types of health problems before people enter under the care of the ECCI teams in order to evaluate some sort of preventive healthcare. Another direction for the future development of the system is the incorporation of Internet of Things (IoT) devices into the home of the people assisted by these ECCI teams in order to provide a better and faster assistance. Deep learning techniques may eventually be applied if enough data is collected thus improving the pattern recognition components of the system.

CONCLUSION

The chapter discusses and presents a system destined to capture geographically marked data about ECCI teams displacements. It describes the main architectural choices, namely in terms of the underlying operating system, virtualization and container technology adoption. It also presents the main choices in terms of programming languages and the related software packages.

The system uses a machine learning software framework to recognize ECCI teams patterns and propose cost optimizations.

Future developments of the system include a more refined approach to the cost estimation problem by usage of better machine learning techniques and an eventual adoption of deep learning technologies.

ACKNOWLEDGMENT

This research was supported by I4E project [grant numbers 0445-4IE-4-P] funded by the Interreg V-A España-Portugal (POCTEP) 2014-2020 program.

REFERENCES

Administração Central do Sistema de Saúde. (2017). *Relatório De Monitorização Da Rede Nacional De Cuidados Continuados Integrados*. doi:10.1021/jp507355t

Browning, J. B., & Alchin, M. (2019). *Pro Python 3*. Apress. doi:10.1007/978-1-4842-4385-5

Django. (2019). *The web framework for perfectionists*. Retrieved from https://www.djangoproject.com/

Docker Inc. (2019a). *Eclipse-mosquitto - Docker Hub*. Retrieved from https://hub.docker.com/_/eclipse-mosquitto/

Docker Inc. (2019b). *Docker Hub*. Retrieved from https://hub.docker.com/

Donat, W. (2018). *Learn Raspberry Pi Programming with Python*. Apress. doi:10.1007/978-1-4842-3769-4

Eclipse Foundation. (2019a). *Eclipse Mosquitto™ An open source MQTT broker.* Retrieved from https://mosquitto.org/

Eclipse Foundation. (2019b). *Eclipse-PAHO – MQTT and MQTT SN software.* Retrieved from http://www.eclipse.org/paho/

GeoDjango. (2019). *GeoDjango, Django documentation.* Retrieved from https://docs.djangoproject.com/en/dev/ref/contrib/gis/

Google. (2019). *Kotlin and Android*. Retrieved from https://developer.android.com/kotlin/

Government, P. (2006). Decreto-Lei 101/2006. Academic Press.

Hagos, T. (2018). *Learn Android Studio 3 with Kotlin*. Manning. doi:10.1007/978-1-4842-3907-0

Hauck, T. (2014). *Scikit-Learn Cookbook.* PACKT PUB.

Hillar, G. C. (2017). *MQTT Essentials - A Lightweight IoT Protocol*. Packt Publishing.

Kata Containers. (2019). Retrieved from https://katacontainers.io/

Juba, S., Vannahme, A., & Volkov, A. (2015). *Learning PostgreSQL*. Packt Publishing.

Larabel. (2019). Benchmarking the Python optimizations of Clear Linux against, Ubuntu, Intel Python. *Phoronix*. Retrieved from https://www.phoronix.com/scan.php?page=news_item&px=Clear-Linux-2019-Python-Perf

Mouat, A. (2015). *Using Docker*. O'Reilly Media, Inc.

Pedregosa, F., Varoquaux, G., Gramfort, A., Michel, V., Thirion, B., Grisel, O., & Duchesnay, E. (2011). Scikit-learn: Machine Learning in Python. *Journal of Machine Learning Research*, *12*, 2825–2830.

Popek, G. J., & Goldberg, R. P. (1974). Formal requirements for virtualizable third generation architectures. *Communications of the ACM*, *17*(7), 412–421. doi:10.1145/361011.361073

PopulationPyramid.net. (2019). *População: Portugal 2016*. Retrieved from https://www.populationpyramid.net/pt/portugal/2016/

Portnoy, M. (2016, August 19). *Virtualization essentials*. John Wiley & Sons Inc.

PyPi. (2019). *paho-mqtt*. Retrieved from https://pypi.org/project/paho-mqtt/

TIOBE Software BV. (2019, July). *TIOBE Index.* Retrieved from https://www.tiobe.com/tiobe-index/

Waveshare. (2019, July). *GSM/GPRS/GNSS HAT - Waveshare Wiki.* Retrieved from https://www.waveshare.com/wiki/GSM/GPRS/GNSSHAT

ADDITIONAL READING

Ashley, W. D. (2019). *Foundations of Libvirt Development.* Apress. doi:10.1007/978-1-4842-4862-1

Bahgat, K. (2015). *Python Geospatial Development Essentials.* Packt Publishing.

Cook, J. (2017). *Docker for Data Science.* Apress; doi:10.1007/978-1-4842-3012-1

Diener, M. (2015). *Python Geospatial Analysis Cookbook.* Packt Publishing.

Dmitry Jemerov, S. I. (2016). *Kotlin in Action.* Manning.

Dua, R., Konduri, S. K., & Kohli, V. (2016). *Learning Docker Networking.* Packt Publishing.

Goasguen, S. (2015). *Docker Cookbook.* O'Reilly UK Ltd.

Graser, A. (2016). *Learning QGIS* (3rd ed.). Packt Publishing.

Hackeling, G. (2014). *Mastering Machine Learning With scikit-learn.* Packt Publishing.

Holla, S. (2015). *Orchestrating Docker.* Packt Publishing.

Ivanov, K. (2017). *KVM Virtualization Cookbook.* Packt Publishing.

Kraft, T. J. (2014). *Postgis Cookbook.* PACKT PUB.

Juba, S., Vannahme, A., & Volkov, A. (2015). *Learning PostgreSQL.* Packt Publishing.

Julian, D. (2016). *Designing Machine Learning Systems with Python.* Packt Publishing.

Kirk, M. (2017). *Thoughtful Machine Learning with Python.* O'Reilly UK Ltd

Lawhead, J. (2015). *QGIS Python Programming Cookbook.* Packt Publishing.

Marquez, A. (2015). *PostGIS Essentials.* Packt Publishing.

Maymala, J. (2015). *PostgreSQL for Data Architects.* Packt Publishing.

McKendrick, R. (2016). *Extending Docker*. Packt Publishing.

Micha Jaworski, T. Z. (2016). *Expert Python Programming* (2nd ed.). Packt Publishing.

Mukhedkar, P., Vettathu, A., & Chirammal, H. D. (2016). *Mastering KVM Virtualization*. Packt Publishing.

Sarkar, D., Bali, R., & Sharma, T. (2018). *Practical Machine Learning with Python*. Apress; doi:10.1007/978-1-4842-3207-1

Shaun. (2014). *PostgreSQL 9 High Availability Cookbook*. PACKT PUB.

Swamynathan, M. (2017). *Mastering Machine Learning with Python in Six Steps*. Packt Publishing; doi:10.1007/978-1-4842-2866-1

Westra, E. (2016). *Python Geospatial Development* (3rd ed.). PACKT PUB.

KEY TERMS AND DEFINITIONS

Container Technology: An operating system level virtualization to develop and deliver software.

Geographical Information System: A system designed to capture store, manipulate, and analyze geographic data.

Machine Learning: The scientific area that studies algorithms and mathematical models that computer systems may use to perform tasks relying on pattern recognition and inference.

Pattern Recognition: The automatic detection of regularities in data using algorithms and the corresponding use of these regularities to perform actions.

Virtual Machine: An emulation of a computer system. Virtual machines provide the functions of a physical machine. They may use special hardware or software to enhance their performance.

Compilation of References

Abad, L. (2014). Media literacy for older people facing the digital divide: The e-inclusion programmes design. *Media Education Research Journal, 21*(42), 173–180.

Abdullrahim, A., & De Coster, R. 2016. *A Framework of E-Health Systems Adoption and Telemedicine Readiness in Developing Countries.* International Conference on Information Society (i-Society). 10.1109/i-Society.2016.7854188

Abellán García, A., Rodríguez-Laso, A., Pujol Rodríguez, R., & Barrios, L. (2017). *12.000 centenarios en 2017 en España, ¿222.000 en 2066?* Retrieved October 15, 2018, from http://envejecimientoenred.es/centenarios_en_espana/

Administração Central do Sistema de Saúde. (2017). *Relatório De Monitorização Da Rede Nacional De Cuidados Continuados Integrados.* doi:10.1021/jp507355t

Agarwal, S., Santra, B., & Mukherjee, D. P. (2018). Anubhav: Recognizing emotions through facial expression. *The Visual Computer, 34*(2), 177–191. doi:10.100700371-016-1323-z

Almeida, A., Fiore, A., Mainetti, L., Mulero, R., Patrono, L., & Rametta, P. (2017). An iot-aware architecture for collecting and managing data related to elderly behavior. *Wireless Communications and Mobile Computing, 2017*, 2017. doi:10.1155/2017/5051915

Alwin, D. F. (2012). Integrating varieties of life course concepts. *The Journals of Gerontology. Series B, Psychological Sciences and Social Sciences, 67*(2), 206–220. doi:10.1093/geronb/gbr146 PMID:22399576

American Diabetes Association. (2019a). Older adults: Standards of medical care in diabetes. *Diabetes Care, 42*(Supplement 1), S139–S147. doi:10.2337/dc19-S012 PMID:30559238

American Diabetes Association. (2019b). Lifestyle Management: Standards of Medical Care in Diabetes - 2019. *Diabetes Care, 42*(Supplement 1), S46–S60. doi:10.2337/dc19-S005 PMID:30559231

American Geriatrics Society Expert Panel on Person-Centered. (2016). Person-Centered Care: A Definition and Essential Elements. *Journal of the American Geriatrics Society, 64*(1), 15–18. doi:10.1111/jgs.13866 PMID:26626262

Amorim, J. S., Leite, R. C., Brizola, R., & Yonamine, C. Y. (2018). Virtual reality therapy for rehabilitation of balance in the elderly: a systematic review and META-analysis. *Advances in Rheumatology, 58.*

Andrew, M. K., Dupuis-Blanchard, S., Maxwell, C., Giguere, A., Keefe, J., Rockwood, K., & St John, P. (2018). Social and societal implications of frailty, including impact on Canadian healthcare systems. *The Journal of Frailty & Aging*, *7*(4), 217–223. doi:10.14283/jfa.2018.30 PMID:30298169

Apóstolo, J., Bobrowicz-Campos, E., Moreno-Casbas, T., Teixeira-Santos, L., Sánchez de Madariag, R., Casado-Ramírez, E., ... ModulEn Consortium (2019). A study protocol for development and validation of a clinical prediction model for frailty (modulen): A new European commitment to tackling frailty. *Translational Medicine @ UniSa*, *19*(6), 36-41.

Apóstolo, J., Cooke, R., Bobrowicz-Campos, E., Santana, S., Marcucci, M., Cano, A., ... Holland, C. (2018). Effectiveness of interventions to prevent pre-frailty and frailty progression in older adults: A systematic review. *JBI Database of Systematic Reviews and Implementation Reports*, *16*(1), 140–232. doi:10.11124/JBISRIR-2017-003382 PMID:29324562

Arbonés, G., Carbajal, A., Gonzalvo, B., González-Gross, M., Joyanes, M., Marques-Lopes, I., ... Vaquero, M. P. (2003). Nutrición y recomendaciones dietéticas para personas mayores. *Nutrición Hospitalaria*, *18*(3), 109–137. PMID:12875088

Armstrong, D. G., Najafi, B., & Shahinpoorc, M. (2017). Potential Applications of Smart Multifunctional Wearable Materials to Gerontology. *Gerontology*, *63*(3), 287–298. doi:10.1159/000455011 PMID:28076861

Arnhold, M., Quade, M., & Kirch, W. (2014). Mobile applications for diabetics: A systematic review and expert-based usability evaluation considering the special requirements of diabetes patients age 50 years or older. *Journal of Medical Internet Research*, *16*(4), 1–18. doi:10.2196/jmir.2968 PMID:24718852

Arsand, E., Muzny, M., Bradway, M., Muzik, J., & Hartvigsen, G. (2015, May). Performance of the First Combined Smartwatch and Smartphone Diabetes Diary Application Study. *Journal of Diabetes Science and Technology, 9*(3), 556–563. doi:10.1177/1932296814567708

Atlam, H., Walters, R., & Wills, G. (2018). Internet of Things: State-of-the-art, Challenges, Applications, and Open Issues. *International Journal of Intelligent Computing Research*, *9*(3), 928–938. doi:10.20533/ijicr.2042.4655.2018.0112

Baez, N. L. X., & Reckziegel, J. (2013). O direito humano fundamental de autodeterminação e os seus limites éticos frente ao princípio da proteção da dignidade humana. *Prisma Juridico*, *12*(1), 225–252. doi:10.5585/prismaj.v12n1.3427

Baig, M. M., GholamHosseini, H., Moqeem, A. A., Mirza, F., & Lindén, M. (2017). A Systematic Review of Wearable Patient Monitoring Systems - Current Challenges and Opportunities for Clinical Adoption. *Journal of Medical Systems*, *41*(7), 115. doi:10.100710916-017-0760-1 PMID:28631139

Bantom, S. A. (2016). *Accessibility to patients' own health information: A case in rural Eastern Cape, South Africa*. Cape Town: Cape Peninsula University of Technology. doi:10.1145/2987491.2987505

Barbosa, H., Castro, A. V., & Carrapatoso, E. (2018). Serious Games and Rehabilitation for Elderly Adults. *Global Scientific Journal, 6*(1), 275–283. Retrieved from http://www.globalscientificjournal.com/researchpaper/Serious-Games-and-Rehabilitation-for-Elderly-Adults.pdf%0Awww.globalscientificjournal.com

Barnaghi, P., Wang, W., Henson, C., & Taylor, K. (2012). Semantics for the Internet of Things: Early progress and back to the future. *International Journal on Semantic Web and Information Systems*, *8*(1), 1–21. doi:10.4018/jswis.2012010101

Baumgartner, P. C., Haynes, R. B., Hersberger, K. E., & Arnet, I. (2018). A Systematic Review of Medication Adherence Thresholds Dependent of Clinical Outcomes. *Frontiers in Pharmacology*, *9*, 1290. doi:10.3389/fphar.2018.01290 PMID:30524276

Beard, J. R. (2019). Moving Beyond Disease-Based Models of Prevention. In J.-P. Michel (Ed.), *Prevention of Chronic Diseases and Age-Related Disability*. Springer. doi:10.1007/978-3-319-96529-1_20

Beard, J. R., Officer, A., De Carvalho, I. A., Sadana, R., Pot, A. M., Michel, J. P., ... Chatterji, S. (2016, May 21). The World report on ageing and health: A policy framework for healthy ageing. *Lancet*, *387*(10033), 2145–2154. doi:10.1016/S0140-6736(15)00516-4 PMID:26520231

Bernabe, J. B., Elicegui, I., Gandrille, E., Gligoric, N., Gluhak, A., Hennebert, C., ... Nati, M. (2017, June). SocIoTal—The development and architecture of a social IoT framework. In *2017 Global Internet of Things Summit (GIoTS)* (pp. 1-6). IEEE.

Bernardi, R. B., & Barros, H. M. T. (2010). Uso de fármacos em idosos. In *Medicamentos na prática clínica* (pp. 142–153). Porto Alegre: Artmed.

Berners-Lee, T. (2017). *Solid vision*. https://solid.mit.edu/

Bernocchi, P., Giordano, A., Pintavalle, G., Galli, T., Ballini Spoglia, E., Baratti, D., & Scalvini, S. (2019). Feasibility and Clinical Efficacy of a Multidisciplinary Home-Telehealth Program to Prevent Falls in Older Adults: A Randomized Controlled Trial. *Journal of the American Medical Directors Association*, *20*(3), 340–346. doi:10.1016/j.jamda.2018.09.003 PMID:30366759

Berrocal, J., Garcia-Alonso, J., Canal, C., & Murillo, J. M. (2016). *Situational-Context: A Unified View of Everything Involved at a Particular Situation.* Springer. Retrieved from https://link.springer.com/10.1007/978-3-319-38791-8

Berrocal, J., Garcia-Alonso, J., Murillo, J. M., Mendes, D., Fonseca, C., & Lopes, M. (2018, jun). Context-aware mobile app for the mul- tidimensional assessment of the elderly. In *2018 13th iberian confer- ence on information systems and technologies (cisti)* (pp. 1–6). IEEE. Retrieved from https://ieeexplore.ieee.org/document/8399239/

Berrocal, J., Garcia-Alonso, J., Canal, C., & Murillo, J. M. (2016, June). Situational-Context: a unified view of everything involved at a particular situation. In *International Conference on Web Engineering* (pp. 476-483). Springer. 10.1007/978-3-319-38791-8_34

Berrocal, J., Garcia-Alonso, J., Murillo, J. M., & Canal, C. (2017). Rich contex- tual information for monitoring the elderly in an early stage of cognitive impairment. *Pervasive and Mobile Computing*, *34*, 106–125. doi:10.1016/j.pmcj.2016.05.001

Berrocal, J., Garcia-Alonso, J., Vicente-Chicote, C., Hern'andez, J., Mikkonen, T., Canal, C., & Murillo, J. M. (2017, February). Early analysis of resource consumption patterns in mobile applications. *Pervasive and Mobile Computing*, *35*, 32–50. doi:10.1016/j.pmcj.2016.06.011

Berry, E. H., & Kirschner, A. (2013). Demography of Rural Aging. In *Rural aging in 21st century America* (pp. 17–36). Dordrecht: Springer Netherlands; Retrieved from http://www.springerlink.com/index/10.1007/978

Bhattacherjee, A. (2012). Social Science Research: Principles, Methods, and Practices (2nd ed.). Tampa: Creative Commons Attribution-NonCommercial-ShareAlike 3.0 Unported License.

Bickmore, T. W., Caruso, L., & Clough-Gorr, K. (2005). Acceptance and usability of a relational agent interface by urban older adults. *CHI '05 Extended Abstracts on Human Factors in Computing Systems - CHI '05*, 1212. doi:10.1145/1056808.1056879

Bickmore, T. W., Pfeifer, L. M., & Paasche-Orlow, M. K. (2007). *Health Document Explanation by Virtual Agents*. Intelligent Virtual Agents. doi:10.1007/978-3-540-74997-4_18

Bickmore, T. W., Caruso, L., Clough-Gorr, K., & Heeren, T. (2005). 'It's just like you talk to a friend' relational agents for older adults. *Interacting with Computers*, *17*(6), 711–735. doi:10.1016/j.intcom.2005.09.002

Bickmore, T. W., Puskar, K., Schlenk, E. A., Pfeifer, L. M., & Sereika, S. M. (2010). Maintaining reality: Relational agents for antipsychotic medication adherence. *Interacting with Computers*, *22*(4), 276–288. doi:10.1016/j.intcom.2010.02.001

Bickmore, T. W., Silliman, R. A., Nelson, K., Cheng, D. M., Winter, M., Henault, L., & Paasche-Orlow, M. K. (2013). A randomized controlled trial of an automated exercise coach for older adults. *Journal of the American Geriatrics Society*, *61*(10), 1676–1683. doi:10.1111/jgs.12449 PMID:24001030

Blaschke, C. M., Freddolino, P. P., & Mullen, E. E. (2009). Ageing and Technology: A Review of the Research Literature. *British Journal of Social Work*, *39*(4), 641–656. doi:10.1093/bjsw/bcp025

Bleijenberg, N., de Man-van Ginkel, J. M., Trappenburg, J. C. A., Ettema, R. G. A., Sino, C. G., Heim, N., ... Schuurmans, M. J. (2018). Increasing value and reducing waste by optimizing the development of complex interventions: Enriching the development phase of the Medical Research Council (MRC) Framework. *International Journal of Nursing Studies*, *79*, 86–93. doi:10.1016/j.ijnurstu.2017.12.001 PMID:29220738

Bloom, D. E., Chatterji, S., Kowal, P., Lloyd-Sherlock, P., McKee, M., Rechel, B., ... Smith, J. P. (2015, February). Macroeconomic implications of population ageing and selected policy responses. *Lancet*, *385*(9968), 649–657. doi:10.1016/S0140-6736(14)61464-1 PMID:25468167

Bobrowicz-Campos, E., Couto, F., Teixeira-Santos, L., & Apóstolo, J. (2019Accepted for publication). Community-led ecosystem - a promising strategy to strengthen person-centered geriatric care in preventing age-related dependency. In C. Fonseca, M. Lopes, D. Mendes, F. Mendes, & J. García-Alonso (Eds.), Handbook of Research on Health Systems and Organizations for an Aging Society. Academic Press.

Bonmati-Carrion, M., Arguelles-Prieto, R., Martinez-Madrid, M., Reiter, R., Hardeland, R., Rol, M., & Madrid, J. (2014). Protecting the Melatonin Rhythm through Circadian Healthy Light Exposure. *International Journal of Molecular Sciences*, *15*(12), 23448–23500. doi:10.3390/ijms151223448 PMID:25526564

Bouznad, S., Chibani, A., Amirat, Y., Lyazid, S., Prestes, E., Sebbak, F., & Fiorini, S. (2017). Context-aware monitoring agents for ambient assisted living applications. In *European conference on ambient intelligence* (pp. 225–240). 10.1007/978-3-319-56997-0_18

Bresnick, J. (2017). *Understanding the Basics of Clinical Decision Support Systems*. Retrieved January 6, 2019, from https://healthitanalytics.com/features/understanding-the-basics-of-clinical-decision-support-systems

Brinkman, S., Voortman, T., Kiefte-de Jong, J., van Rooij, F., Ikram, M., Rivadeneira, F., ... Schoufour, J. (2018). The association between lifestyle and overall health, using the frailty index. *Archives of Gerontology and Geriatrics*, *76*, 85–91. doi:10.1016/j.archger.2018.02.006 PMID:29477949

Brown, S. (2018). *The {C4} Model for Software Architecture*. InfoQ.

Brownie, S. (2006). Why are elderly individuals at risk of nutritional deficiency? *International Journal of Nursing Practice*, *12*(2), 110–118. doi:10.1111/j.1440-172X.2006.00557.x PMID:16529597

Browning, J. B., & Alchin, M. (2019). *Pro Python 3*. Apress. doi:10.1007/978-1-4842-4385-5

Buckingham, D. (2007). Digital media literacies: Rethinking media education in the age of the Internet. *Research in Comparative and International Education*, *2*(1), 43–55. doi:10.2304/rcie.2007.2.1.43

Bucy, E. P. (2000). Social access to the internet. *The Harvard International Journal of Press/Politics*, *5*(1), 50–61. doi:10.1177/1081180X00005001005

Buinhas, S., Cláudio, A. P., Carmo, M. B., Balsa, J., Cavaco, A., Mendes, A., … Guerreiro, M. P. (2019). *Virtual Assistant to Improve Self-care of Older People with Type 2 Diabetes: First Prototype*. doi:10.1007/978-3-030-16028-9_21

Cacciata, M., Stromberg, A., Lee, J. A., Sorkin, D., Lombardo, D., Clancy, S., ... Evangelista, L. S. (2019). Effect of exergaming on health-related quality of life in older adults: A systematic review. *International Journal of Nursing Studies*, *93*, 30–40. doi:10.1016/j.ijnurstu.2019.01.010 PMID:30861452

Camargo, B. V. (2005). Alceste: um programa informático de análise quantitative de dados textuais. In A. S. P. Moreira (Ed.), *Perspectivas teórico-metodológicas em representações sociais* (pp. 511–539). João Pessoa: UFPB/Editora Universitária.

Cane, J., Richardson, M., Johnston, M., Ladha, R., & Michie, S. (2015). From lists of behaviour change techniques (BCTs) to structured hierarchies: Comparison of two methods of developing a hierarchy of BCTs. *British Journal of Health Psychology*, *20*(1), 130–150. doi:10.1111/bjhp.12102 PMID:24815766

Canham, S., Mauro, P., Kaufmann, C., & Sixsmith, A. (2015). Association of Alcohol Use and Loneliness Frequency Among Middle-Aged and Older Adult Drinkers. *Journal of Aging and Health*, *28*(2), 267–284. doi:10.1177/0898264315589579 PMID:26082130

Cano, A., Dargent, G., Carriazo, A., López-Samaniego, L., Apóstolo, J., Bobrowicz-Campos, E., ... Obbia, P. (2018). T ackling frailty and functional decline: Background of the action group A3 of the European innovation partnership for active and healthy ageing. *Maturitas*, *115*, 69–73. doi:10.1016/j.maturitas.2018.06.009 PMID:30049350

CANONICAL. (2020). *OpenStack Docs: Welcome to the OpenStack Charm Guide*. https://docs.openstack.org/charm-guide/latest/

Carneiro, I., De, D. C., & De Souza, R. (2013). *A Etnografia : Um Modo De Entender a Alimentação*. Academic Press.

Center on Technology and Disability. (2018). *Assistive Technology*, *101*. Retrieved from https://www.ctdinstitute.org/sites/default/files/file_attachments/CTD-AT101-V4.pdf

Centers for Disease Control and Prevention. (2017). National Diabetes Statistics Report: Estimates of Diabetes and Its Burden in the United States. Atlanta, GA: Centers for Disease Control and Prevention.

Chang, A.-M., & Kannan, P. K. (2006). Employee Technology Readiness and Adoption of Wireless Technology and Services. *39th Hawaii International Conference on System Sciences*.

Chattopadhyay, S., Li, J., Land, L., & Ray, P. (2008). A Framework for Assessing ICT Preparedness for e-Health Implementations. *10th IEEE International Conference on e-Health Networking, Applications and Service (HEALTHCOM 2008)*. 10.1109/HEALTH.2008.4600122

Chen, N. (2006). *Convention over Configuration*. Academic Press.

Chen, C. C. H., Schilling, L. S., & Lyder, C. H. (2001). A concept analysis of malnutrition in the elderly. *Journal of Advanced Nursing*, *36*(1), 131–142. doi:10.1046/j.1365-2648.2001.01950.x PMID:11555057

Chen, C., Gan, P., & How, C. (2018). Approach to frailty in the elderly in primary care and the community. *Singapore Medical Journal, 59*(5), 240–245. doi:10.11622medj.2018052 PMID:29799055

Chen, L., Pei, J.-H., Kuang, J., Chen, H.-M., Chen, Z., Li, Z.-W., & Yang, H.-Z. (2015). Effect of lifestyle intervention in patients with type 2 diabetes: A meta-analysis. *Metabolism: Clinical and Experimental, 64*(2), 338–347. doi:10.1016/j.metabol.2014.10.018 PMID:25467842

Chen, Y. R., & Schulz, P. J. (2016). The Effect of Information Communication Technology Interventions on Reducing Social Isolation in the Elderly: A Systematic Review. *Journal of Medical Internet Research, 18*(1), e18. doi:10.2196/jmir.4596 PMID:26822073

Chiauzzi, E., Rodarte, C., & DasMahapatra, P. (2015). Patient-centered activity monitoring in the self-management of chronic health conditions. *BMC Medicine, 13*(1), 77. doi:10.118612916-015-0319-2 PMID:25889598

Cho, D.-K., Lee, U., Noh, Y., Park, T., & Song, J. (2015, May). PlaceWalker: An energy-efficient place logging method that con- siders kinematics of normal human walking. *Pervasive and Mobile Computing, 19*, 24–36. Retrieved 2018-02-08, from https://www.sciencedirect.com/science/article/pii/S1574119214000583

Chomutare, T., Fernandez-Luque, L., Årsand, E., & Hartvigsen, G. (2011). Features of Mobile Diabetes Applications: Review of the Literature and Analysis of Current Applications Compared Against Evidence-Based Guidelines. *Journal of Medical Internet Research, 13*(3), e65. doi:10.2196/jmir.1874 PMID:21979293

Cho, N. H., Shaw, J. E., Karuranga, S., Huang, Y., da Rocha Fernandes, J. D., Ohlrogge, A. W., & Malanda, B. (2018). IDF Diabetes Atlas: Global estimates of diabetes prevalence for 2017 and projections for 2045. *Diabetes Research and Clinical Practice, 138*, 271–281. doi:10.1016/j.diabres.2018.02.023 PMID:29496507

Chrvala, C. A., Sherr, D., & Lipman, R. D. (2016). Diabetes self-management education for adults with type 2 diabetes mellitus: A systematic review of the effect on glycemic control. *Patient Education and Counseling, 99*(6), 926–943. doi:10.1016/j.pec.2015.11.003 PMID:26658704

Claudino, R. G., de Lima, L. K. S., de Assis, E. D. B., & Torro, N. (2019, Dec). Facial expressions and eye tracking in individuals with social anxiety disorder: a systematic review. *Psicologia: Reflexào e Crítica, 32*(1), 9. Retrieved from https://prc.springeropen.com/articles/10.1186/s41155-

Cláudio, A. P., Carmo, M. B., Pinto, V., Cavaco, A., & Guerreiro, M. P. (2015). Virtual humans for training and assessment of self-medication consultation skills in pharmacy students. *10th International Conference on Computer Science & Education (ICCSE)*, 175–180. 10.1109/ICCSE.2015.7250238

Clegg, A., Young, J., Iliffe, S., Rikkert, M., & Rockwood, K. (2013). Frailty in elderly people. *Lancet, 381*(9868), 752–762. doi:10.1016/S0140-6736(12)62167-9 PMID:23395245

Coiera, E. (2006). Communication systems in healthcare. *The Clinical Biochemist., 27*(2), 89–98. Retrieved from https://www.ncbi.nlm.nih.gov/pubmed/17077879

Coleman, A., Herselman, M. E., & Potass, D. (2012). *E-Health Readiness Assessment for E-Health Framework for Africa: A Case Study of Hospitals in South Africa*. Malaga: Institute for Computer Sciences, Social Informatics and Telecommunications Engineering.

Conselho Regional De Enfermagem Do Estado De São Paulo (COREN-SP). (2011). *Erros de medicação: definições e estratégias de prevenção. Rede Brasileira de Enfermagem e Segurança do Paciente (REBRAENSP – POLO SÃO PAULO)*. Disponível em: http://inter.coren-sp.gov.br/sites/default/files/erros_de_medicacao-definicoes_e_estrategias_de_prevencao.pdf

Cosco, T., Prina, A., Perales, J., Stephan, B., & Brayne, C. (2014). Operational definitions of successful ageing: A systematic review. *International Psychogeriatrics, 26*(03), 373–381. doi:10.1017/S1041610213002287 PMID:24308764

Council of the European Union. (2012). Council Declaration on the European Year for Active Ageing and Solidarity between Generations (2012): The Way Forward. *European Commission*. Retrieved from http://register.consilium.europa.eu/doc/srv?l=EN&f=ST%2017468%202012%20INIT

Council of the European Union. (2018). Recomendação do Conselho de 22 de maio de 2018 sobre as Competências Essenciais para a Aprendizagem ao Longo da Vida (Texto relevante para efeitos do EEE). *Jornal Oficial da União Europeia, C 189*, 1-13.

Cradock, K. A., ÓLaighin, G., Finucane, F. M., Gainforth, H. L., Quinlan, L. R., & Ginis, K. A. M. (2017). Behaviour change techniques targeting both diet and physical activity in type 2 diabetes: A systematic review and meta-analysis. *The International Journal of Behavioral Nutrition and Physical Activity, 14*(18), 1–17. doi:10.118612966-016-0436-0 PMID:28178985

Cradock, K. A., ÓLaighin, G., Finucane, F., Mckay, R., Quinlan, L. R., Ginis, K. A. M., & Gainforth, H. L. (2017). Diet Behavior Change Techniques in Type 2 Diabetes: A Systematic Review and Meta-analysis. *Diabetes Care, 40*(12), 1800–1810. doi:10.2337/dc17-0462 PMID:29162585

Craig, P., Dieppe, P., Macintyre, S., Michie, S., Nazareth, I., & Petticrew, M. (2008). Developing and evaluating complex interventions: The new Medical Research Council guidance. *BMJ, 337*(a1655), 979–983. doi:10.1136/bmj.a1655

Cui, M., Wu, X., Mao, J., Wang, X., & Nie, M. (2016). T2DM self-management via smartphone applications: A systematic review and meta-analysis. *PLoS One, 11*(11), 1–15. doi:10.1371/journal.pone.0166718 PMID:27861583

Czaja, S. J. (2016). Long-term care services and support systems for older adults: The role of technology. *The American Psychologist, 71*(4), 294–301. doi:10.1037/a0040258 PMID:27159436

D'Avanzo, B., Shaw, R., Riva, S., Apostolo, J., Bobrowicz-Campos, E., Kurpas, D., ... Holland, C. (2017). Stakeholders' views and experiences of care and interventions for addressing frailty and pre-frailty: A meta-synthesis of qualitative evidence. *PLoS One*, *12*(7), e0180127. doi:10.1371/journal.pone.0180127 PMID:28723916

Dalri, Robazzi, & Silva. (2010). Riscos ocupacionais e alterações de saúde entre trabalhadores de enfermagem brasileiros de unidades deurgência e emergência. *Cienc. enferm., Concepción, 16*(2), 69-81. Disponible en http://www.scielo.cl/scielo.php?script=sci_arttext&pid=S0717-95532010000200008&lng=es&nrm=iso

Dantcheva, A., Bilinski, P., Broutart, J. C., Robert, P., & Bremond, F. (2016). *Emotion facial recognition by the means of automatic video analysis. Gerontechnology Journal.*

Daskalopoulou, C., Stubbs, B., Kralj, C., Koukounari, A., Prince, M., & Prina, A. (2018). Associations of smoking and alcohol consumption with healthy ageing: A systematic review and meta-analysis of longitudinal studies. *BMJ Open*, *8*(4), e019540. doi:10.1136/bmjopen-2017-019540 PMID:29666127

Datta, S. K., Bonnet, C., Gyrard, A., Da Costa, R. P. F., & Boudaoud, K. (2015, October). Applying Internet of Things for personalized healthcare in smart homes. In *2015 24th Wireless and Optical Communication Conference (WOCC)* (pp. 164-169). IEEE. 10.1109/WOCC.2015.7346198

Davis, F. D. (1989). Perceived Usefulness, Perceived Ease Of Use, and User Acceptance Of Information Technology. *MIS Quartely*, *13*(3), 319–339. doi:10.2307/249008

Davis, S., Mirick, D., & Stevens, R. (2001). Night Shift Work, Light at Night, and Risk of Breast Cancer. *Journal of the National Cancer Institute*, *93*(20), 1557–1562. doi:10.1093/jnci/93.20.1557 PMID:11604479

de Jong, C. C., Ros, W. J., & Schrijvers, G. (2014). The Effects on Health Behavior and Health Outcomes of Internet-Based Asynchronous Communication Between Health Providers and Patients With a Chronic Condition: A Systematic Review. *Journal of Medical Internet Research*, *16*(1), e19. doi:10.2196/jmir.3000 PMID:24434570

De Rosis, S., & Barsanti, S. (2016). Patient satisfaction, e-health and the evolution of the patient-general practitioner relationship: Evidence from Italian survey. *Health Policy (Amsterdam)*, *120*(11), 1279–1292. doi:10.1016/j.healthpol.2016.09.012 PMID:27836231

Dent, E., Kowal, P., & Hoogendijk, E. (2016). Frailty measurement in research and clinical practice: A review. *European Journal of Internal Medicine*, *31*, 3–10. doi:10.1016/j.ejim.2016.03.007 PMID:27039014

Deshpande, P. R., Rajan, S., Sudeepthi, B. L., & Nazir, A. (2011). Patient-reported outcomes: A new era in clinical research. *Perspectives in Clinical Research*, *2*(4), 137–144. doi:10.4103/2229-3485.86879 PMID:22145124

Diagnostics. (2017). iBreast Exam. *Botswana's Premier Health Journal, 16*, 1-15.

Dias, D., & Cunha, J. (2018). Wearable health devices - vital sign monitoring, systems and technologies. *Sensors (Basel), 18*(8), 2414. doi:10.339018082414 PMID:30044415

DiMaggio, P., Hargittai, E., Celeste, C., & Shafer, S. (2004). From unequal access to differentiated use: a literature review and agenda for research on digital inequality. In K. Neckerman (Ed.), *Social inequality* (pp. 355–400). New York: Russell Sage Foundation.

DiMaria-Ghalili, R. A., & Amella, E. (2005). Nutrition in older adults. *The American Journal of Nursing, 105*(3), 40–50. doi:10.1097/00000446-200503000-00020 PMID:15729041

Django. (2019). *The web framework for perfectionists.* Retrieved from https://www.djangoproject.com/

Dobson, J. (2019). Co-production helps ensure that new technology succeeds. *BMJ (Clinical Research Ed.), 366*, l4833. doi:10.1136/bmj.l4833

Docker Inc. (2019a). *Eclipse-mosquitto - Docker Hub.* Retrieved from https://hub.docker.com/_/eclipse-mosquitto/

Docker Inc. (2019b). *Docker Hub.* Retrieved from https://hub.docker.com/

Dodd, J. C. (2016). *Healthcare IT Transformation : Bridging Innovation, Integration, Interoperability, and Analytics.* CRC Press. doi:10.1201/9781315366876

Donat, W. (2018). *Learn Raspberry Pi Programming with Python.* Apress. doi:10.1007/978-1-4842-3769-4

Dufva, T., & Dufva, M. (2019). Grasping the future of the digital society. *Futures, 107*, 17–28. doi:10.1016/j.futures.2018.11.001

Eclipse Foundation. (2019a). *Eclipse Mosquitto™ An open source MQTT broker.* Retrieved from https://mosquitto.org/

Eclipse Foundation. (2019b). *Eclipse-PAHO – MQTT and MQTT SN software.* Retrieved from http://www.eclipse.org/paho/

ECRI Institution. (2017). *Executive brief: Top 10 Health Technology Hazards for 2018. A Report from Health Devices.* Retrieved from: https://www.ecri.org/Resources/Whitepapers_and_reports/Haz_18.pdf

Eliopoulos, C. (2011). *Enfermagem Gerontológica* (7th ed.). Porto Alegre: Artmed.

EMPATHiE Consortium. (2014). *EMPATHiE - Empowering patients in the management of chronic diseases - Final Summary Report.* Retrieved from https://ehff.eu/wp-content/uploads/2015/10/empathie_frep_en.pdf

Escorpizo, R., Finger, M. E., Glssel, A., Gradinger, F., Lckenkemper, M., & Cieza, A. (2011, June). A systematic review of functioning in vocational rehabilitation using the International Classification of Functioning, Dis- ability and Health. *Journal of Occupational Rehabilitation, 21*(2), 134–146. doi:10.100710926-011-9290-8 PMID:21328062

Esen, M. & Erdogmus, N. (2014). The Effects Of Technology Readiness On Technology Acceptance In E-HRM: Mediating Role Of Perceived Usefulness. *Bilgi Ekonomisi ve Yönetimi Dergisi, 9*(1).

European Commission. (2012). *Commission presents new Rethinking Education strategy. Press Release.* Brussels: European Commission. Retrieved from https://europa.eu/rapid/press-release_IP-12-1233_en.htm

European Commission. (2014). *Population aging in Europe: Facts, implications and policies.* Retrieved from: https://ec.europa.eu/research/social-sciences/pdf/policy_reviews/kina26426enc.pdf

European Commission. (2016). *Europe in a changing world – Inclusive, innovative and reflective societies.* Retrieved from https://ec.europa.eu/programmes/horizon2020/en/h2020-section/europe-changing-world-inclusive-innovative-and-reflective-societies

European Commission. (2017). *Digital Transformation Monitor: Uptake of digital solutions in the healthcare industry.* European Commission. Retrieved from https://ec.europa.eu/growth/tools-databases/dem/

European Commission. (2018). *Communication from the Commission to the European parliament, the council, the European economic and social committee and the committee of the regions on enabling the digital transformation of health and care in the digital single market; empowering citizens and building a healthier society.* Brussels: European Commission. Retrieved from https://eur-lex.europa.eu/legal-content/EN/TXT/?uri=CELEX:52018SC0126

Eurostat. (2019). *Individuals using the internet for interacting with public authorities.* Retrieved from http://appsso.eurostat.ec.europa.eu/nui/mainPage.do

Faber, S., van Geenhuizen, M., & de Reuver, M. (2017). eHealth adoption factors in medical hospitals: A focus on theNetherlands. *International Journal of Medical Informatics, 100*, 77–89. doi:10.1016/j.ijmedinf.2017.01.009 PMID:28241940

Facts About Healthy Aging. (2015, June). Retrieved 2018-02-08, from https://www.ncoa.org/news/resources-for-reporters/get-the- facts/healthy-aging-facts/

Facts and Figures on Healthy Ageing and Long-term Care - EUROPEAN IN- NOVATION PARTNERSHIP - European Commission. (2013, February). Retrieved 2018-02-08, from https://ec.europa.eu/eip/ageing/library/facts-and-figures-healthy-ageing-and-long-term-careen

Favela, J., Castro, L. A., Franco-Marina, F., Sánchez-García, S., Juárez-Cedillo, T., Espinel Bermudez, C., ... García-Peña, C. (2013). Nurse home visits with or without alert buttons versus usual care in the frail elderly: A randomized controlled trial. *Clinical Interventions in Aging, 8*, 85–95. doi:10.2147/CIA.S38618 PMID:23378751

Feil-Seifer, D., & Mataric, M. (2005). Socially Assistive Robotics. *9th International Conference on Rehabilitation Robotics, 2005. ICORR 2005.* doi:10.1109/icorr.2005.1501143

Félix, I. B., Guerreiro, M. P., Cavaco, A., Cláudio, A. P., Mendes, A., Balsa, J., ... Henriques, A. (2019). Development of a Complex Intervention to Improve Adherence to Antidiabetic Medication in Older People Using an Anthropomorphic Virtual Assistant Software. *Frontiers in Pharmacology*, *10*(June), 1–13. doi:10.3389/fphar.2019.00680 PMID:31281256

Fieldhouse, M., & Nicholas, D. (2008). Digital literacy as information savvy: The road to information literacy. In C. Lankshear & M. Knobel (Eds.), *Digital literacies: Concepts, policies and practices* (pp. 47–72). New York: Peter Lang Publishing.

Fielding, R. T. (2000). *Architectural Styles and the Design of Network-based Software Architectures*. Academic Press.

Fineberg, H. V., & Rowe, S. (1998). *Improving Public Understanding : Guidelines for Communicating Emerging Science on Nutririon, Food Safety, and Health*. Academic Press.

Fiore, A., Caione, A., Zappatore, D., Mitri, G. D., & Mainetti, L. (2017). De- ploying Mobile Middleware for the Monitoring of Elderly People with the Internet of Things: A Case Study. In *Cloud Infrastructures, Services, and IoT Systems for Smart Cities* (pp. 29–36). Cham: Springer; doi:10.1007/978-3-319-67636-44

Flores-Martin, D. (2017, November). Meeting IoT Users' Preferences by Emerging Behavior at Run-Time. In *International Conference on Service-Oriented Computing* (pp. 333-338). Springer.

Flores-Martin, D., Pérez-Vereda, A., Berrocal, J., Canal, C., & Murillo, J. M. (2018). *Coordinación de Dispositivos IoT mediante Web Semántica y Ontologías en Situational-Context. JISBD.*

Fonseca, A. (2018). *Boas práticas de Againg in Place. Divulgar para valorizar. Guia de boas práticas.* Lisboa: Fundação Calouste Gulbenkian / Faculdade de Educação e Psicologia — Universidade Católica Portuguesa.

Free, C., Phillips, G., Watson, L., Galli, L., Felix, L., Edwards, P., ... Haines, A. (2013). The Effectiveness of Mobile-Health Technologies to Improve Health Care Service Delivery Processes: A Systematic Review and Meta-Analysis. *PLoS Medicine*, *10*(1), e1001363. doi:10.1371/journal.pmed.1001363 PMID:23458994

Fu, A. S., Gao, K. L., Tung, A. K., Tsang, W. W., & Kwan, M. M. (2015). Effectiveness of Exergaming Training in Reducing Risk and Incidence of Falls in Frail Older Adults With a History of Falls. *Archives of Physical Medicine and Rehabilitation*, *96*(12), 2096–2102. doi:10.1016/j.apmr.2015.08.427 PMID:26360975

Galán-Jiménez, J., Berrocal, J., Garcia-Alonso, J., Canal-Velasco, J. C., & Murillo, J. M. (2017). *Coordinating heterogeneous IoT devices by means of the centralized vision of the SDN controller*. Academic Press.

Gan, Y., Chen, J., & Xu, L. (2019, July). Facial expression recog-nition boosted by soft label with a diverse ensemble. *Pattern Recognition Letters*, *125*, 105–112. doi:10.1016/j.patrec.2019.04.002

Gao, G., & Kerr, M. (2016). Documentation of Patient Problems and Strengths in Electronic Health Records. *Internal Medicine: Open Access*, *6*(3). doi:10.4172/2165-8048.1000221

Garc'ıa-Alonso, J., Berrocal, J., Murillo, J. M., Mendes, D., Fonseca, C., & Lopes, M. (2018). Situational-context for virtually modeling the elderly. *9th international symposium on ambient intelligence.*

Garcia-Alonso, J., Berrocal, J., Murillo, J. M., Mendes, D., Fonseca, C., & Lopes, M. (2019, Jun.). Situational-Context for Virtually Modeling the Elderly. Springer. Retrieved from https://link.springer.com/10.1007/978-3-030-01746-0

Garcia-Alonso, J., Berrocal, J., Murillo, J. M., Mendes, D., Fonseca, C., & Lopes, M. (2018). Situational-Context for Virtually Modeling the Elderly. *International symposium on ambient intelligence.*

García-Pérez, L. E., Álvarez, M., Dilla, T., Gil-Guillén, V., & Orozco-Beltrán, D. (2013). Adherence to therapies in patients with type 2 diabetes. *Diabetes Therapy : Research, Treatment and Education of Diabetes and Related Disorders*, *4*(2), 175–194. doi:10.100713300-013-0034-y PMID:23990497

GeoDjango. (2019). *GeoDjango, Django documentation.* Retrieved from https://docs.djangoproject.com/en/dev/ref/contrib/gis/

George-Walker, L., & Tyler, M. (2014). Connected Older Adults: Conceptualising their Digital Participation. *The Journal of Literacy and Technology*, *15*(2), 200–214.

Gerling, K. M. (2011). Exploring the Potential of Gamification Among Frail Elderly Persons. *Ext Abs CHI*, *2011*, 1–4.

Gilbert, B. J., Goodman, E., Chadda, A., Hatfield, D., Forman, D. E., & Panch, T. (2015). The Role of Mobile Health in Elderly Populations. *Current Geriatrics Reports*, *4*(4), 347–352. doi:10.100713670-015-0145-6

Gillison, F. B., Rouse, P., Standage, M., Sebire, S. J., & Ryan, R. M. (2019). A meta-analysis of techniques to promote motivation for health behaviour change from a self-determination theory perspective. *Health Psychology Review*, *13*(1), 110–130. doi:10.1080/17437199.2018.1534071 PMID:30295176

Gitlow, L. (2014). Technology Use by Older Adults and Barriers to Using Technology. *Physical & Occupational Therapy in Geriatrics*, *32*(3), 271–280. doi:10.3109/02703181.2014.946640

Gobbens, R. J., Luijkx, K. G., Wijnen-Sponselee, M. T., & Schols, J. M. (2010). Towards an integral conceptual model of frailty. *The Journal of Nutrition, Health & Aging*, *14*(3), 175–181. doi:10.100712603-010-0045-6 PMID:20191249

Godfray, H. C. J., Beddington, J. R., Crute, I. R., Haddad, L., Lawrence, D., Muir, J. F., ... Toulmin, C. (2010, February 12). Food security: The challenge of feeding 9 billion people. *Science*, *327*(5967), 812–818. doi:10.1126cience.1185383 PMID:20110467

Golinowska, S., Groot, W., Baji, P., & Pavlova, M. (2016). Health promotion targeting older people. *BMC Health Services Research*, *16*(S5), 345. doi:10.118612913-016-1514-3 PMID:27608680

Golla, A., Muller, T., Wohlfarth, K., Jahn, P., Mattukat, K., & Mau, W. (2018). Home-based balance training using Wii Fit: A pilot randomised controlled trial with mobile older stroke survivors. *Pilot and Feasibility Studies*, *4*(1), 143. doi:10.118640814-018-0334-0 PMID:30155268

Gomes, G. C. V., Simoes, M. D. S., Lin, S. M., Bacha, J. M. R., Viveiro, L. A. P., Varise, E. M., ... Pompeu, J. E. (2018). Feasibility, safety, acceptability, and functional outcomes of playing Nintendo Wii Fit Plus(TM) for frail older adults: A randomized feasibility clinical trial. *Maturitas*, *118*, 20–28. doi:10.1016/j.maturitas.2018.10.002 PMID:30415751

Google. (2019). *Kotlin and Android*. Retrieved from https://developer.android.com/kotlin/

Gouveia, B. R., Gouveia, É. R., Ihle, A., Jardim, H. G., Martins, M. M., Freitas, D. L., & Kliegel, M. (2018). The effect of the ProBalance Programme on health-related quality of life of community-dwelling older adults: A randomised controlled trial. *Archives of Gerontology and Geriatrics*, *74*, 26–31. doi:10.1016/j.archger.2017.08.012 PMID:28941936

Government of Botswana. (2004). *Maitlamo: Botswana's National ICT Policy*. Gaborone: Government of Botswana.

Government of Botswana. Ministry of Health, 2010. Integrated health service plan: A strategy for changing the health sector for a healthy Botswana 2010-2020, Gaborone: Government of Botswana, Ministry of Health.

Government, P. (2006). Decreto-Lei 101/2006. Academic Press.

Goyal, S. J., Upadhyay, A. K., Jadon, R., & Goyal, R. (2018). Real-life facial expression recognition systems: A review. In *Smart computing and informatics* (pp. 311–331). Springer. doi:10.1007/978-981-10-5544-7_31

Graupner, S., Kotov, V., & Trinks, H. (2002). *Resource-Sharing and Service Deployment in Virtual Data Centers*. Academic Press.

Gray, D. E. (2013). *Doing Research in the Real World* (3rd ed.). London: Sage Publications.

Greenhalgh, T., Procter, R., Wherton, J., Sugarhood, P., Hinder, S., & Rouncefield, M. (2015). What is quality in assisted living technology? The ARCHIE framework for effective telehealth and telecare services. *BMC Medicine*, *13*(1), 91. doi:10.118612916-015-0279-6 PMID:25902803

Gubbi, J., Buyya, R., Marusic, S., & Palaniswami, M. (2013, September). Internet of Things (IoT): A vision, architectural elements, and future directions. *Future Generation Computer Systems*, *29*(7), 1645–1660. Retrieved 2018-02-08, from https://www.sciencedirect.com/science/article/pii/S0167739X13000241

Guillen, J., Miranda, J., Berrocal, J., Garcia-Alonso, J., Murillo, J. M., & Canal, C. (2013). People as a service: A mobile-centric model for providing collective sociological profiles. *IEEE Software*, *31*(2), 48–53. doi:10.1109/MS.2013.140

Gwyther, H., Bobrowicz-Campos, E., Apóstolo, J., Marcucci, M., Cano, A., & Holland, C. (2018). A realist review to understand the efficacy and outcomes of interventions designed to minimise, reverse or prevent the progression of frailty. *Health Psychology Review*, *12*(4), 382–404. doi:10.1080/17437199.2018.1488601 PMID:29916302

Gyrard, A., Datta, S. K., Bonnet, C., & Boudaoud, K. (2015, August). Cross-domain Internet of Things application development: M3 framework and evaluation. In *2015 3rd International Conference on Future Internet of Things and Cloud* (pp. 9-16). IEEE.

Hackman, E. M., & Moe, G. L. (1999). Evaluation of newspaper reports of nutrition-related research. *Journal of the American Dietetic Association*, *99*(12), 1564–1566. doi:10.1016/S0002-8223(99)00384-3 PMID:10608952

Haghi, M., Thurow, K., & Stoll, R. (2017). Wearable Devices in Medical Internet of Things: Scientific Research and Commercially Available Devices. *Healthcare Informatics Research*, *23*(1), 4–15. doi:10.4258/hir.2017.23.1.4 PMID:28261526

Hagos, T. (2018). *Learn Android Studio 3 with Kotlin*. Manning. doi:10.1007/978-1-4842-3907-0

Halfon, N., & Hochstein, M. (2002). Life Course Heath Development: An Integrated Framework for Developing Health, Policy, and Research. *The Milbank Quarterly*, *80*(3), 433–479. doi:10.1111/1468-0009.00019 PMID:12233246

Halse, R., Shoneye, C., Pollard, C., Jancey, J., Scott, J., Pratt, I., ... Kerr, D. (2019). Improving Nutrition and Activity Behaviors Using Digital Technology and Tailored Feedback: Protocol for the LiveLighter Tailored Diet and Activity (ToDAy) Randomized Controlled Trial. *JMIR Research Protocols*, *8*(2), e12782. doi:10.2196/12782 PMID:30801257

Haluza, D., & Jungwirth, D. (2015). ICT and the future of health care: Aspects of health promotion. *International Journal of Medical Informatics*, *84*(1), 48–57. doi:10.1016/j.ijmedinf.2014.09.005 PMID:25293532

Hammersley, M., & Atkinson, P. (1994). *Etnografía*. Barcelona: Métodos de Investigación. Paidós.

Hauck, T. (2014). *Scikit-Learn Cookbook*. PACKT PUB.

Heart, T., & Kalderon, E. (2013). Older adults: Are they ready to adopt health-related ICT? *International Journal of Medical Informatics*, *82*(11), e209–e231. doi:10.1016/j.ijmedinf.2011.03.002 PMID:21481631

Helbostad, J., Vereijken, B., Becker, C., Todd, C., Taraldsen, K., Pijnappels, M., ... Mellone, S. (2017). Mobile Health Applications to Promote Active and Healthy Ageing. *Sensors (Basel)*, *17*(3), 622. doi:10.339017030622 PMID:28335475

Helsper, E. (2008). *Digital inclusion: an analysis of social disadvantage and the information society*. London: Department for Communities and Local Government.

Henriques, M. A., Costa, M. A., & Cabrita, J. (2012). Adherence and medication management by the elderly. *Journal of Clinical Nursing*, *21*(21–22), 3096–3105. doi:10.1111/j.1365-2702.2012.04144.x PMID:22882751

Henry, B. L., & Moore, D. J. (2016). Preliminary Findings Describing Participant Experience With iSTEP, an mHealth Intervention to Increase Physical Activity and Improve Neurocognitive Function in People Living With HIV. *J Assoc Nurses AIDS Care*, *27*(4), 495–511. doi:10.1016/j.jana.2016.01.001 PMID:26847379

Herv'as, R., Bravo, J., & Fontecha, J. (2014). An assistive navigation system based on augmented reality and context awareness for people with mild cognitive impairments. *IEEE Journal of Biomedical and Health Informatics*, *18*(1), 368–374. doi:10.1109/JBHI.2013.2266480 PMID:24403436

Higgins, J., & Green, S. (2008). *Cochrane handbook for systematic reviews of interventions*. West Sussex: John Wiley & Sons Ltd. doi:10.1002/9780470712184

Hillar, G. C. (2017). *MQTT Essentials - A Lightweight IoT Protocol*. Packt Publishing.

Hirschberg, J., & Manning, C. D. (2015). Advances in natural language processing. *Science*, *349*(6245), 261–266. doi:10.1126cience.aaa8685 PMID:26185244

Hong, J., Kim, J., Kim, S. W., & Kong, H. J. (2017). Effects of home-based tele-exercise on sarcopenia among community-dwelling elderly adults: Body composition and functional fitness. *Exp Gerontol, 87*(Pt A), 33-39. doi:10.1016/j.exger.2016.11.002

Hoque, R. M., Bao, Y., & Sorwar, G. (2016). Investigating factors influencing the adoption of e-Health in developing countries: A patient's perspective. *Informatics for Health & Social Care*, *§§§*, 1–17. PMID:26865037

Hossain, M. S., & Muhammad, G. (2015). Cloud-assisted speech and face recognition framework for health monitoring. *Mobile Networks and Applications*, *20*(3), 391–399. doi:10.100711036-015-0586-3

Hou, C., Carter, B., Hewitt, J., Francisa, T., & Mayor, S. (2016). Do Mobile Phone Applications Improve Glycemic Control (HbA1c) in the Self-management of Diabetes? A Systematic Review, Meta-analysis, and GRADE of 14 Randomized Trials. *Diabetes Care*, *39*(11), 2089–2095. doi:10.2337/dc16-0346 PMID:27926892

Hsieh, N. (2015). *Ontology Based Integration of Residential Care of the Elderly System in Long-Term Care Institutions*. doi:10.12720/jait.6.3.96-102

Hung, E. S., Chen, S. C., Chang, F. C., Shiao, Y., Peng, C. W., & Lai, C. H. (2019). Effects of Interactive Video Game-Based Exercise on Balance in Diabetic Patients with Peripheral Neuropathy: An Open-Level, Crossover Pilot Study. *Evidence-based complementary and alternative medicine: eCAM, 2019*, 4540709. doi:10.1155/2019/4540709

Hung, J. W., Yu, M. Y., Chang, K. C., Lee, H. C., Hsieh, Y. W., & Chen, P. C. (2016). Feasibility of Using Tetrax Biofeedback Video Games for Balance Training in Patients With Chronic Hemiplegic Stroke. *PM & R*, *8*(10), 962–970. doi:10.1016/j.pmrj.2016.02.009 PMID:26968609

Ichikawa, D., Kashiyama, M., & Ueno, T. (2017). Tamper-Resistant Mobile Health Using Blockchain Technology. *JMIR mHealth and uHealth*, *5*(7), e111. doi:10.2196/mhealth.7938 PMID:28747296

INE. (2006). *Sociedade da informação e do conhecimento - Inquérito à utilização de tecnologias da informação e da comunicação pelas famílias: 2006*. INE.

INE. (2014). Proyección de la Población de España 2014-2064: Notas de prensa. In Instituto Nacional de Estadística (INE). doi:10.1017/CBO9781107415324.004

INE. (2015). *Sociedade da Informação e do Conhecimento - Inquérito à Utilização de Tecnologias da Informação e da Comunicação pelas Famílias*. INE.

INE. (2018). Encuesta continua de hogares. *Instituto Nacional de Estadística (INE).* https://www.ine.es/dyngs/INEbase/es/operacion.htm?c=Estadistica_C&cid=1254736176952&menu=ultiDatos&idp=1254735572981

Instituto de Mayores y Servicios Sociales (IMSERSO). (2015). *Informe 2014*. Las Personas Mayores en España.

International Diabetes Federation. (2017). *IDF Diabetes Atlas* (8th ed.). Retrieved from https://diabetesatlas.org/

IronPaper. (2015). *Ironpaper*. https://www.ironpaper.com/webintel/articles/internet-things-market-statistics-2015/

Islam, S., Daehan, K., Kabir, M., Hossain, M., & Kyung-Sup, K. (2015). The Internet of Things for Health Care: A Comprehensive Survey. *IEEE Access : Practical Innovations, Open Solutions*, *3*, 678–708. doi:10.1109/ACCESS.2015.2437951

JBI. (2011). *Joanna Briggs Institute Reviewers' Manual*. Adelaide: The Joanna Briggs Institute. University of Adelaide.

Jenkins, H., Purushotma, R., Weigel, M., Clinton, K., & Robison, A. (2009). *Confronting the Challenges of Participatory Culture. Media education for the 21st Century*. Massachusetts Institute of Technology. doi:10.7551/mitpress/8435.001.0001

Jodelet, D. (2001). Representações sociais: um domínio em expansão. In As representações sociais. Rio de Janeiro: EdUERJ.

Juba, S., Vannahme, A., & Volkov, A. (2015). *Learning PostgreSQL*. Packt Publishing.

Kalyani, R. R., Golden, S. H., & Cefalu, W. T. (2017). Diabetes and aging: Unique considerations and goals of care. *Diabetes Care*, *40*(4), 440–443. doi:10.2337/dci17-0005 PMID:28325794

Kamińska, M. S., Miller, A., Rotter, I., Szylińska, A., & Grochans, E. (2018). The effectiveness of virtual reality training in reducing the risk of falls among elderly people. *Clinical Interventions in Aging*, *13*, 2329–2338. doi:10.2147/CIA.S183502 PMID:30532523

Kata Containers. (2019). Retrieved from https://katacontainers.io/

Kebede, M. M., Liedtke, T. P., Möllers, T., & Pischke, C. R. (2017). Characterizing Active Ingredients of eHealth Interventions Targeting Persons With Poorly Controlled Type 2 Diabetes Mellitus Using the Behavior Change Techniques Taxonomy: Scoping Review. *Journal of Medical Internet Research*, *19*(10), e348. doi:10.2196/jmir.7135 PMID:29025693

Kgasi, M. R. (2014). *Assessment of e-health readiness in rural South Africa*. Pretoria: Tshwane University Of Technology.

Kgasi, M. R., & Kalema, B. M. (2014). Assessment E-health Readiness for Rural South African Areas. *Journal of Industrial and Intelligent Information*, *2*(2), 131–135. doi:10.12720/jiii.2.2.131-135

Khatun, F., Heywood, A. E., Ray, P. K., Bhuiya, A., & Liawa, S.-T. (2016). Community readiness for adopting mHealth in rural Bangladesh: Aqualitative exploration. *International Journal of Medical Informatics*, *93*, 49–56.

Khatun, F., Heywood, A. E., Ray, P. K., Hanifi, S., Bhuiya, A., & Liawa, S.-T. (2015). Determinants of readiness to adopt mHealth in a rural community of Bangladesh. *International Journal of Medical Informatics*, *84*, 847–856.

Khosravi, P., Rezvani, A., & Wiewiora, A. (2016). The impact of technology on older adults' social isolation. *Computers in Human Behavior*, *63*, 594–603. doi:10.1016/j.chb.2016.05.092

Kiberu, V. M. (2016). E-Health Readiness Assessment in Uganda: Integration of Telemedicine services into Public Healthcare System. IEEE Computer Society.

Kim, B. Y., & Lee, J. (2017). Smart Devices for Older Adults Managing Chronic Disease: A Scoping Review. *JMIR mHealth and uHealth*, *5*(5), e69. doi:10.2196/mhealth.7141 PMID:28536089

Kim, J., Yun, J., Choi, S. C., Seed, D. N., Lu, G., Bauer, M., ... Song, J. (2016). Standard-based IoT platforms interworking: Implementation, experiences, and lessons learned. *IEEE Communications Magazine*, *54*(7), 48–54. doi:10.1109/MCOM.2016.7514163

King, N. (2003). Smart Home –A Definition. *Housing Learning & Improvement Network*, 1–6. Retrieved from http://www.housinglin.org.uk/_library/Resources/Housing/Housing_advice/Smart_Home_-_A_definition%5C_September_2003.pdf

King, A. C., Campero, I., Sheats, J. L., Castro Sweet, C. M., Garcia, D., Chazaro, A., ... Bickmore, T. (2017). Testing the comparative effects of physical activity advice by humans vs. computers in underserved populations: The COMPASS trial design, methods, and baseline characteristics. *Contemporary Clinical Trials*, *61*(April), 115–125. doi:10.1016/j.cct.2017.07.020 PMID:28739541

Kobayashi, L., & Steptoe, A. (2018). Social Isolation, Loneliness, and Health Behaviors at Older Ages: Longitudinal Cohort Study. *Annals of Behavioral Medicine*, *52*(7), 582–593. doi:10.1093/abm/kax033 PMID:29860361

Ko, P., Kientz, J., Choe, E., Kay, M., Landis, C., & Watson, N. (2015). Consumer Sleep Technologies: A Review of the Landscape. *Journal of Clinical Sleep Medicine*, *11*(12), 1455–1461. doi:10.5664/jcsm.5288 PMID:26156958

Krejcie, R. V., & Morgan, D. W. (1970). Determining sample size for research activities. *Educational and Psychological Measurement*, *30*(3), 607–610.

Kuh, D. (2019). A Life Course Approach to Healthy Ageing. In J.-P. Michel (Ed.), *Prevention of Chronic Diseases and Age-Related Disability* (pp. 1–9). Springer. doi:10.1007/978-3-319-96529-1_1

Kuiper, J., Zuidersma, M., Zuidema, S., Burgerhof, J., Stolk, R., Oude Voshaar, R., & Smidt, N. (2016). Social relationships and cognitive decline: A systematic review and meta-analysis of longitudinal cohort studies. *International Journal of Epidemiology*. doi:10.1093/ije/dyw089 PMID:27272181

Kulkarni, A., Shendge, A., Varma, V., & Kimmatkar, N. V. (2018). *Intelligent emotion detection system using facial images*. Academic Press.

Kuo, K. M., Liu, C. F., & Ma, C. C. (2013). An investigation of the effect of nurses' technology readiness on the acceptance of mobile electronic medical record systems. *Medical Informatics and Decision Making*, *13*(1), 88. doi:10.1186/1472-6947-13-88 PMID:23938040

Kusumastuti, S., Derks, M. G. M., Tellier, S., Di Nucci, E., Lund, R., Mortensen, E. L., & Westendorp, R. G. J. (2016). Successful ageing: A study of the literature using citation network analysis. *Maturitas*, *93*, 4–12. doi:10.1016/j.maturitas.2016.04.010 PMID:27156006

Kvaavik, E. (2010). Influence of Individual and Combined Health Behaviors on Total and Cause-Specific Mortality in Men and Women. *Archives of Internal Medicine*, *170*(8), 711. doi:10.1001/archinternmed.2010.76 PMID:20421558

Lang, P., Michel, J., & Zekry, D. (2009). Frailty Syndrome: A Transitional State in a Dynamic Process. *Gerontology*, *55*(5), 539–549. doi:10.1159/000211949 PMID:19346741

Larabel. (2019). Benchmarking the Python optimizations of Clear Linux against, Ubuntu, Intel Python. *Phoronix*. Retrieved from https://www.phoronix.com/scan.php?page=news_item&px=Clear-Linux-2019-Python-Perf

Lassila, O., & Swick, R. R. (1998). *Resource description framework (RDF) model and syntax specification*. Academic Press.

Lavie, C. J., Johannsen, N., Swift, D., Sénéchal, M., Earnest, C., Church, T., ... Blair, S. N. (2014). Exercise is Medicine—The Importance of Physical Activity, Exercise Training, Cardiorespiratory Fitness, and Obesity in the Prevention and Treatment of Type 2 Diabetes. *European Endocrinology*, *10*(1), 18–22. doi:10.17925/EE.2014.10.01.18 PMID:29872459

Leape, L. L., Bates D. W., Cullen, D. J., & Cooper, J. (1995). System analysis of adverse drug events. JAMA, 274(1), 35-43.

Lee, J. (2005). *The Adoption Gap: Health Information Technology In Small Physician Practices.* The People to People Health Foundation.

Lee, J., Cain, C., Young, S., Chockley, N., & Burstin, H. (2005). The Adoption Gap: Health Information Technology In Small Physician Practices. The People toPeople Health Foundation.

Lee, C.-H., Kim, Y., & Lee, B.-H. (2014). Augmented reality-based postural control training improves gait function in patients with stroke: Randomized controlled trial. *Hong Kong Physiotherapy Journal*, *32*(2), 51–57. doi:10.1016/j.hkpj.2014.04.002

Leedy, P. D., & Ormrod, J. E. (2010). *Practical Research: Planning and Design* (9th ed.). Boston: Pearson Education International.

Lee, J.-A., Choi, M., Lee, S. A., & Jiang, N. (2018). Effective behavioral intervention strategies using mobile health applications for chronic disease management: A systematic review. *BMC Medical Informatics and Decision Making*, *18*(1), 12. doi:10.118612911-018-0591-0 PMID:29458358

Lee, P. G., & Halter, J. B. (2017). The pathophysiology of hyperglycemia in older adults: Clinical considerations. *Diabetes Care*, *40*(4), 444–452. doi:10.2337/dc16-1732 PMID:28325795

Lesauskaitė, V., Damulevičienė, G., Knašienė, J., Kazanavičius, E., Liutkevičius, A., & Janavičiūtė, A. (2019). Older Adults—Potential Users of Technologies. *Medicina*, *55*(6), 253. doi:10.3390/medicina55060253 PMID:31181673

Li, H., Buenaposada, J. M., & Baumela, L. (2008). Real-time facial expression recognition with illumination-corrected image sequences. In *Automatic face & gesture recognition, 2008. fg'08. 8th IEEE international conference on* (pp. 1–6). IEEE.

Li, J., Ray, P., Seale, H., & MacIntyre, R. (2012). An E-Health Readiness Framework For Public Health Services-Pandemic Perspective. In *System Science (HICSS), 2012 45th Hawaii International Conference*. IEEE. 10.1109/HICSS.2012.95

Livingstone, S. (2004). What is media literacy? *Intermedia*, *32*(3), 18–20.

Li, W., Liu, K., Yang, H., & Yu, C. (2014). Integrated clinical pathway management for medical quality improvement - Based on a semiotically inspired systems architecture. *European Journal of Information Systems*, *23*(4), 400–417. doi:10.1057/ejis.2013.9

Lowrie, I. (2018). Algorithms and Automation: An Introduction. *Cultural Anthropology*, *33*(3), 349–359. doi:10.14506/ca33.3.01

Lowsky, D., Olshansky, S., Bhattacharya, J., & Goldman, D. (2013). Heterogeneity in Healthy Aging. *The Journals of Gerontology. Series A, Biological Sciences and Medical Sciences*, *69*(6), 640–649. doi:10.1093/gerona/glt162 PMID:24249734

Lozano-Monasor, E., López, M. T., Vigo-Bustos, F., & Fernández-Caballero, A. (2017). Facial expression recognition in ageing adults: From lab to ambient assisted living. *Journal of Ambient Intelligence and Humanized Computing*, *8*(4), 567–578. doi:10.100712652-017-0464-x

Lumme-Sandt, K. (2011). Images of ageing in a 50+ magazine. *Journal of Aging Studies*, *25*(1), 45–51. doi:10.1016/j.jaging.2010.08.013

Lustria, M. L. A., Noar, S. M., Cortese, J., Van Stee, S. K., Glueckauf, R. L., & Lee, J. (2013). A meta-analysis of web-delivered tailored health behavior change interventions. *Journal of Health Communication*, *18*(9), 1039–1069. doi:10.1080/10810730.2013.768727 PMID:23750972

Lv, J.-J., Shao, X.-H., Huang, J.-S., Zhou, X.-D., & Zhou, X. (2017, March). Data augmentation for face recognition. *Neurocomputing*, *230*, 184–196. doi:10.1016/j.neucom.2016.12.025

Madden, R., Sykes, C., & Ustun, B. T. (n.d.). *World Health Organization Family of International Classifications: definition, scope and purpose*. Retrieved from https://www.who.int/classifications/en/FamilyDocument2007.pdf?ua=1

Magalhaes, A. M. M., Riboldi, C. O., & Dall'Agnol, C. M. (2009). Planejamento de recursos humanos de enfermagem: desafio para as lideranças. *Rev. bras. enferm., Brasília*, *62*(4), 608-612. Available from http://www.scielo.br/scielo.php?script=sci_arttext&pid=S0034-71672009000400020&lng=en&nrm=iso

Magalhaes, K. A., Giacomin, K. C., dos Santos, W. J., & Firmo, J. O. (2015). A visita domiciliária do agente comunitário de saúde a famílias com idosos frágeis. *Ciencia & Saude Coletiva*, *20*(12), 3787–3796. doi:10.1590/1413-812320152012.07622014 PMID:26691803

Maheshwar, M., Narender, K., Balakrishna, N., & Rao, D. (2018). Teenagers Understanding and Influence of Media Content on their Diet and Health- Related Behaviour. *Journal of Clinical Nutrition & Dietetics*, *04*(02). doi:10.4172/2472-1921.100071

Mainetti, L., Patrono, L., Secco, A., & Sergi, I. (2016, July). An IoT-aware AAL system for elderly people. In *2016 International Multidisciplinary Conference on Computer and Energy Science (SpliTech)* (pp. 1-6). IEEE. 10.1109/SpliTech.2016.7555929

Majumder, S., Aghayi, E., Noferesti, M., Memarzadeh-Tehran, H., Mondal, T., Pang, Z., & Deen, M. (2017). Smart Homes for Elderly Healthcare—Recent Advances and Research Challenges. *Sensors (Basel)*, *17*(11), 2496. doi:10.339017112496 PMID:29088123

Malcolm, M., Frost, H., & Cowie, J. (2019). Loneliness and social isolation causal association with health-related lifestyle risk in older adults: A systematic review and meta-analysis protocol. *Systematic Reviews*, *8*(1), 48. doi:10.118613643-019-0968-x PMID:30732659

Mansour, E., Sambra, A. V., Hawke, S., Zereba, M., Capadisli, S., Ghanem, A., ... Berners-Lee, T. (2016, April). A demonstration of the solid platform for social web applications. In *Proceedings of the 25th International Conference Companion on World Wide Web* (pp. 223-226). International World Wide Web Conferences Steering Committee. 10.1145/2872518.2890529

Marek, K. D., Stetzer, F., Adams, S. J., Popejoy, L. L., & Rantz, M. (2012). Aging in place versus nursing home care: Comparison of costs to Medicare and Medicaid. *Research in Gerontological Nursing*, *5*(2), 123–129. doi:10.3928/19404921-20110802-01 PMID:21846081

Martens, H. (2010). Evaluating media literacy education: Concepts, theories and future directions. *The National Association for Media Literacy Education's Journal of Media Literacy Education*, *2*(1), 1–22.

Martin, A. (2008). Digital Literacy and the "Digital Society". In C. Lankshear & M. Knobel (Eds.), *Digital literacies: Concepts, policies and practices* (pp. 151–176). New York: Peter Lang Publishing.

Martínez-Alcalá, C., Rosales-Lagarde, A., Alonso-Lavernia, M., Ramírez-Salvador, J., Jiménez-Rodríguez, B., Cepeda-Rebollar, R., ... Agis-Juárez, R. A. (2018). Digital inclusion in older adults: A comparison between face-to-face and blended digital literacy workshops. *Frontiers in ICT*, *5*, 21. doi:10.3389/fict.2018.00021

Martinez-Nicolas, A., Madrid, J., García, F., Campos, M., Moreno-Casbas, M., Almaida-Pagán, P., ... Rol, M. (2018). Circadian monitoring as an aging predictor. *Scientific Reports*, *8*(1), 15027. doi:10.103841598-018-33195-3 PMID:30301951

Martin, S. A., & Sinsky, C. A. (2016). The map is not the territory: Medical records and 21st century practice. *Lancet*, *388*(10055), 2053–2056. doi:10.1016/S0140-6736(16)00338-X PMID:27125861

Matias, R., Paixão, V., Bouça, R., & Ferreira, J. (2017). A Perspective on Wearable Sensor Measurements and Data Science for Parkinson's Disease. *Frontiers in Neurology*, *8*, 677. doi:10.3389/fneur.2017.00677 PMID:29312115

Matos, A. P., Festas, M. I., & Seixas, A. M. (2016). Digital media and the challenges for media education. *Applied Technologies and Innovations*, *12*(2), 43–53. doi:10.15208/ati.2016.04

Matthew-Maich, N., Harris, L., Ploeg, J., Markle-Reid, M., Valaitis, R., Ibrahim, S., ... Isaacs, S. (2016). Designing, Implementing, and Evaluating Mobile Health Technologies for Managing Chronic Conditions in Older Adults: A Scoping Review. *JMIR mHealth and uHealth*, *4*(2), e29. doi:10.2196/mhealth.5127 PMID:27282195

Mayron, L. M. (2015, May). Biometric Authentication on Mobile Devices. *IEEE Security and Privacy*, *13*(3), 70–73. doi:10.1109/MSP.2015.67

Mazzotta, I., Novielli, N., & De Carolis, B. (2009). Are ECAs more persuasive than textual messages? In Lecture Notes in Computer Science (Vol. 5773, pp. 527–528). Springer. doi:10.1007/978-3-642-04380-2_75

McAuley, A. (2014). Digital health interventions: Widening access or widening inequalities? *Public Health*, *128*(12), 1118–1120. doi:10.1016/j.puhe.2014.10.008 PMID:25458115

McCormack, B. (2004). Person-centredness in gerontological nursing: An overview of the literature. *Journal of Clinical Nursing*, *13*(s13a), 31–38. doi:10.1111/j.1365-2702.2004.00924.x PMID:15028037

McPhail, S. M. (2016, July). Multimorbidity in chronic dis- ease: impact on health care resources and costs. *Risk Management and Healthcare Policy, 9*, 143–156. Retrieved 2018-02-08, from https://www.ncbi.nlm.nih.gov/pmc/articles/PMC4939994/

MEASURE Evaluation. (2018). MEASURE Evaluation Organisation. Retrieved 05 22, 2018, from https://www.measureevaluation.org/his-strengthening-resource-center/country-profiles/botswana

Medical Research Council. (2000). *A Framework for Development and Evaluation of RCTs for Complex Interventions to Improve Health.* Author.

Melanson, D. (2010). *Sanofi-Aventis debuts iBGStar blood glucose meter for iPhone.* Retrieved October 15, 2018, from https://www.engadget.com/2010/09/21/sanofi-aventis-debuts-ibgstar-blood-glucose-meter-for-iphone/?guccounter=1

Mendes, D. (2014). *Clinical Practice Knowledge Acquisition and Interrogation using Natural Language.* Universidade de Évora. https://www.rdpc.uevora.pt/bitstream/10174/12553/1/dissertation_Dm_PhDi.pdf

Mendes, D. J. M., Rodrigues, I. P., & Fonseca, C. (n.d.). *Clinical Decision Support Systems Question and Answering.* doi:10.4018/978-1-5225-4944-4.ch009

Mendes, D., Rodrigues, I., Fonseca, C., Lopes, M. J., García-alonso, J. M., & Berrocal, J. (2018). *Anonymized distributed PHR using Blockchain for openness and non- repudiation guarantee.* Academic Press.

Mendes, D., & Rodrigues, I. P. (2013). OGCP - A new ontology for clinical practice knowledge representation and a proposal for automated population. *Proceedings of JIUE 2013 - Jornadas Do Departamento de Informática Da Universidade de Évora - Évora, Portugal.*

Metcalf, D., Milliard, S. T., Gomez, M., & Schwartz, M. (2016). Wearables and the internet of things for health: Wearable, interconnected devices promise more efficient and comprehensive health care. *IEEE Pulse, 7*(5), 35–39. doi:10.1109/MPUL.2016.2592260 PMID:28113167

Miasso, A. I., Silva, A. E. B. C., Cassiani, S. H. B., & Grou, C. R. (2006). O processo de preparo e administração de medicamentos: identificação de problemas para propor melhorias e prevenir erros de medicação. *Rev Latino-Am Enfermagem, Ribeirão Preto, 14*(3), 354-63. Available from http://www.scielo.br/scielo.php?script=sci_arttext&pid=S0104-11692006000300008&lng=en&nrm=iso

Michie, S., Atkins, L., & West, R. (2014). The Behavior Change Wheel: A Guide To Designing Interventions. London: Silverback Publishing.

Michie, S., Johnston, M., Francis, J., Hardeman, W., & Eccles, M. (2008). From Theory to Intervention: Mapping Theoretically Derived Behavioural Determinants to Behaviour Change Techniques. *Applied Psychology, 57*(4), 660–680. doi:10.1111/j.1464-0597.2008.00341.x

Michie, S., Richardson, M., Johnston, M., Abraham, C., Francis, J., Hardeman, W., ... Wood, C. E. (2013). The behavior change technique taxonomy (v1) of 93 hierarchically clustered techniques: Building an international consensus for the reporting of behavior change interventions. *Annals of Behavioral Medicine*, *46*(1), 81–95. doi:10.100712160-013-9486-6 PMID:23512568

Michie, S., van Stralen, M. M., & West, R. (2011). The behaviour change wheel: A new method for characterising and designing behaviour change interventions. *Implementation Science; IS*, *6*(42), 1–11. doi:10.1186/1748-5908-6-42 PMID:21513547

Micoulaud-Franchi, J. A., Sagaspe, P., De Sevin, E., Bioulac, S., Sauteraud, A., & Philip, P. (2016). Acceptability of embodied conversational agent in a health care context. Lecture Notes in Computer Science, 10011, 416–419. doi:10.1007/978-3-319-47665-0_45

Migneault, J. P., Farzanfar, R., Wright, J. A., & Friedman, R. H. (2006). How to write health dialog for a talking computer. *Journal of Biomedical Informatics*, *39*(5), 468–481. doi:10.1016/j.jbi.2006.02.009 PMID:16564749

Milner, C., van Norman, K., & Milner, J. (2012). The Media's Portrayal of Ageing. In J. Beard, S. Biggs, D. Bloom, L. Fried, P. Hogan, A. Kalache, & J. Olshansky (Eds.), *Global Population Ageing: Peril or Promise?* (pp. 28-31). World Economic Forum.

Ministry of Health, Government of Botswana. (2010). Integrated Health Service Plan: A Strategy for Changing the Health Sector For Healthy Botswana 2010-2020. Gaborone: Government of Botswana.

Moahi, K. H., & Bwalya, K. J. (2017). Knowledge Sharing for Healthcare and Medicine in Developing Countries: Opportunities, Issues, and Experiences. In K. H. Moahi, K. J. Bwalya, & P. M. I. Sebina (Eds.), *Health Information Systems and the Advancement of Medical Practice in Developing Countries* (pp. 60–77). Hershey, PA: IGI Global. doi:10.4018/978-1-5225-2262-1.ch004

Moguel, E., Berrocal, J., Murillo, J. M., Garcia-Alonso, J., Mendes, D., Fonseca, C., & Lopes, M. (2018). *Enriched elderly virtual profiles by means of a multidimensionalidad integrated assessment platform*. Academic Press.

Moguel, E., Berrocal, J., Murillo, J. M., Garc'ıa-Alonso, J., Mendes, D., Fonseca, C., & Lopes, M. (2018, January). Enriched elderly virtual profiles by means of a multidimensional integrated assessment plat- form. *Procedia Computer Science*, *138*, 56–63. doi:10.1016/j.procs.2018.10.009

Moloi, J., & Mutula, S. (2007). E-records management in an e-government setting in Botswana. *Information Development*, *23*(4), 290–306.

Monkaresi, H., Calvo, R. A., Pardo, A., Chow, K., Mullan, B., & Lam, M., ... Cook, D. I. (2013). Intelligent Diabetes Lifestyle Coach. *Fifth International Workshop on Smart Healthcare and Wellness Applications (SmartHealth'13)*, 1–4.

Monteserin, R., Brotons, C., Moral, I., Altimir, S., San Jose, A., Santaeugenia, S., ... Padrós, J. (2010). Effectiveness of a geriatric intervention in primary care: A randomized clinical trial. *Family Practice*, *27*(3), 239–245. doi:10.1093/fampra/cmp101 PMID:20053673

Moore, L., Britten, N., Lydahl, D., Naldemirci, O., Elam, M., & Wolf, A. (2017). Barriers and facilitators to the implementation of person-centred care in different healthcare contexts. *Scandinavian Journal of Caring Sciences*, *31*(4), 662–673. doi:10.1111cs.12376 PMID:27859459

Morales Suárez-Varela, M. T. (2009, April). la utilidad del pastillero para mejorar el terapéutico. *Atencion Primaria*, *41*(4), 185–191. doi:10.1016/j.aprim.2008.07.003 PMID:19328598

Morley, J. E., & Silver, A. J. (1995, dec). Nutritional Issues in Nursing Home Care. *Annals of Internal Medicine*, *123*(11), 850. Retrieved from http://annals.org/article.aspx?doi=10.7326/0003-4819-123-

Mota-Pinto, A., Rodrigues, V., Botelho, A., Veríssimo, M. T., Morais, A., Alves, C., ... de Oliveira, C. R. (2010). A socio-demographic study of aging in the Portuguese population: The EPEPP study. *Archives of Gerontology and Geriatrics*, *52*(3), 304–308. doi:10.1016/j.archger.2010.04.019 PMID:20510469

Mouat, A. (2015). *Using Docker*. O'Reilly Media, Inc.

Mshali, H., Lemlouma, T., Moloney, M., & Magoni, D. (2018). A survey on health monitoring systems for health smart homes. *International Journal of Industrial Ergonomics*, *66*, 26–56. doi:10.1016/j.ergon.2018.02.002

Mugo, D. M., & Nzuki, D. (2014). Determinants of Electronic Health in Developing Countries. *International Journal of Arts and Commerce*, *3*(3), 49–60.

Munshi, M. (2019). *Treatment of type 2 diabetes mellitus in the older patient - UpToDate*. Retrieved September 16, 2019, from https://www.uptodate.com/contents/treatment-of-type-2-diabetes-mellitus-in-the-older-patient

Nagykaldi, Z. J., Tange, H., & De Maeseneer, J. (2018). Moving from problem-oriented to goal-directed health records. *Annals of Family Medicine*, *16*(2), 155–159. doi:10.1370/afm.2180 PMID:29531108

Ndlovu, K., Mauco, K. L., & Littman-Quinn, R. (2017). Telemedicine in Low Resource Settings: A Case for Botswana. In K. H. Moahi, K. J. Bwalya, & P. M. I. Sebina (Eds.), *Health Information Systems and the Advancement of Medical Practice in Developing Countries* (pp. 129–148). Hershey, PA: IGI Global. doi:10.4018/978-1-5225-2262-1.ch008

Niess, J., & Diefenbach, S. (2016). Communication Styles of Interactive Tools for Self-Improvement. *Psychology of Well-Being*, *6*(1), 3. doi:10.118613612-016-0040-8 PMID:27335769

Nieuwlaat, R., Wilczynski, N., Navarro, T., Hobson, N., Jeffery, R., Keepanasseril, A., ... Haynes, R. (2014). Interventions for enhancing medication adherence [Review]. *Cochrane Database of Systematic Reviews*, (11), 1–730. doi:10.1002/14651858.CD000011.pub4 PMID:25412402

Ni, Q., Hernando, A., & Cruz, I. (2015). The Elderly's Independent Living in Smart Homes: A Characterization of Activities and Sensing Infrastructure Survey to Facilitate Services Development. *Sensors (Basel), 15*(5), 11312–11362. doi:10.3390150511312 PMID:26007717

Nkwe, N. (2011). State of Information Technology Auditing in Botswana. *Asian Journal of Finance & Accounting, 3*(1), 125–137. doi:10.5296/ajfa.v3i1.894

Nkwe, N. (2012). E-Government: Challenges and Opportunities in Botswana. *International Journal of Humanities and Social Science, 2*(17), 39–48.

Nóbrega, S. M., & Coutinho, M. P. L. (2011). O teste de associação livre de palavras. In M. P. L. Coutinho (Ed.), *Métodos de pesquisa em psicologia social: perspectivas qualitativas e quantitativas* (pp. 95–106). João Pessoa: Editora Universitária.

Nolan, M. R., Davies, S., Brown, J., Keady, J., & Nolan, J. (2004). Beyond 'person-centred' care: A new vision for gerontological nursing. *Journal of Clinical Nursing, 13*(s1), 45–53. doi:10.1111/j.1365-2702.2004.00926.x PMID:15028039

Nordrum, A. (2016). The internet of fewer things. *IEEE Spectrum, 53*(10), 12–13. doi:10.1109/MSPEC.2016.7572524

Núñez, C. A. V., Mendoza, P. S., Hernández, K. A., & Molinares, D. J. (2016). Internet de las cosas y la salud centrada en el hogar. *Salud Uninorte, 32*(2).

Nweke, H. F., Teh, Y. W., Mujtaba, G., & Al-garadi, M. A. (2019). Data fusion and multiple classifier systems for human activity detection and health monitoring: Review and open research directions. *Information Fusion, 46*, 147–170. doi:10.1016/j.inffus.2018.06.002

Nwosu, A. C., Quinn, C., Samuels, J., Mason, S., & Payne, T. R. (2018). Wearable smartwatch technology to monitor symptoms in advanced illness. *BMJ Supportive & Palliative Care, 8*(2), 237. doi:10.1136/bmjspcare-2017-001445 PMID:29101119

OECD/EU. (2018). *Health at a Glance: Europe 2018*. Summary in Spanish. doi:10.1787/fd41e65f-es

Officer, A., & de la Fuente-Núñez, V. (2018). A global campaign to combat ageism. *Bulletin of the World Health Organization, 96*(4), 295–296. doi:10.2471/BLT.17.202424 PMID:29695887

Ojo, S. O., Olugbara, O. O., Ditsa, G., Adigun, M. O., & Xulu, S. S. (2007). Formal Model for e-Healthcare Readiness Assessment in Developing Country Context. Dubai: 4th International Conference in Innovations in Information Technology, 2007. IIT '07.IEEE.

op den Akker, R., Klaassen, R., & Nijholt, A. (2016). Virtual Coaches for Healthy Lifestyle. In *Toward Robotic Socially Believable Behaving Systems - Volume II. Modeling Social Signals* (Vol. 106). doi:10.1016/j.neulet.2006.07.043

op den Akker, R., Klaassen, R., Lavrysen, T., Geleijnse, G., van Halteren, A., Schwietert, H., & van der Hout, M. (2011). A Personal Context-aware Multi-device Coaching Service That Supports a Healthy Lifestyle. *Proceedings of the 25th BCS Conference on Human-Computer Interaction*, 443–448. Retrieved from https://dl.acm.org/citation.cfm?id=2305316.2305397

Open Access King, R. C., Villeneuve, E., White, R. J., Sherratt, R. S., Holderbaum, W., & Harwin, W. S. (2017). Application of data fusion techniques and technologies for wearable health monitoring. *Medical Engineering & Physics*, *42*, 1–12. doi:10.1016/j.medengphy.2016.12.011 PMID:28237714

Organisation for Economic Co-operation and Development. (2015a). *Adults, Computers and Problem Solving: What's the Problem?* Paris: OECD Publishing. doi:10.1787/9789264236844-

Organisation for Economic Co-operation and Development. (2015b). *Health data governance: Privacy, monitoring and research.* Paris: OECD Publishing. doi:10.1787/9789264244566-

Organisation for Economic Co-operation and Development. (2017). *Preventing Ageing Unequally.* Paris: OECD Publishing. doi:10.1787/9789264279087-

Organisation for Economic Co-operation and Development. (2019). *How's life in the Digital Age?: Opportunities and risks of the digital transformation for people's well-being.* Paris: OECD Publishing. doi:10.1787/9789264311800

Organization for Economic Co-operation and Development. (2017). *Economic Survey of Portugal.* Available from: https://www.oecd.org/eco/surveys/Portugal-2017-OECD-economic-survey-overview.pdf

Padala, K. P., Padala, P. R., Lensing, S. Y., Dennis, R. A., Bopp, M. M., Parkes, C. M., ... Sullivan, D. H. (2017). Efficacy of Wii-Fit on Static and Dynamic Balance in Community Dwelling Older Veterans: A Randomized Controlled Pilot Trial. *Journal of Aging Research*, *4653635*, 1–9. doi:10.1155/2017/4653635 PMID:28261500

Paiva, D., Silva, S., Severo, M., Moura-Ferreira, P., Lunet, N., & Azevedo, A. (2017). Limited Health Literacy in Portugal Assessed with the Newest Vital Sign Prevalência de Literacia em Saúde Inadequada em Portugal Medida com o Newest Vital Sign. *Acta Medica Portuguesa*, *30*(12), 861–869. doi:10.20344/amp.9135 PMID:29364799

Pal, K., Eastwood, S. V., Michie, S., Farmer, A. J., Barnard, M. L., Peacock, R., ... Murray, E. (2013). Computer-based diabetes self-management interventions for adults with type 2 diabetes mellitus. *Cochrane Database of Systematic Reviews*, (3). doi:10.1002/14651858.CD008776.pub2 PMID:23543567

Pandi-Perumal, S., Moscovitch, A., Srinivasan, V., Spence, D., Cardinali, D., & Brown, G. (2009). Bidirectional communication between sleep and circadian rhythms and its implications for depression: Lessons from agomelatine. *Progress in Neurobiology*, *88*(4), 264–271. doi:10.1016/j.pneurobio.2009.04.007 PMID:19454302

Parasuraman, A. (2000). Technology Readiness Index (TRI): A Multiple-Item Scale to Measure Readiness to Embrace New Technologies. *Service Research*, *2*(4), 307–320. doi:10.1177/109467050024001

Patnaik, S., & Patnaik, A. N. (2015). E-Health For All - Is India Ready? *National Journal of Community Medicine*, *6*(4), 633–638.

Patton, D. E., Hughes, C. M., Cadogan, C. A., & Ryan, C. A. (2017). Theory-Based Interventions to Improve Medication Adherence in Older Adults Prescribed Polypharmacy: A Systematic Review. *Drugs & Aging*, *34*(2), 97–113. doi:10.100740266-016-0426-6 PMID:28025725

Pedregosa, F., Varoquaux, G., Gramfort, A., Michel, V., Thirion, B., Grisel, O., & Duchesnay, E. (2011). Scikit-learn: Machine Learning in Python. *Journal of Machine Learning Research*, *12*, 2825–2830.

Peek, C., Higgins, I., Milson-Hawke, S., McMillan, M., & Harper, D. (2007). Towards innovation: The development of a person centred model of care for older people in acute care. *Contemporary Nurse*, *26*(2), 164–176. doi:10.5172/conu.2007.26.2.164 PMID:18041967

Pels, F., & Kleinert, J. (2016). Loneliness and physical activity: A systematic review. *International Review of Sport and Exercise Psychology*, *9*(1), 231–260. doi:10.1080/1750984X.2016.1177849

Peral-Peral, B., Arenas-Gaitán, J., & Villarejo-Ramos, A.-F. (2015). From digital divide to psycho-digital divide: Elders and online social networks. *Media Education Research Journal*, *23*(45), 57–64.

Perera, C. (2012). The Evolution of E-Health – Mobile Technology and mHealth. *Journal of Mobile Technology in Medicine*, *1*(1), 1–2. doi:10.7309/jmtm.1

Perera, C., Zaslavsky, A., Christen, P., & Georgakopoulos, D. (2014). Context Aware Computing for the Internet of Things: A survey. *IEEE Communications Surveys and Tutorials*, *16*(1), 414–454. doi:10.1109/SURV.2013.042313.00197

Pettigrew, S., Worrall, C., Biagioni, N., Talati, Z., & Jongenelis, M. (2017). The role of food shopping in later life. *Appetite*, *111*, 71–78.

Pinto, S., Cabral, J., & Gomes, T. (2017, March). We-care: An IoT-based health care system for elderly people. In *2017 IEEE International Conference on Industrial Technology (ICIT)* (pp. 1378-1383). IEEE. 10.1109/ICIT.2017.7915565

Pirlich, M., & Lochs, H. (2001). Nutrition in the elderly. *Best Practice & Research. Clinical Gastroenterology*, *15*(6), 869–884. doi:10.1053/bega.2001.0246 PMID:11866482

Popek, G. J., & Goldberg, R. P. (1974). Formal requirements for virtualizable third generation architectures. *Communications of the ACM*, *17*(7), 412–421. doi:10.1145/361011.361073

PopulationPyramid.net. (2019). *População: Portugal 2016*. Retrieved from https://www.populationpyramid.net/pt/portugal/2016/

Portnoy, M. (2016, August 19). *Virtualization essentials*. John Wiley & Sons Inc.

Prazeres, F., & Santiago, L. (2015). Prevalence of multimorbidity in the adult population attending primary care in Portugal: A cross-sectional study. *BMJ Open*, *5*(9), e009287. doi:10.1136/bmjopen-2015-009287 PMID:26408832

Prensky, M. (2001). Digital natives, digital immigrants. *On the Horizon*, *9*(5), 1–6. doi:10.1108/10748120110424816

Puts, M. T. E., Toubasi, S., Andrew, M. K., Ashe, M. C., Ploeg, J., Atkinson, E., ... McGilton, K. (2017). Interventions to prevent or reduce the level of frailty in community-dwelling older adults: A scoping review of the literature and international policies. *Age and Ageing*, *46*(3), 383–392. doi:10.1093/ageing/afw247 PMID:28064173

PyPi. (2019). *paho-mqtt*. Retrieved from https://pypi.org/project/paho-mqtt/

Quan-Haase, A., Williams, C., Kicevski, M., Elueze, I., & Wellman, B. (2018). Dividing the grey divide: Deconstructing myths about older adults' online activities, skills and attitudes. *The American Behavioral Scientist*, *62*(9), 1207–1228. doi:10.1177/0002764218777572

Rahmani, A. M., Thanigaivelan, N. K., Gia, T. N., Granados, J., Negash, B., Liljeberg, P., & Tenhunen, H. (2015, January). Smart e-health gateway: Bringing intelligence to internet-of-things based ubiquitous healthcare systems. In *2015 12th Annual IEEE Consumer Communications and Networking Conference (CCNC)* (pp. 826-834). IEEE.

Rahman, S. A., Taghizadeh, S. K., Ramayah, T., & Alam, M. M. D. (2017). Technology acceptance among micro-entrepreneurs in marginalized social strata: The case of social innovation in Bangladesh. *Technological Forecasting and Social Change*, *118*, 236–245. doi:10.1016/j.techfore.2017.01.027

Rantala, L., & Suoranta, J. (2008). Digital Literacy Policies in the EU - Inclusive Partnership as the Final Stage of Governmentality? In C. Lankshear & M. Knobel (Eds.), *Digital literacies: Concepts, policies and practices* (pp. 91–117). New York: Peter Lang Publishing.

Rezai-Rad, M., Vaezi, R., & Nattagh, F. (2012). E-Health Readiness Assessment Framework in Iran. *Iranian Journal of Public Health*, *41*(10), 43–51. PMID:23304661

Ring, L., Utami, D., & Bickmore, T. (2014). The right agent for the job? The effects of agent visual appearance on task domain. Lecture Notes in Computer Science, 8637, 374–384. doi:10.1007/978-3-319-09767-1_49

RNAO. (2007). *Falls Prevention. Building the Foundations for Patient Safety. Self-Learning Package*. Ontario: Nurses' Association of Ontario.

Robles, R., & Tai-hoon, K. (2010). Applications, Systems and Methods in Smart Home Technology: A Review. *International Journal of Advanced Science and Technology*, *15*, 37–48.

Rockwood, K., Fox, R. A., Stolee, P., Robertson, D., & Beattie, B. L. (1994). Frailty in elderly people: An evolving concept. *Canadian Medical Association Journal*, *150*(4), 489–495. PMID:8313261

Rodrigues, R., Huber, M., & Lamura, G. (2012). *Facts and figures on healthy ageing and long-term care*. Vienna: European Centre for Social Welfare Policy and Research.

Roman, R., Zhou, J., & Lopez, J. (2013). On the features and challenges of security and privacy in distributed internet of things. *Computer Networks*, *57*(10), 2266–2279. doi:10.1016/j.comnet.2012.12.018

Roukos, S. (2008). Natural Language Understanding. Springer Handbooks. doi:10.1007/978-3-540-49127-9_31

Rozanova, J., Northcott, H., & McDaniel, S. (2006). Seniors and Portrayals of Intra-generational and Inter-generational Inequality in the Globe and Mail. *Canadian Journal of Aging*, *25*(4), 373-386.

Sadana, R., & Michel, J.-P. (2019). Healthy Ageing: What Is It and How to Describe It? In J.-P. Michel (Ed.), *Prevention of Chronic Diseases and Age-Related Disability* (pp. 11–24). Springer. doi:10.1007/978-3-319-96529-1_2

Saleh, S., Khodor, R., Alameddine, M., & Baroud, M. (2016). Readiness of healthcare providers for eHealth: The case from primary healthcare centers in Lebanon. *BMC Health Services Research*, *16*(644), 1–11. doi:10.118612913-016-1896-2 PMID:27832788

Sánchez López, M. A., Fernández Alemán, J. L., Toval, A., & Carrillo de Gea, J. M. (2015). *Teléfonos inteligentes para la tercera edad: una revisión de aplicaciones móviles de salud.* Academic Press.

Santos, G. O. R., Wolf, R., Silva, M. M., Rodacki, A. L. F., & Pereira, G. (2019). Does exercise intensity increment in exergame promote changes in strength, functional capacity and perceptual parameters in pre-frail older women? A randomized controlled trial. *Experimental Gerontology*, *116*, 25–30. doi:10.1016/j.exger.2018.12.009 PMID:30553026

Sapkota, S., Brien, J. A. E., Greenfield, J. R., & Aslani, P. (2015). A systematic review of interventions addressing adherence to anti-diabetic medications in patients with type 2 diabetes - Components of interventions. *PLoS One*, *10*(2), 1–17. doi:10.1371/journal.pone.0118296 PMID:26053004

Saraiva, E. R. A., Coutinho, M. P. L., & Miranda, R. S. (2011). O emprego do software Alceste e o desvendar do mundo lexical em pesquisa documental. In *Métodos de pesquisa em psicologia social: perspectivas qualitativas e quantitativas* (pp. 67–94). João Pessoa: Editora Universitária.

Saunders, M., Lewis, P., & Thornhill, A. (2016). *Research Methods For Business Students* (7th ed.). Harlow: Pearson.

Scheibe, C., & Rogow, F. (2012). *The teacher's guide to media literacy: Critical thinking in a multimedia world.* Thousand Oaks, CA: Corwin. doi:10.4135/9781483387581

Schmidhuber, J., & Tubiello, F. N. (2007). Global food security under climate change. *Proceedings of the National Academy of Sciences of the United States of America*, *104*(50), 19703–19708. doi:10.1073/pnas.0701976104 PMID:18077404

Schneider, M. (2006). Public health and the aging population. In *Introduction to public health* (2nd ed.). Academic Press.

Schreurs, K., Quan-Haase, A., & Martin, K. (2017). Problematizing the Digital Literacy Paradox in the Context of Older Adults' ICT Use: Aging, Media Discourse, and Self-Determination. *Canadian Journal of Communication*, *42*(2), 359–377. doi:10.22230/cjc.2017v42n2a3130

Sebina, P. M., & Grand, B. (2017). Records Management and Open Data in Healthcare Provision in Africa: Reflections and Lessons for Botswana. In K. H. Moahi, K. J. Bwalya, & P. M. Sebina (Eds.), *Health Information Systems and the Advancement of Medical Practice in Developing Countries* (pp. 1–13). Hershey: IGI Global.

Seiler, W. O. (1999). Nutritional status of ill elderly patients. *Zeitschrift für Gerontologie und Geriatrie*, *32*(S1), I7–I11. doi:10.1007003910050174 PMID:10441797

Self Care Forum. (2016). *What do we mean by self care and why is it good for people?* Retrieved September 16, 2019, from http://www.selfcareforum.org/about-us/what-do-we-mean-by-self-care-and-why-is-good-for-people/

Serakan, U., & Bougie, R. (2013). *Research Methods for Business:A Skill-Building Approach* (6th ed.). West Sussex: Wiley and sons.

Shrestha, N., Kubler, S., & Främling, K. (2014, August). Standardized framework for integrating domain-specific applications into the IoT. In *2014 International Conference on Future Internet of Things and Cloud* (pp. 124-131). IEEE. 10.1109/FiCloud.2014.29

Sirin, E., & Parsia, B. (2007, June). SPARQL-DL: SPARQL Query for OWL-DL. In OWLED (Vol. 258). Academic Press.

Skjaeret, N., Nawaz, A., Morat, T., Schoene, D., Helbostad, J. L., & Vereijken, B. (2016). Exercise and rehabilitation delivered through exergames in older adults: An integrative review of technologies, safety and efficacy. *International Journal of Medical Informatics*, *85*(1), 1–16. doi:10.1016/j.ijmedinf.2015.10.008 PMID:26559887

Slawomirski, L., Auraaen, A., & Klazinga, N. (2017). The economics of patient safety: Strengthening a value-based approach to reducing patient harm at national level. *OECD Health Working Paper, 96*. Retrieved from: https://www.oecd-ilibrary.org/docserver/5a9858cd-en.pdf?expires=1562940862&id=id&accname=guest&checksum=1E1B38EC433983A757038ADADA17CA82

Smith, J., & Gerstorf, D. (2006). Ageing differently: potential and limits. In S. Daatland & S. Biggs (Eds.), *Ageing and diversity: Multiple pathways and cultural migrations* (pp. 13–28). Policy Press.

Sociedade Portuguesa de Diabetologia. (2016). Relatório Anual do Observatório Nacional da Diabetes 2016. In *Letra Soluvel - Publicidade e Marketing, Lda* (Vol. 1). Retrieved from https://www.clinicadadiabetes.pt/assets/docs/relatorio_anual_Diabetes_2016/

Son, M., & Han, K. (2011). Beyond the technology adoption: Technology readiness effects on post-adoption behavior. *Journal of Business Research*, *64*(11), 1178–1182. doi:10.1016/j.jbusres.2011.06.019

Sousa, A. M. D. (2013). *Valiação da cultura de segurança do doente num centro hospitalar da zona centro* (Dissertação). Faculdade de Economia da Universidade de Coimbra, Coimbra, Portugal.

Sousa, L. M., Firmino, C. F., Marques-Vieira, C. M., Severino, S., & Pestana, H. C. (2018). Revisões da literatura científica: Tipos, métodos e aplicações em enfermagem. *Revista Portuguesa de Enfermagem de Reabilitação, 1*(1), 46–55.

Srinidhi, N., Dilip Kumar, S., & Venugopal, K. (2019). Network optimizations in the Internet of Things: A review. *Engineering Science And Technology. International Journal (Toronto, Ont.), 22*(1), 1–21. doi:10.1016/j.jestch.2018.09.003

Stenholm, S., Head, J., Kivimäki, M., Kawachi, I., Aalto, V., Zins, M., ... Vahtera, J. (2016). Smoking, physical inactivity and obesity as predictors of healthy and disease-free life expectancy between ages 50 and 75: A multicohort study. *International Journal of Epidemiology, 45*(4), dyw126. doi:10.1093/ije/dyw126 PMID:27488415

Stergiou, C., Psannis, K. E., Kim, B.-G., & Gupta, B. (2018). Secure integration of IoT and cloud computing. *Future Generation Computer Systems, 78*, 964–975. doi:10.1016/j.future.2016.11.031

Straudi, S., Severini, G., Sabbagh Charabati, A., Pavarelli, C., Gamberini, G., Scotti, A., & Basaglia, N. (2017). The effects of video game therapy on balance and attention in chronic ambulatory traumatic brain injury: An exploratory study. *BMC Neurology, 17*(1), 86–86. doi:10.118612883-017-0871-9 PMID:28490322

Suk, M., & Prabhakaran, B. (2014). Real-time mobile facial expression recognition system a case study. In *Proceedings of the IEEE conference on computer vision and pattern recognition workshops* (pp. 132–137). 10.1109/CVPRW.2014.25

Suzman, R., Beard, J. R., Boerma, T., & Chatterji, S. (2015). Health in an ageing world - What do we know? *Lancet, 385*(9967), 484–486. doi:10.1016/S0140-6736(14)61597-X PMID:25468156

Swetina, J., Lu, G., Jacobs, P., Ennesser, F., & Song, J. (2014). Toward a standardized common M2M service layer platform: Introduction to oneM2M. *IEEE Wireless Communications, 21*(3), 20–26.

Szilagyi, I., & Wira, P. (2016, October). Ontologies and Semantic Web for the Internet of Things-a survey. In *IECON 2016-42nd Annual Conference of the IEEE Industrial Electronics Society* (pp. 6949-6954). IEEE. 10.1109/IECON.2016.7793744

Szturm, T., Betker, A. L., Moussavi, Z., Desai, A., & Goodman, V. (2011). Effects of an interactive computer game exercise regimen on balance impairment in frail community-dwelling older adults: A randomized controlled trial. *Physical Therapy, 91*(10), 1449–1462. doi:10.2522/ptj.20090205 PMID:21799138

Taivalsaari, A., & Mikkonen, T. (2017). A roadmap to the programmable world: Software challenges in the IoT era. *IEEE Software, 34*(1), 72–80. doi:10.1109/MS.2017.26

Takayuki, M. (1999). Human Rights, the Right of Self-Determination and the Right to Freedom - Munakata Takayuki; The International Journal for Peace Studies. *International Journal of Peace Studies*, *4*(1). Retrieved from http://www.gmu.edu/programs/icar/ijps/vol4_1/takayuki.htm

Tanskanen, J., & Anttila, T. (2016). A Prospective Study of Social Isolation, Loneliness, and Mortality in Finland. *American Journal of Public Health*, *106*(11), 2042–2048. doi:10.2105/AJPH.2016.303431 PMID:27631736

Task Force on Research and Development for Technology to Support Aging Adults. (2019). *Emerging Technologies to Support an Aging Population*. Washington, DC: Committee on Technology of the National Science & Technology Council.

Teddlie, C., & Yu, F. (2007). Mixed methods sampling: A typology with examples. *Journal of Mixed Methods Research*, *1*(1), 77–100. doi:10.1177/1558689806292430

The Enterprice Of Healthcare Magazine. (2010). *e-Health, The Enterprice Of HealthCare*. Available at: https://ehealth.eletsonline.com/2010/04/paperless-hospital-in-africa-offers-prototype-for-new-model-of-care/

Thomas, D. R., & Hodges, I. D. (2010). *Designing and managing your research project: core skills for social and health research*. Sage Publications. doi:10.4135/9781446289044

Thomas, E., Battaglia, G., Patti, A., Brusa, J., Leonardi, V., Palma, A., & Bellafiore, M. (2019). Physical activity programs for balance and fall prevention in elderly: A systematic review. *Medicine*, *98*(27), e16218. doi:10.1097/MD.0000000000016218 PMID:31277132

Thompson, D., Callender, C., Gonynor, C., Cullen, K. W., Redondo, M. J., Butler, A., & Anderson, B. J. (2019). Using Relational Agents to Promote Family Communication Around Type 1 Diabetes Self-Management in the Diabetes Family Teamwork Online Intervention: Longitudinal Pilot Study. *Journal of Medical Internet Research*, *21*(9), e15318. doi:10.2196/15318 PMID:31538940

TIOBE Software BV. (2019, July). *TIOBE Index*. Retrieved from https://www.tiobe.com/tiobe-index/

Tirado-Morueta, R., Aguaded-Gómez, J. I., & Hernando-Gómez, A. H. (2018). The socio-demographic divide in Internet usage moderated by digital literacy support. *Technology in Society*, *55*, 47–55. doi:10.1016/j.techsoc.2018.06.001

Topaz, M., Golfenshtein, N., & Bowles, K. H. (2014). The Omaha System: A systematic review of the recent literature. *Journal of the American Medical Informatics Association*, *21*(1), 163–170. doi:10.1136/amiajnl-2012-001491 PMID:23744786

Tsikriktsis, N. (2004). A Technology Readiness–Based Taxonomy of Customers:A Replication and Extension. *Journal of Service Research*, *7*(1), 42–52. doi:10.1177/1094670504266132

Tucker, A. T., Maass, A., Bain, D. S., Chen, L. H., Azzam, M., Dawson, H., & Johnston, A. (2010). Augmentation of venous, arterial and microvascular blood supply in the leg by isometric neuromuscular stimulation via the peroneal nerve. *The International Journal of Angiology*, *19*(1), 31–37. doi:10.1055-0031-1278361 PMID:22477572

Tur, G., Celikyilmaz, A., He, X., Hakkani-Tür, D., & Deng, L. (2018). Deep Learning in Conversational Language Understanding. In *Deep Learning in Natural Language Processing* (pp. 23–48). Springer Singapore. doi:10.1007/978-981-10-5209-5_2

Tziraki-Segal, Ch., de Luca, V., Santana, S., Romano, R., Tramontano, G., Scattola, P., ... Illario, M. (2019). Creating a Culture of Health in Planning and Implementing Innovative Strategies Addressing Non-communicable Chronic Diseases. *Frontiers in Sociology*, *4*, 9. doi:10.3389/fsoc.2019.00009

União Européia. (2008). *Direção-Geral da Saúde e da Segurança dos Alimentos da Comissão Européia*. Disponível em: https://ec.europa.eu/health/patient_safety/policy/index_pt.htm

União Européia. (2012). *Comissão ao Parlamento Europeu. Sobre a segurança dos pacientes, incluindo a prevenção e o controlo de infecções associadas aos cuidados de saúde(2009/C 151/01)*. Disponível em: https://ec.europa.eu/health/patient_safety/docs/council_2009_report_pt.pdf

Upatising, B., Hanson, G. J., Kim, Y. L., Cha, S. S., Yih, Y., & Takahashi, P. Y. (2013). Effects of home telemonitoring on transitions between frailty states and death for older adults: A randomized controlled trial. *International Journal of General Medicine*, *6*, 145–151. doi:10.2147/IJGM.S40576 PMID:23525664

Valenzuela, T., Okubo, Y., Woodbury, A., Lord, S. R., & Delbaere, K. (2018). Adherence to Technology-Based Exercise Programs in Older Adults: A Systematic Review. *Journal of Geriatric Physical Therapy*, *41*(1), 49–61. doi:10.1519/JPT.0000000000000095 PMID:27362526

Van der Elst, M., Schoenmakers, B., Duppen, D., Lambotte, D., Fret, B., Vaes, B., & De Lepeleire, J. (2018). Interventions for frail community-dwelling older adults have no significant effect on adverse outcomes: A systematic review and meta-analysis. *BMC Geriatrics*, *18*(1), 249. doi:10.118612877-018-0936-7 PMID:30342479

van Deursen, A., Courtois, C., & van Dijk, J. (2014). Internet skills, sources of support and benefiting from internet use. *International Journal of Human-Computer Interaction*, *30*(4), 278–290. doi:10.1080/10447318.2013.858458

van Deursen, A., Helsper, E., Eynon, R., & van Dijk, J. (2017). The compoundness and sequentiality of digital inequality. *International Journal of Communication*, *11*, 452–473.

van Deursen, A., & van Dijk, J. (2010). Internet skills and the digital divide. *New Media & Society*, *13*(6), 893–911. doi:10.1177/1461444810386774

van Dijk, J. A. (2012). The evolution of digital divide. The digital divide turns to inequality of skills and usage. In J. Bus, M. Crompton, M. Hildebrandt, & G. Metakides (Eds.), Digital Enlightenment - Yearbook 2012 (pp. 57-74). Amsterdam: IOSS Press.

van Dijk, J. A. (2005). *The deepening divide: Inequality in the information society*. SAGE Publications.

van Wissen, A., Vinkers, C., & van Halteren, A. (2016). Developing a Virtual Coach for Chronic Patients: A User Study on the Impact of Similarity, Familiarity and Realism. In A. Meschtscherjakov, B. De Ruyter, V. Fuchsberger, M. Murer, & M. Tscheligi (Eds.), *Persuasive Technology* (pp. 263–275). Cham: Springer International Publishing. doi:10.1007/978-3-319-31510-2_23

Vanhaecht, K. (2007). *The impact of Clinical Pathways on the organisation of care processes.* Katholieke Universiteit Leuven.

Vaportzis, E., Clausen, M. G., & Glow, A. (2017). Older Adults Perceptions of Technology and Barriers to Interacting with Tablet Computers: A Focus Group Study. *Frontiers in Psychology*, *8*, 1687. doi:10.3389/fpsyg.2017.01687 PMID:29071004

Velasco, H., & Díaz de Rada, A. (2006). *La Lógica de La Investigación Etnográfica*. Madrid: Trotta.

Vilelas, J. (2017). *Investigação. O processo de construção do conhecimento*. Lisboa: Edições Sílabo.

Wachter, R. M. (2013). *Compreendendo a segurança do paciente* (2nd ed.). Porto Alegre: AMGH.

Walczuch, R., Lemmink, J., & Streukens, S. (2007). The effect of service employees' technology readiness on technology acceptance. *Information & Management*, *44*(2), 206–215. doi:10.1016/j.im.2006.12.005

Wallace, S., Graham, C., & Saraceno, A. (2013). Older adults' use of technology. *Perspectives on Gerontology*, *18*(2), 50–59. doi:10.1044/gero18.2.50

Wang, A., Pruksachatkun, Y., Nangia, N., Singh, A., Michael, J., Hill, F., . . . Bowman, S. R. (2019). *SuperGLUE: A Stickier Benchmark for General-Purpose Language Understanding Systems*. https://arxiv.org/abs/1905.00537

Wang, Q., Com, B., Myers, M., & Sundaram, D. (2013). Digital natives and digital immigrants: Towards a model of digital fluency. *Business & Information Systems Engineering*, *6*(6), 409–419. doi:10.100712599-013-0296-y

Wang, Z., Yang, Z., & Dong, T. (2017). A Review of Wearable Technologies for Elderly Care that Can Accurately Track Indoor Position, Recognize Physical Activities and Monitor Vital Signs in Real Time. *Sensors (Basel)*, *17*(2), 341. doi:10.339017020341 PMID:28208620

Waveshare. (2019, July). *GSM/GPRS/GNSS HAT - Waveshare Wiki*. Retrieved from https://www.waveshare.com/wiki/GSM/GPRS/GNSSHAT

Webb, T. L., Joseph, J., Yardley, L., & Michie, S. (2010). Using the Internet to promote health behavior change: A systematic review and meta-analysis of the impact of theoretical basis, use of behavior change techniques, and mode of delivery on efficacy. *Journal of Medical Internet Research*, *12*(1), e4. doi:10.2196/jmir.1376 PMID:20164043

WHO. (2015). *World report on ageing and health.* Geneve: World Health Organization.

Wildenbos, G. A., Peute, L., & Jaspers, M. (2018). Aging barriers influencing mobile health usability for older adults: A literature based framework (MOLD-US). *International Journal of Medical Informatics*, *114*, 66–75. doi:10.1016/j.ijmedinf.2018.03.012 PMID:29673606

Williams, J. L. S., Walker, R. J., Smalls, B. L., Campbell, J. A., & Egede, L. E. (2014). Effective interventions to improve medication adherence in Type 2 diabetes: A systematic review. *Diabetes Management*, *4*(1), 29–48. doi:10.2217/dmt.13.62 PMID:25214893

Wolf, P., Schmidt, A., & Klein, M. (2008, July). *SOPRANO-An extensible, open AAL platform for elderly people based on semantical contracts.* In 3rd Workshop on Artificial Intelligence Techniques for Ambient Intelligence (AITAmI'08), 18th European Conference on Artificial Intelligence (ECAI 08), Patras, Greece.

Wong, R. (2018). A new strategic approach to successful ageing and healthy ageing. *Geriatrics*, *3*(4), 86. doi:10.3390/geriatrics3040086 PMID:31011121

Wook, M., Yusof, Z. M., & Nazri, M. Z. A. (2017). Educational data mining acceptance among undergraduate students. *Education and Information Technologies*, *22*(3), 1195–1216. doi:10.100710639-016-9485-x

World Health Organization – Regional Office for Europe. (2017). *Age-friendly environments in Europe. A handbook of domains for policy action.* Copenhagen: World Health Organization.

World Health Organization Regional Office for Africa. (2014). *World Health Organization Regional Office for Africa.* Available at. http://www.aho.afro.who.int/profiles_information/index.php/Botswana:Health_information,_research,_evidence_and_knowledge

World Health Organization. (2003). *Diet, nutrition and the prevention of chronic diseases.* Geneva: WHO.

World Health Organization. (2004). *World Aliance for Patient Safety: Forward Programme.* Geneva: WHO Press.

World Health Organization. (2015). Chapter 3: Health in Older Age. In World Report on Ageing and Health (pp. 43–63). WHO.

World Health Organization. (2015). *World Report on Ageing and Health*. Geneva, Switzerland: World Health Organization.

World Health Organization. (2017). *Global strategy and action plan on ageing and health.* Geneva: World Health Organization.

World Health Organization. (2017). *Global strategy and action plan on ageing and health.* Retrieved from https://apps.who.int/bookorders

World Health Organization. (2018). *Ageing and health.* Geneva, Switzerland: World Health Organization.

World Health Organization. (2019). *WHO guideline Recommendations on Digital Interventions for Health System Strengthening*. Retrieved from https://www.ncbi.nlm.nih.gov/pubmed/31162915

Wu, C.-C., Zeng, Y.-C., & Shih, M.-J. (2015, Jun). Enhancing retailer marketing with an facial recognition integrated recommender system. In *2015 IEEE international conference on consumer electronics* (pp. 25–26). IEEE. Retrieved from https://ieeexplore.ieee.org/document/7216881/

Wu, Q., Zhao, W., & Jacopo, T. (2018, may). Towards Ob jective Assessment of Movie Trailer Quality Using Human Electroencephalogram and Facial Recognition. In *2018 IEEE international conference on electro/information technology* (pp. 0449–0452). IEEE. Retrieved from https://ieeexplore.ieee.org/document/8500283/

Wu, R. C., Morra, D., Quan, S., Lai, S., Zanjani, S., Abrams, H., & Rossos, P. G. (2010). The use of smartphones for clinical communication on internal medicine wards. *Journal of Hospital Medicine*, *5*(9), 553–559. doi:10.1002/jhm.775 PMID:20690190

Wu, R., Rossos, P., Quan, S., Reeves, S., Lo, V., Wong, B., & Morra, D. (2011). An evaluation of the use of smartphones to communicate between clinicians: A mixed-methods study. *Journal of Medical Internet Research*, *13*(3), e59. doi:10.2196/jmir.1655 PMID:21875849

Xiang, J., & Stanley, S. J. (2017). From online to offline: Exploring the role of e-health consumption,patient involvement, and patient-centered communication on perceptions of health care quality. *Computers in Human Behavior*, *70*, 446–452. doi:10.1016/j.chb.2016.12.072

Yang, W. C., Wang, H. K., Wu, R. M., Lo, C. S., & Lin, K. H. (2016). Home-based virtual reality balance training and conventional balance training in Parkinson's disease: A randomized controlled trial. *Journal of the Formosan Medical Association*, *115*(9), 734–743. doi:10.1016/j.jfma.2015.07.012 PMID:26279172

Ye, Q., Khan, U., Boren, S. A., Simoes, E. J., & Kim, M. S. (2018). An Analysis of Diabetes Mobile Applications Features Compared to AADE7™: Addressing Self-Management Behaviors in People With Diabetes. *Journal of Diabetes Science and Technology*, *12*(4), 808–816. doi:10.1177/1932296818754907 PMID:29390917

Yu, B., Ndumu, A., Liu, J., & Fan, Z. (2016). E-inclusion or digital divide: An integrated model of digital inequality. *Proceedings of the Association for Information Science and Technology*, *53*(1), 1–5. doi:10.1002/pra2.2016.14505301099

Yuehong, Y. I. N., Zeng, Y., Chen, X., & Fan, Y. (2016). The internet of things in healthcare: An overview. *Journal of Industrial Information Integration*, *1*, 3–13. doi:10.1016/j.jii.2016.03.004

Yusif, S., & Soar, J. (2014). Preparedness for e-Health in developing countries: The case of Ghana. *Journal of Health Informatics in Developing Countries*, *8*(2), 18–37.

Yusif, S., Soar, J., & Hafeez-Baig, A. (2016). Older people, assistive technologies, and the barriers to adoption: A systematic review. *International Journal of Medical Informatics*, *94*, 112–116. doi:10.1016/j.ijmedinf.2016.07.004 PMID:27573318

Zainab, N., & Naz, H. (2017). Daily living functioning, social engagement and wellness of older adults. *Psychology, Community & Health*, *6*(1), 93–102. doi:10.5964/pch.v6i1.213

Zheng, Y., Ley, S. H., & Hu, F. B. (2018). Global aetiology and epidemiology of type 2 diabetes mellitus and its complications. *Nature Reviews. Endocrinology*, *14*(2), 88–98. doi:10.1038/nrendo.2017.151 PMID:29219149

Zilidou, V., Douka, S., Ziagkas, E., Romanopoulou, E., & Politopoulos, N. (2018). Technology's Role on Physical Activity for Elderly People. In M. Auer & T. Tsiatsos (Eds.), *Interactive Mobile Communication Technologies and Learning. IMCL 2017. Advances in Intelligent Systems and Computing* (Vol. 725). Cham: Springer. doi:10.1007/978-3-319-75175-7_66

About the Contributors

David José Murteira Mendes, born in Évora (Portugal) in the 4th of July of 1966, achieved a PhD degree in Computer Science in Universidade de Évora (Portugal) in 2014. Previously he owns a MSc in Applied Artificial Intelligence also from the same University, an MBA from Universidad de Extremadura (Badajoz, Spain) a BSc in Computer Science from Universidade Nova de Lisboa (Portugal). He has developed a Software Engineer career from 1989 and developed mainly software for government organizations in particular for Hospitals intended both for management and clinical support. He acted as IT coordinator near the Mozambican Health Ministry after having designed the national Health Information System according to the governments memorandum "Health Strategic Program 2009/14". Currently as of 2020 he is R&D Manager for DECSIS, SA where he maintains the relations with academia regarding ICT applied to Healthy Ageing Environments. He has special interest in scuba diving being an active PADI instructor and underwater photographer.

José García-Alonso has a PhD in Information Technology from the University of Extremadura since 2014, and a lecturer in the Department of Computer Systems and Telematics Engineering at the same university since 2010, since 2016 as Associate Professor. During his career he has made numerous publications in various prestigious conferences and magazines. Also noteworthy is its transfer work, which has been carried out with the participation in various research projects and contracts with companies and through the creation of two technology-based companies.

* * *

Maria de Lurdes Almeida, PhD in Nursing Sciences, MSc in Nursing Sciences, is coordinator of the Scientific-Pedagogical Unit of Nursing in ESEnfC.

João Luis Alves Apostolo has an aggregation degree in Nursing Sciences (2017), Postdoctoral program in Nursing Sciences (2013), PhD in Nursing Sciences (2008), master's degree in addictions and psychosocial pathologies (2000), postgraduate study in health service administration (2000), degree in nursing (1998) with a specialization in mental health and psychiatric nursing (1997). Is Coordinating Professor in Nursing School of Coimbra, Vice coordinator of The Health Sciences Research Unit: Nursing (UICISA: E) and Director of The Portugal Centre for Evidence Based Practice: A Joanna Briggs Institute (JBI) Centre of Excellence (PCEBP). Published 141 articles in journals. Has 8 section(s) of books and 4 book(s). Organized 21 event(s). Participated in 77 event(s). Supervised 8 PhD thesis(es) e co-supervised 1. Supervised 7 MSc dissertation(s). Has received 14 awards and/or honors. Participates and/or participated as Principal Investigator in 5 funded project(s). In his professional activities interacted with 794 collaborator(s) co-authorship of scientific papers.

João Balsa is Assistant Professor at the Informatics Department of the Faculty of Sciences of the University of Lisbon. Research interest: Artificial Intelligence, Multi-Agent Based Simulation, Intelligent Virtual Assistants, Natural Language Processing.

Javier Berrocal received the Ph.D. degree in computer science from the University of Extremadura, Spain, in 2014. In 2016, he obtained an Associate position in the University of Extremadura. His main research interests are mobile computing, context awareness, pervasive systems, crowd sensing, the Internet of Things, and fog computing. He is a cofounder of the company Gloin, which is a software-consulting company.

Elzbieta Bobrowicz-Campos has a PhD in Psychology (Psychological Assessment) by Faculty of Psychology and Educational Sciences - University of Coimbra (FPCEUC). Specialist in Clinical and Health Psychology with Advanced Specialty in Neuropsychology. Researcher at the Faculty of Psychology and Educational Sciences, Centre of 20th Century Interdisciplinary Studies (CEIS20) - University of Coimbra, and at the Health Sciences Research Unit: Nursing (UICISA: E) of Nursing School of Coimbra (ESEnfC).

David Caballero is a professor at the Nursing School of the University of Extremadura.

Maria Beatriz Carmo is graduated in Mathematics from the Faculty of Sciences of the University of Lisbon (FCUL), Portugal. She holds a PhD in Informatics from the same University. She is assistant professor at the Department of Informatics of FCUL and a researcher of the Agent and Systems Modelling group (MAS) of the Biosystems & Integrative Sciences Institute (BioISI). Her main research interests are in the areas of Visualization, Computer Graphics, Virtual and Augmented Reality, and Digital Heritage. She lectures graduation and master courses in these areas. She is also the coordinator of the Master Programme in Informatics of FCUL.

Joshua Chukwuere is an Associate Professor in the Department of Information Systems, North-West University (NWU), South Africa. His research area includes social media, e-learning, smart city, e-health, Internet of things (IoT) and many more. He has published a number of accredited journals, and conference papers and has presented papers in local and international conferences.

Ana Paula Cláudio is an Assistant Professor at the Informatics Department of the Faculty of Sciences of the University of Lisbon (FCUL), and a Researcher in BioISI- Biosystems & Integrative Sciences Institute (BioISI). She holds a Mathematics degree from FCUL and a PhD in Informatics from the same University. Her main research interests are on Computer Graphics in general, Serious Games, 3D modeling, Virtual and Augmented Reality, Digital Heritage, and she teaches undergraduate and graduate courses covering these topics. She is also the coordinator of the Bachelor Programme in Information Technology of FCUL.

Adriana Raquel Neves Coelho. Ph.D. in Nursing Sciences the Institute of Biomedical Sciences Abel Salazar, University of Porto (2019). Degree in Nursing (2007). Postgraduate in Nurse Attention in Palliative Care (2012). Master in Palliative and Supportive Care (2013). Master's in health research (2015). Associate researcher at the Portugal Centre for Evidence-Based Practice: A Joanna Briggs Institute Centre of Excellence, Health Sciences Research Unit: Nursing (UICISA: E - ESEnfC). Guest Adjunct Professor at the Nursing School of Coimbra, Portugal. Peer reviewer for 4 international scientific journals. She has published 18 articles in international scientific journals and 23 papers in conference proceedings. She has received 3 awards and/or honors.

Daniel Flores-Martin is a PhD student first-year at the University of Extremadura, Spain. He belongs to the Quercus Software Engineering group, where he is developing his doctoral thesis on interconnection and adaptation of IoT devices based on context, in a dynamic way. His main interests are Internet of Things, Social and Pervasive Computing, Internet of People (IoP) and Services from mobile devices.

Isabel Gil is an Adjunct Professor, The Health Sciences Research Unit: Nursing, Nursing School of Coimbra, Portugal.

Margarida Goes holds a BSc in Nursing from Polytechnic Institute of Beja and an MSc in Human Ecology from University of Évora, Portugal. She even holds a

BSc in Business Organization and Management from Modern University of Lisbon. She is finishing her PhD in Nursing. See lectures Nursing Sciences in Health School of Polytechnic Institute of Beja, Portugal, where she is Assistant Professor. Her research interests include mainly Aging, Quality of Life, International Classification of Functionality, Disability and Health and Epidemiology.

Maria Adriana Henriques, PhD, RN, is coordinator professor at the Escola Superior de Enfermagem de Lisboa (ESEL) (Nursing School of Lisbon).She has a Master's degree in epidemiology. She is member of the Technical-Scientific Council and the General Council of the ESEL. She is a member of Scientific Committee of Doctoral Programme in Nursing of the University of Lisbon. Her research interest is in older people with chronic condition and supervises PhD thesis and master dissertations. Last years she participated in the ESSEnCE-project (University Exeter), in "NURSE – LEAD-Nursing Leadership Educational Program for Doctoral Nursing Students and Postdoctoral Nurses" and in VaSelfCare-project, Portugal 2020.

José Jasnau Caeiro was born the 15th of March 1963. B.Sc. Physics Engineering and Materials Science, Faculdade de Ciências e Tecnologia/Universidade Nova de Lisboa, 1986; MSc. in Electrical and Computer Engineering, Instituto Superior Técnico/Universidade de Lisboa, 1993; PhD. in Electrical and Computer Engineering, Instituto Superior Técnico/Universidade de Lisboa, 2010. Assistant professor of computer science at the Instituto Politécnico de Beja since 1997, and invited researcher at INESC-ID Lisboa since 1988.

Lorenzo Juárez is a Senior Lecturer. Doctor in Social and Cultural Anthropology. Member of The International Commission on the Anthropology of Food and Nutrition (ICAF).

Armanda P. M. Matos is Assistant Professor at the Faculty of Psychology and Sciences of Education of Coimbra University, Portugal, and has a PhD in Sciences of Education (Psychology of Education), from the same University. Researcher at the Centre for 20th Century Interdisciplinary Studies (CEIS 20) - University of Coimbra. Her research interests are in the area of media education/media literacy, in which she has been developing much of her teaching activities, as well as writings and scientific projects. She leads the Portuguese team of the Red Interuniversitaria Euroamericana de Investigación ALFAMED, and is currently leading the research project "Digital and media literacy competencies in Portugal – COMEDIG (PTDC/CED-EDG/32560/2017)".

Enrique Moguel is a Software Engineer at Quercus Software Engineering Group.

Henrique Oliveira holds a PhD in Electrical and Computer Engineering, from Instituto Superior Técnico (IST), Lisbon, Portugal. He joined the Multimedia Signal Processing Group of Lisbon's lab of Instituto de Telecomunicações. He lectures in Escola Superior de Tecnologia e Gestão – Instituto Politécnico de Beja, Portugal, where he is Assistant Professor in the Engineering Department. His research interests include image processing, pattern recognition, geographic information systems and remote sensing.

Vitor Sérgio de Oliveira Parola. Ph.D. in Nursing Sciences the Institute of Biomedical Sciences Abel Salazar, University of Porto (2019). Degree in Nursing (2007). Postgraduate in Nurse Attention in Palliative Care (2012). Master in Palliative and Supportive Care (2013). Master's in health research (2015). Associate researcher at the Portugal Centre for Evidence-Based Practice: A Joanna Briggs Institute Centre of Excellence, Health Sciences Research Unit: Nursing (UICISA: E - ESEnfC). Guest Adjunct Professor at the Nursing School of Coimbra, Portugal. Peer reviewer for 9 international scientific journals. He has published 20 articles in international scientific journals and 27 papers in conference proceedings, and 1 chapter book. He has received 2 awards and/or honors.

Patrícia Pereira, MSc, Nursing – Specialization in Rehabilitation Nursing; Hospital Espírito Santo de Évora, Portugal.

Alejandro Pérez-Vereda works at the Languages and Computer Science Department of the University of Malaga. My research interests are Mobile Computing, Context Awareness, Pervasive Systems, Crowd Sensing and Internet of Things.

Gorete Reis, PhD, Nursing Sciences; Professor at University of Évora, Portugal; Filiation to Comprehensive Health Research Centre (CHRC). Researcher in POCTEP 0445_4IE_4_P, Portugal. ID orcid 000-003-1001-4142.

Borja Rivero Jiménez is Scientific Research Staff of the University of Extremadura, 4IE Project.

Jorge Manuel Azevedo Santos holds a Ph.D. in Applied Mathematics and is an assistant tenured professor at the Mathematics Department of University of Évora. His teaching areas are Statistics and Operations Research at both under and post-graduate levels He is responsible for several subjects ranging from the bachelors to Ph.D. degree in the areas of statistics and Operations Research. He is a Founding Member of the EURO Working Group on Stochastic Optimization and member of several international societies He is an active member of the Centro de Investigação em Matemática e Aplicações (CIMA) in the Research group of Statistics, Stochastic Processes and Applications. He has published 5 articles in specialized journals, has 9 chapters of books and 1 book published. He has 3 technical production items. He works in the areas of exact sciences with emphasis on computer science and information.

Paulo Silva, MSc, Nursing – Specialization in Rehabilitation Nursing. Unidade Local de Saúde do Baixo Alentejo, Portugal, Beja. ID orcid 0000-0001-7383-7651.

Margarida Sim-Sim, PhD, Psycology; Professor at University of Évora, Portugal; Filiation to Comprehensive Health Research Centre (CHRC). ID orcid 0000-0002-0028-2664.

Luís Sousa has a PhD in Nursing from the Portuguese Catholic University (UCP). Master's in human resource development policies from the University Institute of Lisbon (ISCTE-IUL). Specialization in Rehabilitation Nursing by the Lisbon School of Nursing (ESEL). Graduated in Health Management from the Atlantic University. Adjunct Professor, University of Évora (UÉ), nursing department.

Luísa Teixeira-Santos is a PhD student in Nursing Sciences at ICBAS/UP - Institute for the Biomedical Sciences Abel Salazar / Porto University. Have a master's degree in Mental Health and Psychiatry Nursing and is a Research Grant Holder at the Health Sciences Research Unit: Nursing of the Nursing School of Coimbra (Portugal).

Filipa Ventura is a Junior Researcher at Health Sciences Research Unit: Nursing (UICISA: E). PhD in Health Care Sciences, Specialist nurse in Oncological Care, RN.

Index

I

K

L

M

N

O

P

Q

R

S

T

V

W

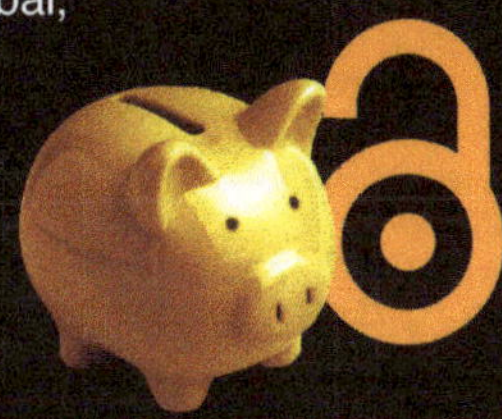

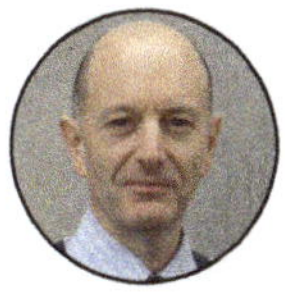

www.ingramcontent.com/pod-product-compliance
Lightning Source LLC
LaVergne TN
LVHW080858300926
849162LV00003B/467
9781799819370